T0212900

Lecture Notes in Computer Science 9072

Commenced Publication in 1973
Founding and Former Series Editors:
Gerhard Goos, Juris Hartmanis, and Jan van Leeuwen

More information about this series at http://www.springer.com/series/7409

Thomas MacTavish · Santosh Basapur (Eds.)

Persuasive Technology

10th International Conference, PERSUASIVE 2015
Chicago, IL, USA, June 3–5, 2015
Proceedings

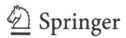 Springer

Editors
Thomas MacTavish
IIT Institute of Design
Chicago
USA

Santosh Basapur
IIT Institute of Design
Chicago
USA

ISSN 0302-9743   ISSN 1611-3349   (electronic)
Lecture Notes in Computer Science
ISBN 978-3-319-20305-8   ISBN 978-3-319-20306-5   (eBook)
DOI 10.1007/978-3-319-20306-5

Library of Congress Control Number: 2015940763

LNCS Sublibrary: SL3 – Information Systems and Applications, incl. Internet/Web and HCI

Springer Cham Heidelberg New York Dordrecht London
© Springer International Publishing Switzerland 2015

Printed on acid-free paper

Springer International Publishing AG Switzerland is part of Springer Science+Business Media
(www.springer.com)

Preface

Persuasive technology is an interdisciplinary research field that focuses on the design and development of technologies aimed at changing users' attitudes or behaviors through persuasion and social influence, but not through coercion or deception. PERSUASIVE, the International Conference on Persuasive Technology, is the leading venue to meet and discuss the latest theories and applications of persuasive technology in a growing number of domains, including personal healthcare, environmentally sustainable behaviors, and public and industrial safety. Previous PERSUASIVE conferences were held in Padua, Sydney, Linköping, Columbus, Copenhagen, Claremont, Oulu, Palo Alto, and Eindhoven.

This volume collects the papers presented at the 10th edition of the conference that took place in Chicago, USA, during June 2015. On June 2, a doctoral consortium and co-design workshop was held. On June 3, tutorials and workshops were held and during June 4-5 the formal single-track conference proceedings were held. The general chairs for the conference were Patrick Whitney and Tom MacTavish. The organizing chairs were Tom MacTavish and Santosh Basapur. The conference benefited from the collaboration of 50 scholars who were members of the Scientific Committee. In addition to the themes of persuasive technology addressed in previous editions of the conference, this event highlighted the special theme of "Personal Empowerment Through Persuasive Design" to acknowledge the rising trend of consumers with intelligent devices (e.g., smartphones and wearables) and personal data ubiquitously available in large data sets (currently referred to as "the cloud") and the empowerment that will occur as well-designed applications provide personally impactful, data-driven support to people at opportune moments.

The papers in this volume were selected after a thorough selection process. The papers submitted to the conference for oral presentation were examined by at least two experts on the topics of the paper in a double-blind review process. Based on these evaluations, 46% of the 41 of the submitted papers were accepted as full (12 page) papers and 9% were accepted as short (6 pages) papers. All accepted papers underwent a second round of revisions before being included in this volume. We would like to thank all the experts who carefully read the submissions and generously gave of their time to provide advice to the authors. Also, we would like to thank the authors for the effort that they made in this iterative revision process to achieve high-quality results.

In addition to the papers included in this volume, the conference also featured a poster session, a doctoral consortium, workshops, and tutorials. This resulted in contributions that are available in separately published proceedings. Persuasive 2015 offered two international workshops: (1) the Third International Workshop on Behavior Change and (2) Mobile Urban Persuasion. In addition, the conference offered two tutorials: (1) Service Design for Health Behaviors and (2) Mobile Persuasion Design.

The conference received papers from contributors in 20 countries from the continents of Asia, Australia, Europe, North America, and South America.

The conference organization benefited from advice from organizers from prior conferences, in particular Harri Oinas-Kukkonen. Also, it benefited from the guidance of our industrial advisory council comprised of representatives from the companies: Accenture, Connected Health, Datu Health, DigitasLBi, FCB Global, higi, IA Collaborative, Pathfinder Solutions, RTC, and Walgreens. We appreciate the support and enthusiasm shown by all members of the Organizing and Scientific Committees.

May 2015

Thomas MacTavish
Santosh Basapur

Organization

General Chairs

Tom MacTavish	IIT Institute of Design, Illinois, USA
Patrick Whitney	IIT Institute of Design, Illinois, USA

Organizing Committee

Santosh Basapur	IIT Institute of Design, Illinois, USA
Ashley Lukasik	IIT Institute of Design, Illinois, USA
Tom MacTavish	IIT Institute of Design, Illinois, USA
Jaime Rivera	IIT Institute of Design, Illinois, USA
Margo Schwartz	IIT Institute of Design, Illinois, USA

Organizing Committee – Sub-Committees

Doctoral Consortium Committee

Sriram Iyengar	Texas A & M University, Houston, Texas, USA
Sahiti Myneni	University of Texas, Health School of Biomedical Informatics, Houston, Texas, USA
Hanna Schraffenberger	LIACS, Leiden University, The Netherlands

Poster Sessions Committee

Jaime Rivera	IIT Institute of Design, Illinois, USA
Tomoko Ichikawa	IIT Institute of Design, Illinois, USA

Social Media and Communications Committee

Rita Orji	Yale University, Connecticut, USA
Raina Russ	IIT Institute of Design, Illinois, USA
Agnis Stibe	MIT Media Lab, Massachusetts, USA

Workshops and Tutorials

Santosh Basapur	IIT Institute of Design, Illinois, USA
Khan Siddiqui	Johns Hopkins University, Maryland, USA

Conference Awards Committee

Harri Oinas-Kukkonen	University of Oulu, Finland

Scientific Committee Members

Johan Åberg	Linköping University, Sweden
Magnus Bang	Linköping University, Sweden
Shlomo Berkovsky	National ICT, Australia
Timothy Bickmore	Northeastern University, Massachusetts, USA
Robert Biddle	Carleton University, Canada
Winslow Burleson	New York University, New York, USA
Cheryl Campanella Bracken	Cleveland State University, Ohio, USA
Samir Chatterjee	Claremont Graduate University, California, USA
Luca Chittaro	University of Udine, Italy
Janet Davis	Grinnell College, Iowa, USA
Berardina De Carolis	University of Bari, Italy
Peter de Vries	University of Twente, The Netherlands
Sebastian Deterding	Rochester Institute of Technology, New York, USA
Alexander Felfernig	Graz University of Technology, Austria
B.J. Fogg	Stanford University, California, USA
Jill Freyne	CSIRO, Australia
Carlo Galimberti	Università Cattolica di Milano, Italy
Luciano Gamberini	University of Padua, Italy
Mark Gilzenrat	CNN Digital, Georgia, USA
Floriana Grasso	University of Liverpool, UK
Ulrike Gretzel	University of Wollongong, Australia
Marco Guerini	Trento-RISE, Italy
Jaap Ham	Eindhoven University of Technology, The Netherlands
Curtis P. Haugtvedt	Ohio State University, Ohio, USA
Stephen Intille	Northeastern University, Massachusetts, USA
Sriram Iyengar	Texas A & M University, Houston, Texas, USA
Giulio Jacucci	Helsinki Institute for Information Technology, Finland
Anthony Jameson	German Research Center for Artificial Intelligence, Germany
Antti Jylha	University of Helsinki, Finland
Maurits Kaptein	Radboud University, The Netherlands
Sarvnaz Karimi	CSIRO, Australia
Rilla Khaled	IT University of Copenhagen, Denmark
Sitwat Langrial	University of Oulu, Finland
Dan Lockton	Helen Hamlyn Centre for Design, Royal College of Art, UK
Tom MacTavish	Illinois Institute of Technology, Illinois, USA
Judith Masthoff	University of Aberdeen, UK
Cees Midden	Eindhoven University of Technology, The Netherlands
Harri Oinas-Kukkonen	Oulu University, Finland
Rita Orji	Yale University, Massachusetts, USA

Andreas Riener	Johannes Kepler University, Austria
Peter Ruijten	Eindhoven University of Technology, The Netherlands
Juan Salamanca	Universidad ICESI, Columbia
Hanna Schraffenberger	LIACS, Leiden University, The Netherlands
Anna Spagnolli	University of Padua, Italy
Agnis Stibe	Massachusetts Institute of Technology, Massachusetts, USA
Oliviero Stock	FBK-IRST, Italy
Manfred Tscheligi	ICT&S Center, University of Salzburg, Austria
Julita Vassileva	University of Saskatchewan, Canada
Frank Verberne	Eindhoven University of Technology, The Netherlands
Kyung-Hyan Angie Yoo	William Paterson University, New Jersey, USA

Sponsoring Institutions

IIT Institute of Design
Datu Health
DigitasLBi
Steelcase

Sponsors

We would like to recognize our sponsors for their support.

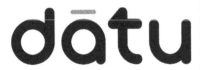

Datu Health -- Leading healthcare systems use the Dātu digital encounter platform to deliver continuous, personalized care for community members, aligned to clinical evidence and to consumer needs. http://datuhealth.com

DigitasLBi

DigitasLBi – is a global marketing and technology agency that transforms businesses for the digital age. They exist to help brands embrace the creative and technological changes revolutionizing all aspects of their business. http://digitaslbi.com

Steelcase

For over 100 years, Steelcase Inc. has helped create great experiences for the world's leading organizations, across industries. We demonstrate this through our family of brands – including Steelcase®, Coalesse®, Designtex®, Details®, PolyVision® and Turnstone®. Together, they offer a comprehensive portfolio of architecture, furniture and technology products and services designed to unlock human promise and support social, economic and environmental sustainability. We are globally accessible through a network of channels, including over 800 dealer locations. Steelcase is a global, industry-leading and publicly traded company with fiscal 2015 revenue of $3.1 billion. http://steelcase.com

Contents

Understanding Individuals

Empowering Individuals

Understanding Communities

Empowering Communities

Understanding Individuals

Involvement as a Working Mechanism for Persuasive Technology

Saskia M. Kelders[✉]

Faculty of Behavioural, Management and Social Sciences, Department of Psychology, Health and Technology, University of Twente, Enschede, The Netherlands
s.m.kelders@utwente.nl

Abstract. Internet interventions have been shown to be effective for treatment of mental health complaints. Although non-adherence poses a problem, persuasive technology might be a solution. However, there is limited insight in how and why technology may lead to more adherence and effectiveness. This study explores the role of involvement in a Behavior Change Support System (BCSS) for treatment of depression. Involvement is seen as an important factor in the success of treatment, but has received little research attention. This study expands on an earlier study and uses self-reported data to explore differences between versions of the BCSS on involvement. The results show that involvement and adherence are related, but involvement outperforms adherence as predictor for effectiveness. This underlines the importance of involvement: it may be a working mechanism of persuasive technology and may be used as an early measure to assess whether the intervention is likely to reach its goals.

Keywords: Persuasive technology · Behavior change support system · Health · Adherence · Involvement

1   Introduction

Internet interventions have been shown to be effective for treatment and management of a range of (mental) health complaints [1, 2]. However, substantial non-adherence (participants not using the Internet intervention as intended, for example by not completing all modules) is often observed, especially when interventions are not part of a strict research protocol and when there is no counselor involved [3]. This non-adherence poses a problem for the effectiveness of Internet interventions because of the 'dose-response' relationship: the more the intervention is used, the more positive effects participants experience [4].

To overcome this problem, persuasive technology can be employed to increase both adherence and effectiveness. Internet interventions for mental health can be seen as Behavior Change Support Systems (BCSSs). A BCSS is defined as 'a sociotechnical information system with psychological and behavioral outcomes designed to form, alter or reinforce attitudes, behaviors or an act of complying without using coercion or deception' [5]. In these systems, different features can be used to increase the persuasiveness. The Persuasive System Design-model (PSD-model) describes four

© Springer International Publishing Switzerland 2015
T. MacTavish and S. Basapur (Eds.): PERSUASIVE 2015, LNCS 9072, pp. 3–14, 2015.
DOI: 10.1007/978-3-319-20306-5_1

categories of features: primary task support, dialogue support, credibility support and social support [6]. Although many of these features have been used in health BCSSs, most research focusses on the effects of the system as a whole, instead of focusing on the added value of features or categories of features [5]. This 'black-box'-approach has resulted in limited insight into the role of these persuasive system design features. Besides limited insight in *what* persuasive technology can do in health BCSSs, there is limited insight in *how* and *why* technology may lead to more adherence and effectiveness. These working mechanisms may be important in understanding why persuasive technology leads to positive results in some cases (e.g. in certain context and for certain people) and not in other cases.

Involvement may be such a working mechanism. In 'offline' therapeutic interventions, the importance of involvement is well known. Studies have shown that more involvement of clients in therapy is beneficial for a better therapeutic relationship [7], which in turn is an important predictor of the effectiveness of therapy [8]. Moreover, it seems that involvement may even be a prerequisite for an intervention to be effective [9]. In many of the theories that are the foundation of BCSSs [5], personal involvement is seen as closely related to the motivation to change behavior, although this has received little research attention. In BCSSs for mental health, it may well be that the way technology is persuasive, e.g. making working with the intervention easier, more fun, more interesting or more relevant, may well be captured by measuring how involved participants are.

In this study, we investigate the role of involvement in a BCSS for the treatment of depression. Different versions of this intervention were created to investigate the influence of persuasive technology on adherence and effectiveness. These results are presented in a different paper [10] and show that persuasive technology did not directly result in increased adherence and effectiveness. However, there were significant differences between variations of the intervention and involvement. This paper builds on these earlier results and uses new analysis of the existing data to further explore these differences and their role in explaining adherence and effectiveness.

2   Methods

2.1   Experimental Design

This paper presents further analyses of data collected within a fractional factorial randomized controlled trial on a web-based intervention for the treatment of people with mild to moderate depressive symptomatology. For the study, different versions of the intervention were created. Five components were chosen (support, text messages, experience through technology, tailoring of success stories, and personalization) of which two levels were created (automated support and human support; text messages and no text messages; high and low experience through technology; high and low tailoring of success stories; high and low personalization). These components were chosen based on research into the design of this intervention (these were the features that deemed to be important to the target group to keep using the intervention [11]). Moreover, these components have been shown to be important for the effectiveness or adherence of online interventions [6, 12-15]. For the fractional factorial design, eight intervention arms were created where each level of each component was present in half of the intervention arms. A more detailed description of this study design is presented in [10].

2.2   Intervention

The web-based intervention 'Living to the full' included nine chronological lessons and is based on Acceptance and Commitment Therapy. Each module included text, online and offline exercises, and metaphors. Participants were instructed to complete one lesson per week, but had twelve weeks in total to complete the nine lessons. The intervention was developed using a human centered design [11]. The intervention was proven effective compared to a waiting list and active control group [16]. Following is the description of the five components of which two levels were created.

Support. Participants randomized in the human support condition, received their weekly feedback from a human counselor. Participants randomized in the automated support condition, received weekly automatically generated feedback. The human counselors were psychology Masters students of the University of Twente, supervised by a clinical psychologist. The counselors were instructed to write a weekly feedback message containing the key learning points and goal of the completed lesson; the key exercises and feedback on at least the core exercise; feedback on the mindfulness exercise; and a preview of the following lesson. The automatically generated feedback contained the same elements, where the feedback on the core exercise and the mindfulness exercise was tailored based on the multiple choice responses of the participants to the question which was added to both exercises. An example question that was added after a core exercise was: 'Was writing down your 'bag of sorrow' confronting to you?'. Feedback messages in both conditions were presented in the same manner: under 'feedback' in the personal home screen, accompanied by a picture of the counselor. In the automated support condition, a picture of a clinical psychologist was placed who was not directly involved in the study. We have chosen to include a picture in both conditions to ensure comparability, but also as an effort to humanize our system [17] and to increase the persuasiveness. Participants were aware of whether their counselor was human or automated to ensure that the system complies to the openness postulate of the PSD-model [6]. Apart from the source of the feedback message, there were two differences between the conditions. Participants in the human support condition had the opportunity to ask questions to their counselor. Questions were elicited when participants completed a lesson, but could also be asked at any time. Participants in the automated support condition, received one additional instant feedback message per lesson. This was an automatically generated message tailored to the multiple choice response of the participant on a different exercise than the core-exercise and was presented as a pop-up accompanied by the picture of the counselor.

Text messages. Participants in the condition that included text messages, had the opportunity to turn the SMS-coach on. This SMS-coach sent three pre-designed text messages each week to a mobile phone number provided by the participant. The timing of the text messages was different each week, but all messages were sent between 9AM and 9PM. Each week one message contained a motivational message (e.g. "Do you realize you have taken the first step to learn to 'live to the full'? Congratulations and keep going!"), one message contained a mindfulness trigger (e.g. "How mindful are you today?") and one message reflected on the content of that week (e.g. "Avoidance is like scratching an itch. It only works for a short time."). This way, the text messages served both as reminders and as suggestion [6]. The timing and content of the messages were based upon the results of the development study [11], to make the system as unobtrusive as possible. All text messages were presented in the 'text message' tab of the application, independent of whether the SMS-coach was turned on or off, but only for the participants in the condition that included text messages.

Experience Through Technology. This component is about the persuasive experience participants have when using the intervention. The high experience condition offers a more immersive and interactive experience than the low experience condition due to two differences. In eight of the nine lessons, a short movie was added to the high experience condition, in which the writer of the course or an experienced clinical psychologist explains the key points of the lesson. The movie does not contain other information than the text, but the information is presented in a different, more immersive way. The second difference was that the high experience condition contained an interactive exercise or multimedia presentation of an exercise or metaphor in seven of the nine lessons, whereas in the low experience condition the exercises and metaphors were presented as text.

Tailoring of Success Stories. The intervention contained a success story for each of the lessons of the intervention that became available at the same time as the lessons. The participants accessed these stories from the personal home screen, under 'experiences of others'. The stories were fictional, but based on experiences of participants in an earlier study on the self-help book version of the intervention and served as the persuasive principle recognition [6]. For the high tailored condition, each success story was tailored on four of the following aspects: gender, age, marital status, daily activity, most prominent symptom and the reason for participating in the web-based intervention. In the low tailored condition a standard success story was presented each week. Attention was paid to vary these stories on the aspects that were used for tailoring in the high tailored condition.

Personalization. Personalization was implemented according to the definition of Knutov et al. 2009 [18], where it is seen as consisting of adaptation (automatic, implicit personalization) and adaptability (the system provides the opportunity to the user for personalization) of the content, presentation, navigation and user input. However, we were only able to personalize a small part of the intervention. Independent of condition, all respondents were addressed with their (reported) first name when logging on to the intervention in a welcome message (e.g. Welcome Saskia, you are at part 1 of lesson 4). Additionally, the high personalization condition showed the self-chosen picture and motto of the participant on the personal home screen as soon as this was chosen in lesson one; and showed the self-chosen most important values on the personal home screen (from lesson seven onwards). Furthermore, in this condition, participants had the opportunity to create their own 'top 5' of things from the course that they found most important. This top 5 was also shown on the personal home screen. The low personalization condition did not provide these options.

2.3   Procedure

Participants were recruited through advertisements in Dutch newspapers. Interested people visited the study website and could register for the study and intervention on this website after reading online information and giving informed consent. A total of 239 respondents fulfilled the inclusion criteria, completed the online baseline questionnaire and were automatically randomized to one of eight intervention arms. Participants received an emailed link to the online post-intervention questionnaire three months after the start of the intervention period. Six months after the start of the intervention period, participants received an emailed link to the online follow-up questionnaire. Up to two automated email reminders were sent to the participants when not filling out a questionnaire.

2.4   Participants

Participants in this intervention were people aged 18 years or older with self-reported mild to moderate depressive symptomatology (>9 and <39 on the Center of Epidemiological Studies – depression scale; CES-D)[19]. Exclusion criteria were receiving psychological or psycho-pharmacological treatment within the last three months, having less than three hours per week time to spend on the web-based intervention and poor Dutch language skills. For this paper, only data was used of participants that have actually started using the intervention, because only then can the participants form an opinion on the intervention and the included persuasive technology. Additionally, only the data from participants that also filled out the post-intervention questionnaire was used, because involvement was assessed at this post-intervention questionnaire. We have chosen not to impute missing data on involvement, because we have no theoretical basis on which to impute these values. Table 1 presents the characteristics of the 134 participants that were included in this study. Significant differences show that within the included participants, there is a higher percentage of females and people with a higher education. Furthermore, participants included in this analysis are more often adherers and have reached a higher lesson in the intervention. These differences in adherence and lesson reached are inherent to our inclusion criteria: a large group of non-adherers was excluded because they did not start using the intervention (n = 33), and drop-out (e.g. participants not filling out questionnaires) and adherence are interrelated [20].

Table 1. Participant characteristics

	All participants	Included	Test value	p
Age Mean (s.d.)	44.9 (12.3)	46.1 (12.0)	$F_{1, 237} = 2.912$	.089
Gender % (no.)			$\chi^2_1 = 7.013$	.008
Male	29.3 (70)	22.4 (30)		
Female	70.7 (169)	77.6 (104)		
Education level % (no.)			$\chi^2_2 = 11.771$	.003
High	66.1 (158)	74.6 (100)		
Middle	26.4 (63)	21.6 (29)		
Low	7.5 (18)	3.7 (5)		
CES-D Mean (s.d.)	25.0 (7.0)	24.4 (7.1)	$F_{1, 237} = 2.088$	.150
Adherence % (no.)			$\chi^2_1 = 97.310$	<.001
Yes	49.4 (118)	77.6 (104)		
No	50.6 (121)	22.4 (30)		
Lesson reached Mean (s.d.)	5.92 (3.59)	8.25 (1.75)	$F_{1, 237} = 278.605$	<.001

2.5   Measurements

Depressive symptoms were measured at baseline, post intervention and follow-up with the CES-D (a self-report questionnaire with 20 items, score 0-60; higher scores mean more depressive symptoms) [19, 21]. Involvement was measured at post intervention with the short version of the Personal Involvement Inventory (10 items, mean score 1-7, higher score means more involvement) [22]. This is a self-report questionnaire formulated as "To me the online course 'Living tot the full' is ...", with a bipolar adjective scale (i.e. for each item participants were asked to rate whether the intervention was e.g. unimportant – important, or boring – interesting). Adherence was measured objective through system log files. The log files contained a record of actions taken by each participant. One of the actions that was logged was starting a new lesson. Each lesson could only be started when the previous lesson was finished and feedback was received. Adherence was defined as a participant starting lesson 9, because the intervention is intended to be used during the nine lessons. Furthermore, the highest lesson reached was recorded (1 to 9) to measure the degree of adherence.

2.6   Data Analysis

Statistical analyses were done using SPSS 20 (IBM, USA). All tests were two-tailed. First, differences on involvement and lesson reached between variations of the technology were investigated using oneway Anova's. Second, the relationship between involvement and adherence was investigated using a oneway Anova to assess whether there were differences on involvement between adherers and non-adherers. The relationship between adherence and involvement was also studied by using a linear regression to investigate the predictive value of lesson reached (i.e. the degree of adherence) on involvement. Third, to investigate the influence of involvement on outcome measures, blockwise regression analyses were used with the clinical outcomes (CES-D on post intervention and follow-up) as dependent variables. Clinical baseline values and adherence or lesson reached were entered in the first block, because of their expected influence on outcome measures. Involvement was entered second in the model, to assess the added value of involvement as predictor.

3   Results

3.1   Involvement and Adherence

There were differences between how the participants who received the different variations scored on involvement and lesson reached (Table 2). On support and on text messages, the variations show significant differences on involvement, where human support and the inclusion of text messages lead to higher scores on involvement. On interaction, the high interaction variant shows higher involvement, although this difference is not significant (p = .08). On tailoring and personalization, no difference between the variations is discernible. On lesson reached, there are no significant differences between the variations of the intervention. Moreover, adherers score significantly higher on involvement than non-adherers, and lesson reached is a significant predictor for involvement. The model including the constant and lesson reached explains 15.5% of the variance in involvement (Table 3).

Table 2. Mean values and differences on involvement and lesson reached

	Mean (s.d.) involvement*	Test value, p	Mean (s.d.) lesson reached	Test value, p
Support		$F_{1, 132}$ =		$F_{1, 132}$ = 2.955,
Automated (n = 62)	5.50 (1.16)	4.411,	7.97 (2.14)	p = .088
Human (n = 72)	5.90 (1.00)	p = .038	8.49 (1.31)	
Text messages		$F_{1, 132}$ =		$F_{1, 132}$ = 0.001,
No (n = 64)	5.51 (1.12)	4.415,	8.25 (1.65)	p = .981
Yes (n = 70)	5.90 (1.04)	p = .038	8.24 (1.85)	
Experience through tech.		$F_{1, 132}$ = 3.116,		$F_{1, 132}$ = 0.185, p = .668
Low (n = 54)	5.51 (1.27)	p = .080	8.17 (2.04)	
High (n = 80)	5.85 (0.94)		8.30 (1.55)	
Tailoring success stories		$F_{1, 132}$ = 1.024,		$F_{1, 132}$ = 0.621, p = .432
Low (n = 82)	5.79 (1.04)	p = .313	8.34 (1.58)	
High (n = 52)	5.59 (1.17)		8.10 (2.00)	
Personalisation		$F_{1, 132}$ =		$F_{1, 132}$ = 2.770,
Low (n = 72)	5.65 (1.09)	0.468,	8.01 (1.87)	p = .098
High (n = 62)	5.78 (1.10)	p = .495	8.52 (1.58)	
Adherence		$F_{1, 132}$ =		-**
Adherers (n = 104)	5.88 (0.96)	10.946,	9.00 (0.00)	
Non-adherers (n = 30)	5.15 (1.34)	p = .001	5.63 (2.24)	

* These results are also presented in [10].

** Difference not tested because the categories are different by definition.

Table 3. Linear regression lesson reached and involvement

Variable	B (SE)	Beta	p
Constant	3.69 (0.42)		<.001
Lesson reached	0.25 (0.05)	0.39	<.001

Note $R^2 = 0.155$, adjusted $R^2 = 0.149$. Model $F_{1, 132} = 24.223$, $P < .001$

3.2 Predictive Value of Involvement

Table 4 and 5 present the results of linear regressions to predict clinical outcomes, i.e. CES-D on post-intervention (Table 4) and on follow-up (Table 5). The signs of the B-values show that increased baseline CES-D predicts higher CES-D scores on post-intervention and follow-up, whereas increased adherence and involvement predict lower CES-D scores on post-intervention and follow-up. Both analysis show that including the variable involvement in step 2 increases the explanatory value of the model (on post-intervention the explained variance increases from 10% to 16% and on follow-up the explained variance increases from 6% to 9% when including involvement). Furthermore, adherence is only a significant predictor in the first step of predicting clinical outcomes on post-intervention. Both analysis show that when including involvement as a predictor, the predictive value of adherence disappears. Lastly, the predictive value of involvement is comparable to that of CES-D on baseline (Beta CES-D 0.28 and 0.22 and Beta involvement -0.29 and -0.23 on post-intervention and follow-up, respectively). Analyses using lesson reached as predictor instead of adherence show similar results (data not shown).

4 Conclusions and Discussion

The results of this study show that differences in the intervention can lead to differences in how involved participants are with the intervention. Significant differences were found between automated and human support, where human support led to more involvement. This may not be a surprising finding, because literature shows that increased counselor interaction leads to increased adherence [3]. It may be more surprising that the difference between automated and human support is similar as the difference between the in- or exclusion of text messages and not larger than that difference. It may be that the way automated support was implemented (e.g. employing virtual presence [23], a social role [6], and a more humanized version of the system [17]) accounts for this relative small difference. It may also be that some of the participants were not complete aware that their counselor was virtual. The picture may have made the counselor too real, although participants were told that their counselor was virtual. This may have made the virtual counselor more effective, but thereby violated the openness postulate of the PSD-model [6]. However, due to the design of the study, this hypothesis cannot be tested. The other significant difference on involvement was seen between the in- and exclusion of text messages, where the inclusion of these messages led to more involvement. The positive effects of reminders are well documented

Table 4. Linear regression predicting CES-D on post-intervention

Step	Variable	B (SE)	Beta	p
1	Constant	12.30 (2.99)		<.001
	CES-D baseline	0.35 (0.11)	0.28	.001
	Adherence	-3.69 (1.81)	-0.17	.044
2	Constant	24.52 (4.54)		<.001
	CES-D baseline	0.36 (0.10)	0.28	<.001
	Adherence	-1.95 (1.81)	-0.09	.283
	Involvement	-2.42 (0.69)	-0.29	.001

Note Model step 1: $R^2 = 0.10$, adjusted $R^2 = 0.09$. Model $F_{2, 131} = 7.337$, $P = .001$; Model step 2: $R^2 = 0.18$, adjusted $R^2 = 0.16$. Model $F_{3, 130} = 9.378$, $P < .001$

Table 5. Linear regression predicting CES-D on follow-up

Step	Variable	B (SE)	Beta	p
1	Constant	11.56 (3.10)		<.001
	CES-D baseline	0.27 (0.11)	0.21	.014
	Adherence	-3.03 (1.88)	-0.14	.109
2	Constant	21.22 (4.78)		<.001
	CES-D baseline	0.28 (0.11)	0.22	.010
	Adherence	-1.65 (1.91)	-0.08	.389
	Involvement	-1.91 (0.73)	-0.23	0.10

Note Model step 1: $R^2 = 0.06$, adjusted $R^2 = 0.05$. Model $F_{2, 131} = 4.212$, $P = .017$; Model step 2: $R^2 = 0.11$, adjusted $R^2 = 0.09$. Model $F_{3, 130} = 5.208$, $P = .002$

(e.g. [24]). However, in this study, reminders did not lead to increased adherence or effectiveness, but only to increased involvement. A reason for not finding an effect on adherence or effectiveness may be the optional nature of the SMS coach: the default state of the coach was off and participants had to change this to turn it on. Analysis of the log-data of the intervention showed that only few participants turned the SMS coach on [25]. On experience through technology, a non-significant difference was seen where high experience led to slightly higher involvement. Although this is not a significant difference, it resonates with literature on the positive effects of increased interaction and on Fogg's functional triad of persuasive technology where creating an experience through technology is one of the ways to increase the persuasiveness of technology [26]. There were no differences on involvement between the levels of tailoring of success stories and personalization, which is contrary to what was expected based on literature of the positive effects of tailoring and personalization. However, this may be explained through the implementation of these variations: the success stories were only a small part of the intervention and a study of the usage of the intervention showed that these success stories were hardly read [25]; the differences on personalization were small and the 'top 5' was implemented in a way that was hard to use for participants. Moreover, the difference between the implementation of tailoring and personalization in this study was small, which may have caused the lack of difference. Nonetheless, the results show that, although there was no difference on adherence and lesson reached between the variations in technology, there were differences on involvement. This shows that involvement may be a more proximal outcome of changes within the technology which is more sensitive to change.

Moreover, scores on involvement were different between participants who adhered to the intervention and participants who did not adhere, where adherers showed the higher involvement scores. Additionally, the more lessons participants complete, the higher their involvement. However, due to the timing of the involvement measure (post-intervention) we cannot say that higher involvement leads to a higher reached lesson, only that the two variables are related. These results were expected and confirm the importance of involvement [7, 9].

The results do show the predictive value of involvement on clinical outcomes. Although this may be expected, it is striking that the predictive value of involvement is on par with the predictive value of clinical baseline scores. However, interpretation of these results should be done with caution, because it may also be that because participants experience more positive results, they are more involved with the intervention. Nonetheless, this cannot account for the differences observed between the variations of technology, because these did not lead to differences in effectiveness [10].

Additionally, the results show that when including involvement as a predictor for clinical outcomes, adherence disappeared as a predictor. The earlier mentioned results about the relationship between involvement and adherence show that these two concepts are related, but they are not the same. A difference is that involvement seems to outperform adherence as a predictor for effectiveness. Other studies have showed that adherence or increased usage of an intervention may not always be a good predictor of effectiveness [27]. It may be that participants have different reasons to adhere, and some reasons (e.g. intrinsic motivation) are more beneficial for the effectiveness of interventions than other reasons (e.g. the feeling that you 'have to' finish the intervention to please someone else) [28]. This study is novel in that it suggests that adherence as a measure does not make a distinction between the different reasons, whereas involvement seems to be closely related to intrinsic motivation, which may be a reason to adhere that is predictive for the success of an intervention for an individual. Therefore, involvement may be a more valuable measure for the working mechanism of an intervention than adherence per se.

A limitation of this study is that only the data of a specific sup-group of participants are used, i.e. participants who started using the intervention and who filled out the post-intervention questionnaire. These participants were more likely to be female and higher educated than participants not included in this study, so the results should be interpreted with caution. Additionally, the included participants were more often adherers and reached a higher lesson, which makes the difference in lesson reached between adherers and non-adherers smaller. A second limitation is that involvement was measured post-intervention and was self-reported. Because of this, the involvement scores may be influenced by the experienced effectiveness of the intervention. However, the predictive value of involvement on effectiveness in this study warrants further research into this area. In future studies, it may be beneficial to measure involvement at different time-points, e.g. early, halfway through and at the end of the intervention period, to see whether involvement changes over time. Furthermore, more implicit ways to measure involvement (e.g. using an Implicit Association Test [29]), may be beneficial because it is seen as more objective.

Future research could benefit from this earlier measure of involvement: it can be used to find out for whom the intervention may not be suitable (as indicated by low involvement scores) and redirect these participants to a different (kind of) intervention. It could also be used as an early assessment of the added value of persuasive technology: if the technology does not lead to higher involvement scores, it may be a good idea to reassess whether the technology is persuasive in the way that it is supposed to be. Lastly, the importance of involvement could be used as a starting point for design: what persuasive elements and techniques can be used to create a behavior change support system that leads to higher involvement.

References

1. Barak, A., et al.: A comprehensive review and a meta-analysis of the effectiveness of internet-based psychotherapeutic interventions. Journal of Technology in Human Services 26(2-4), 109–160 (2008)
2. Webb, T., et al.: Using the internet to promote health behavior change: a systematic review and meta-analysis of the impact of theoretical basis, use of behavior change techniques, and mode of delivery on efficacy. Journal of Medical Internet Research 12(1), e4 (2010)
3. Kelders, S.M., et al.: Persuasive system design does matter: a systematic review of adherence to web-based interventions. Journal of Medical Internet Research 14(6) (2012)
4. Donkin, L., et al.: A systematic review of the impact of adherence on the effectiveness of e-therapies. Journal of Medical Internet Research 13(3) (2011)
5. Oinas-Kukkonen, H.: A foundation for the study of behavior change support systems. Personal and Ubiquitous Computing 17(6), 1223–1235 (2013)
6. Oinas-Kukkonen, H., Harjumaa, M.: Persuasive systems design: Key issues, process model, and system features. Communications of the Association for Information Systems 24(1), 28 (2009)
7. Hill, C.E.: Therapist techniques, client involvement, and the therapeutic relationship: Inextricably intertwined in the therapy process. Psychotherapy: Theory, Research, Practice, Training 42(4), 431 (2005)
8. Lambert, M.J., Barley, D.E.: Research summary on the therapeutic relationship and psychotherapy outcome. Psychotherapy: Theory, Research, Practice, Training 38(4), 357 (2001)
9. Lyubomirsky, S., et al.: Becoming Happier Takes Both a Will and a Proper Way: An Experimental Longitudinal Intervention To Boost Well-Being. Emotion 11(2), 391–402 (2011)
10. Kelders, S.M., et al.: Comparing human and automated support for depression: fractional factorial randomized controlled trial. under review
11. Kelders, S.M., et al.: Development of a web-based intervention for the indicated prevention of depression. BMC Medical Informatics and Decision Making 13, 26 (2013)
12. Furmark, T., et al.: Guided and unguided self-help for social anxiety disorder: randomised controlled trial. British Journal of Psychiatry 195(5), 440–447 (2009)
13. Hurling, R., Fairley, B.W., Dias, M.B.: Internet-based exercise intervention systems: Are more interactive designs better? Psychology & Health 21(6), 757–772 (2006)

14. Strecher, V.J., et al.: Web-based smoking-cessation programs: results of a randomized trial. Am. J. Prev. Med. 34(5), 373–381 (2008)
15. Webb, T.L., et al.: Using the internet to promote health behavior change: a systematic review and meta-analysis of the impact of theoretical basis, use of behavior change techniques, and mode of delivery on efficacy. Journal of Medical Internet Research 12(1), e4 (2010)
16. Pots, W.T.M., et al.: Acceptance and Commitment Therapy as a web-based intervention for depressive symptomatology: Randomised Controlled Trial. British Journal of Psychiatry (in press)
17. Oinas-Kukkonen, H., Oinas-Kukkonen, H.: Humanizing the web: change and social innovation. Palgrave Macmillan (2013)
18. Knutov, E., De Bra, P., Pechenizkiy, M.: AH 12 years later: a comprehensive survey of adaptive hypermedia methods and techniques. New Review of Hypermedia and Multimedia 15(1), 5–38 (2009)
19. Radloff, L.S.: The CES-D scale: A self-report depression scale for research in the general population. Applied Psychological Measurement 1(3), 385–401 (1977)
20. Christensen, H., Griffiths, K.M., Farrer, L.: Adherence in Internet interventions for anxiety and depression: Systematic review. Journal of Medical Internet Research 11(2) (2009)
21. Haringsma, R., et al.: The criterion validity of the Center for Epidemiological Studies Depression Scale (CES-D) in a sample of self-referred elders with depressive symptomatology. International Journal of Geriatric Psychiatry 19(6), 558–563 (2004)
22. Zaichkowsky, J.L.: The Personal Involvement Inventory - Reduction, Revision, and Application to Advertising. Journal of Advertising 23(4), 59–70 (1994)
23. Baylor, A.L.: Promoting motivation with virtual agents and avatars: role of visual presence and appearance. Philos. Trans. R. Soc. Lond. B: Biol. Sci. 364(1535), 3559–3565 (2009)
24. Langrial, S., Oinas-Kukkonen, H.: Less fizzy drinks: A multi-method study of persuasive reminders. In: Bang, M., Ragnemalm, E.L. (eds.) PERSUASIVE 2012. LNCS, vol. 7284, pp. 256–261. Springer, Heidelberg (2012)
25. Kelders, S.M., Bohlmeijer, E.T., van Gemert-Pijnen, J.E.: Participants, Usage, and Use Patterns of a Web-Based Intervention for the Prevention of Depression Within a Randomized Controlled Trial. Journal of Medical Internet Research 15(8) (2013)
26. Fogg, B.J.: Persuasive technology: Using computers to change what we think and do. The Morgan Kaufmann series in interactive technologies 2003, xxviii, 283 p. Morgan Kaufmann Publishers, Boston (2003)
27. Donkin, L., et al.: Rethinking the dose-response relationship between usage and outcome in an online intervention for depression: randomized controlled trial. Journal of Medical Internet Research 15(10) (2013)
28. Donkin, L., Glozier, N.: Motivators and motivations to persist with online psychological interventions: a qualitative study of treatment completers. Journal of Medical Internet Research 14(3) (2012)
29. Nosek, B.A., Greenwald, A.G., Banaji, M.R.: The Implicit Association Test at age 7: A methodological and conceptual review. In: Automatic Processes in Social Thinking and Behavior, pp. 265–292 (2007)

Understanding Persuasion and Motivation in Interactive Stroke Rehabilitation

A Physiotherapists' Perspective on Patient Motivation

Michelle Pickrell[1(✉)], Bert Bongers[1], and Elise van den Hoven[1,2]

[1] Faculty of Design, Architecture and Building, University of Technology,
Sydney, Australia
[2] Industrial Design, Eindhoven University of Technology, Eindhoven, The Netherlands
Michelle.Pickrell@student.uts.edu.au,
{Bert.Bongers,Elise.vandenHoven}@uts.edu.au

Abstract. For the research reported in this paper ethnographic research methodologies were used to explore patient motivation, feedback and the use of interactive technologies in the ward. We have conducted in-depth interviews with physiotherapists, who work closely with stroke patients to help them regain movement and function. From this research, a set of design guidelines have been developed which can be applied in the design of interactive rehabilitation equipment.

Keywords: Rehabilitation · Stroke · Healthcare · Feedback · Design research

1 Introduction

Stroke patients often deal with changes in motivation during rehabilitation. There are a number of reasons for this, including the physical change to the brain resulting from the stroke, psychological issues such as depression as well as improvements and setbacks in their mobility as they complete their rehabilitation. The use of persuasion, both in the interactions between the patient and the physiotherapist and the equipment in the rehabilitation gym is important to help patients succeed with rehabilitation. To explore this topic, we have completed observations of the ward and interviewed physiotherapists. These interviews explored the physiotherapists' perspective on patient motivation as well as patient feedback and the use of technology in the ward.

The research presented in this paper is one part of a larger research initiative into developing equipment that helps stroke patients with their rehabilitation. This research will inform the user centered design approach we will use. This approach will include the researchers, the patients and the physiotherapists working together to design suitable equipment.

© Springer International Publishing Switzerland 2015
T. MacTavish and S. Basapur (Eds.): PERSUASIVE 2015, LNCS 9072, pp. 15–26, 2015.
DOI: 10.1007/978-3-319-20306-5_2

The goals for the study presented in this research paper are:

1. To understand patient motivation from the perspective of the physiotherapist.
2. To understand what types of feedback physiotherapists provide patients during rehabilitation.
3. To understand the day-to-day use of technology used by physiotherapists in the rehabilitation gym..

The objective of this paper is to provide researchers and designers in the field of Human-Computer Interaction (HCI) with the information they need to understand stroke patient motivation as well as a set of guidelines for designing rehabilitation equipment for stroke patients.

2   Background

Whilst this paper focuses on motivation in the context of stroke rehabilitation, the following topics are relevant to acquire an understanding of this multi-faceted area of research. Alongside motivation, the topics of persuasive technology, stroke and stroke rehabilitation are important as well as an understanding of previous work in this area.

2.1   Motivation

The definition of motivation for this study is 'any primary cause of behaviour' [1], however there is an understanding in the physiotherapy domain that motivation is a personality trait that a person either does or does not have [2]. Motivation is a multi-faceted topic that is affected by an understanding of needs and goals. This will be explored through Maslow's 'hierarchy of needs' and goal setting theory.

Basic human motivations result from basic human needs. This is most clearly described through Maslow's 'hierarchy of needs' [3]. Maslow segments human needs into five types - in order of importance – physiological needs, safety needs, social needs, esteem needs and self- actualisation. Maslow also states that needs which have been satisfied no longer motivate. Patients completing their rehabilitation in Sydney hospitals have their physiological needs such as food, air, water and shelter accommodated. However, for patients, lacking safety needs can affect a patient's willingness to complete rehabilitation. For example, patients often fear falling over, due to losing feeling in one leg as a result of their stroke.

As well as the 'hierarchy of needs', there are a range of different motivation theories. The theory that we focus on for this research is goal-setting theory that proposes that goal setting and task performance are directly related. This theory proposes that goals need to be small, specific and clear. It is also important that goals are achievable as setting unachievable goals can be detrimental to motivation. Goals must also be realistic and challenging to increase motivation. Research into goal-setting in stroke rehabilitation [4, 5, 6] has identified that goal setting is a significant factor for successful rehabilitation. However, in a day to day clinical environment, patients do not always have input into their goal setting and therefore do not have a sense of ownership over their rehabilitation and progress [7].

2.2   Persuasive Technology

Persuasive technology is the study of using computing technology to aid behaviour change. Persuasive technology can most commonly be seen in the design of applications for weight loss and giving up smoking. It has been identified that ambitious persuasive technology often fails as a result of taking on too great a behavioural change in one step [8]. It has also been observed that creating a behaviour that is simple, easy and can be done by anyone has a higher chance to yield success. An example of a simple task for stroke patients would be for them to do the same exercise with both hands at the same time. This allows patient to mimic between one hand and the other. As they see improvement, a second task could be introduced. However, it is important that this information or second skill is offered to the patient at the right time [9]. If the patient is bombarded or becomes overwhelmed it may cause them to give up on the system, regardless of how simple.

The introduction of persuasive technology to a rehabilitation setting is likely to have a positive role. However, it is important to carefully design the human computer interaction to reduce any sense of bombardment or belittling of the patient. Instead it should be used as a way of empowering the patient to stay motivated whilst tracking improvements in their performance.

2.3   Stroke and Stroke Rehabilitation

An understanding of the physiology of stroke is essential to understanding the physical and psychological changes to the body that are caused by stroke. A stroke is caused by an interruption to the blood supply to the brain, either by a blockage (ischaemic stroke) or bleeding (haemorrhagic stroke) [10]. A patient's conditions following a stroke vary depending on the severity and location of the stroke. Whilst some patients only suffer minor symptoms that can be rehabilitated quickly, others can have significant impacts on mobility, speech, vision and behavioural changes.

Stroke rehabilitation is a labour intensive process that includes extensive interaction between a patient and their therapist [11]. Two factors that negatively impact the outcome of rehabilitation are lacking motivation and patients not understanding the reasons for doing their rehabilitation exercises [12].

The materials used in the rehabilitation gym include, styrofoam cups, paddle pop sticks, wooden blocks and tape which are manipulated by patients in the process of rehabilitation. Whilst these materials are rudimentary, they can be used with success. However, they do not provide the patient with feedback about the small improvements in their limb movements.

The Nintendo Wii Fit including the Wii Balance Board, and the Xbox Kinect have been introduced to hospitals with mixed results. Some issues with using this technology in a rehabilitation setting are the short length of the games alongside the mapping limitations between the physical interface and game console parameters [13].

2.4   Related Work

This section outlines existing work in the area of designing for stroke rehabilitation, as well as research into the physiotherapist perspective of patients' motivation. These publications come from a range of different research backgrounds, including HCI, technology and clinical research.

In HCI, studies have been completed [14, 15] focusing on tailored rehabilitation solutions for home-based patients. These studies utilise a user centered design process, including extensive research into individual user needs. The designed solutions focused on individual patients, therefore they may not be translatable in a rehabilitation gym context for use by a wider patient audience.

Other research focuses on solutions that can be used by a wider audience. In many cases, researchers have developed their own games by integrating sensors into rehabilitation equipment and designing relevant interfaces for patients. This allows for simple interfaces that can be understood by patients alongside rich and varied feedback, such as those found in video games [13].

The potential of existing gaming consoles for use in rehabilitation context has also been explored in a number of different studies [16, 17]. This research particularly focusses on the Xbox (Kinect) and the Nintendo Wii (fit). Both games have proven useful for patients who are cognitively able and who have a good range of motion, however as they are designed for able-bodied people, they are not able to be used successfully by all patients [18].

The perspective of physiotherapists on patient motivation is not a widely researched topic. A similar study in this area of research looks at physiotherapists attitudes towards motivation and their definition of motivation. As a result motivation is widely seen by physiotherapist as a personality trait [2].

3 Study Design

From our previous work on a set of sensor floor tiles and a sensor sleeve [19], we identified that it is important to understand patient motivation in detail. This includes understanding the causes of increases and decreases in motivation as well as how interaction with computer interfaces adds to or hinders motivation. The following section outlines the study design for this project.

3.1 Participants and Recruitment

All participants work as physiotherapists at the Bankstown Lidcombe Hospital, in the greater Sydney area. The six physiotherapists who were recruited for this study focus primarily on stroke rehabilitation. Physiotherapists were initially contacted via email. The email included an invitation to contribute to the study as well as information about the interviews.

The small sample size of this study is due to the ethics approval under which this study is being completed limiting the study's sample size to the stroke specific physiotherapists at the Bankstown-Lidcombe hospital. This hospital was chosen due to the long-standing relationship between the hospital and the university. As a result of these factors, it must be noted that this may bias the results as different stroke wards throughout the world operate differently and the adoption of technology can vary.

3.2   Observations and Interviews

Physiotherapists were observed completing their day to day work for over 40 hours over a ten week period. The researcher took a fly on the wall approach for the majority of the observations, but at times the researcher would follow the physiotherapists through 'walk-throughs' as they completed their work.

Of the six physiotherapists interviewed, two were senior physiotherapists, two physiotherapists, one a physiotherapist assistant and one a physiotherapist manager. These physiotherapists work directly with stroke patients and have between 5 weeks and 27 years of experience. The interviews had the aims of understanding the physiotherapist perspective on types of patient feedback, patient motivation and the use of interactive technologies in the ward.

3.3   Setting

All interviews took place in the physiotherapist office at the Bankstown-Lidcombe Hospital. This setting was chosen, as it is a quiet location where the interview would not be disturbed. All interviews explored the physiotherapy activities that are conducted at the Stroke and Aged care rehabilitation gymnasium at the Bankstown-Lidcombe Hospital. The equipment used in the gymnasium includes height-adjustable beds, tilt tables which tilt from horizontal to vertical, a treadmill, a Nintendo Wii Fit, Balance Tiles, a set of stairs as well as a range of smaller materials for rehabilitation including styrofoam cups, wooden blocks, clothes pegs, balls and tape.

4   Results

This section presents the combined results from the observations and the interview with the six physiotherapists. Thematic analysis [20] was used to identify the themes and affinity diagramming was used to review and further define these themes.

4.1   Importance of Motivation

All physiotherapist commented that motivation is not essential to patient rehabilitation but in most cases results in better outcomes. It was commented that patient motivation makes a physiotherapist's job easier as they do not have to repeatedly remind and encourage the patients to do their rehabilitation exercises. "(Motivation) makes my job easier, but I wouldn't say that it is essential, people can still get better without being highly motivated, but to get really good results I would say it is important" (Participant 5).

The signs of motivation were also explored. 'Engagement' was the word most commonly used by the physiotherapists to describe patients who were motivated. It was commented that these patients were eager to come down to the gym and would exercise in their rooms outside of their time at the gym. In contrast, unmotivated patients were described as "having a lack of interest" (Participant 1).

4.2   Factors Affecting Motivation

There are a range of different factors which can affect the motivation of a patient. These findings have been grouped into positive factors and negative factors.

The *positive factors* that affect motivation include changes to the patient's ability over time, understanding of improvement, support from family and friends and lifestyle factors before stroke.

During the interviews, all physiotherapists commented that changes to the patient's ability over time are important for changes to motivation. Physiotherapists commented, "When they start seeing a bit of improvement, they kind of just get more motivation and they want to come down to the gym" (Participant 6). However, it was also commented that if the patient is not improving or instead sees declines in their ability, they can lose motivation. "It does change when their function either improves or declines" (Participant 6).

The patients understanding of their improvement is also a factor in their motivation. Physiotherapists commented, "it's all about tracking. You track their improvements for them" (Participant 4). This was explained in the context of one patient who did not recognize and celebrate their improvements, even though they were improving on a weekly basis.

'Family' was discussed as being a motivator in two ways. One was the support provided by family members whilst the patient was completing rehabilitation. The other was that they represent an incentive for the patient to get home. It was observed that patients who were completing their rehabilitation with the support of family members were, in many cases, more motivated to continue doing their repetitions. The second type of motivation that was explored during the interviews was the patient's motivation to return home to live with family, especially when they have family who are dependent on them. In some cases this was a pet such as a dog or a cat.

Lifestyle factors that impact stroke rehabilitation include the patient's level and frequency of exercise before the stroke. During the interviews, physiotherapists commented that patients who have "been intentionally very physically active" (Participant 1) before their stroke usually have more success in the gym.

Negative factors that affect patients' motivation include pain, sickness and psychological issues, difficulties with communication and environmental factors.

During the interviews, 'pain and sickness' were discussed as common factors that result in a change of motivation. Physiotherapists commented that the most common issue affecting confidence was patient falls during the night. The effect of psychological issues on patient motivation was also explored. Physiotherapists commented that a patient's willingness to complete their rehabilitation often has to do with their emotions and mood. "It has a lot to do with their mood and how they are feeling and their emotions about everything that has happened" (Participant 3).

Communication difficulties are another factor that affects motivation. Physiotherapists commented that patients who do not speak English often struggle with motivation as communicating with and understanding the physiotherapist is difficult.

Environmental factors were also discussed as affecting patient motivation in a negative way. "Little distractions stop patients from doing their exercises" (Participant 5) was a comment by one of the physiotherapists when discussing the factors which impede patients from completing the numbers of repetitions they are prescribed.

4.3   Understanding Feedback

In HCI, feedback is defined as 'any form of information from a system, the environment, or a person in response to an action of a person on that system' [21]. During the interviews, feedback was described as "Communication of any type of knowledge of performance back to the patient" (Participant 2). The interviews explored feedback given to the patient during their exercise and following their exercise.

The types of feedback that are given to the patient during their exercise include feedback given by the physiotherapist and feedback given by external factors. It was observed that physiotherapist feedback is usually in the form of verbal or visual feedback. This can be broken into motivational feedback where physiotherapists tell the patient that they are doing a good job, or simply smile at them. The other type of feedback is knowledge of performance where the physiotherapist communicates to the patient what they need to do to complete the exercise correctly or manipulates the patient's limbs.

Feedback given by external factors was identified during the observations. Types of external feedback include the feedback from games such as the Nintendo Wii and the stepping tiles, as well as feedback from the manual hand counters telling the patients how many repetitions of the exercise they have completed. Other feedback includes visual cues that are usually in the form of pieces of tape, set up by the physiotherapists to tell the patients where they need to reach for an exercise. There can also be audio cues such as walking in time with music.

When discussing these external forms of feedback with the physiotherapists, we explored the level of feedback offered by games such as the Nintendo Wii and balance tiles. Physiotherapists commented that games such as the Wii would still require that patients have one-on-one attention from the physiotherapist as these exercises allow for adaptive compensation, meaning that the patient does not have to complete the exercise correctly to receive positive feedback and therefore can be completing the exercise incorrectly without knowing. In many cases, this is due to the technology not being designed to accommodate "spatial relationships, for example where someone is in space" (Participant 1). Feedback following exercise was also explored. Physiotherapists commented that "measurement is really important so there is some concrete example of how patient's movement has changed" (Participant 1).

4.4   Personalisation of Feedback

Observations of the physiotherapists in the rehabilitation ward showed that physiotherapists give different types of feedback depending on the patient and the exercise. The idea of personalisation of feedback was also explored in the physiotherapist interviews. Factors such as age, patient motivation, severity of stroke, cognitive issues and patient goals were discussed as being reasons for giving patients different types of feedback. Physiotherapists also consider the type and amount of feedback provided.

During the interviews, age and patient motivations were explored particularly in relation to the types of exercises performed by different patients. This exploration focused on use of interactive technologies such as the Nintendo Wii. Physiotherapists commented that "It's a lot easier for the younger patients in their 20s, 30s, or even 40s...whereas patients who are in their 70s, 80s and 90s will sort of think that it is a game rather than something that can help them in terms of their rehabilitation" (Participant 2).

Severity of the patient's stroke or a patient's cognitive issues also affect the type of feedback physiotherapists use. Physiotherapists commented that verbal feedback is most commonly used for patients with cognitive issues. They also commented that complex feedback such as that provided by the Wii, often does not work for these patients.

Physiotherapists commented that "setting goals whilst you are practicing is important" (Participant 6). In particular, it is important to set smaller day to day goals which relate to the patient's larger rehabilitation goals. One physiotherapist commented, "I try to give feedback about their broader goals as well as feedback about specific movements" (Participant 1).

The amount and type of information was discussed with the overall consensus that too much information can compromise the patients understanding of what they are meant to do. This can also have a negative effect on their confidence.

5   Discussion

In this section we will discuss the results of the study in relation to the research goals.

Research goal 1 - To understand patient motivation from the physiotherapist perspective.

The results of this study show that there are many different factors affecting patient motivation. These include positive factors such as improvements in performance and support from family. They also include negative factors such as pain, sickness and psychological issues. It was found that whilst motivation is important for patient rehabilitation outcomes, it is not always a necessity for a positive outcome.

Some existing research that focuses on interviewing patients about their perception of rehabilitation, aligns with our results as well as contributing additional findings which were not found in our study. This research aligns with the understanding that a physiotherapist's relationship with a patient can effect their motivation [14]. The additional research findings include patients not understanding the role of the physiotherapist or what is required to reach their goals. This misunderstanding of how to reach goals is exemplified in existing solutions designed for encouraging healthy eating [22] and physical activity [23].

Other existing research that aligns with our findings explores the possibility of the hospital being a demotivating place. This existing research focuses on environmental considerations such as lack of autonomy and comparisons with other patient's rehabilitation [24].

The effect of this on the design of equipment for stroke rehabilitation is that whilst it is important to design to motivate patients, it is not the only or most important factor. Other factors that may be important include correct feedback and the design of equipment that is easy to use and allows for personalisation.

Another factor that needs to be taken into account is that in the context of the rehabilitation ward, physiotherapists motivate patients. However, the importance of motivation may be different for patients who have left the rehabilitation ward and are an outpatient completing their rehabilitation at home. Whilst not covered in this study, this is an important consideration.

Research goal 2 - To understand what types of feedback physiotherapists provide to patients during rehabilitation.

Physiotherapists commented that the types of feedback they use differs depending on the patient, alongside factors such as severity of the stroke, cognitive issues, patient goals and the patients personality traits. It was identified that there are a range of different feedback types used in the gym. These include verbal, visual and physical feedback from physiotherapists, carers and technologies. The relationship between feedback, especially long term feedback, and motivation was also discussed.

Existing research also identifies that feedback is important to act as encouragement and motivation over time. An area of feedback which is covered by this existing research but was not identified during the interviews was the intrinsic (internal) feedback patients receive from their bodies when completing a movement [25].

The effect of this on designing rehabilitation equipment for patients is the need to personalize feedback. It was identified that there are limitations to the technology currently used in the rehabilitation ward, particularly the Nintendo Wii. Physiotherapists identified the short falls of this technology as being the lack of appropriate feedback as well as the ability for patients to use compensatory movements by using the wrong muscles when doing their exercises. Alongside this was the comments that older patients perceive the Wii as a game for children which will not help them with their rehabilitation.

Research goal 3 - To understand physiotherapists day-to-day use of technology in the rehabilitation gym.

We found that physiotherapists use the balance tiles and the Nintendo Wii Fit with patients in the rehabilitation gym because it is set-up and accessible. Physiotherapists commented that whilst the balance tiles can be useful for patients and give appropriate feedback in the form of knowledge of results, the Wii is limited in the useful information that can be provided to the patient. We also found that the majority of the physiotherapists we interviewed would not call themselves 'technically knowledgeable' as they are not required to use complex technology in their day to day work.

Existing research that looks at the feasibility of the Wii for stroke rehabilitation also identifies these short falls. This research discusses the poor patterning and bad selectivity of muscles that is referred to in our interviews as 'adaptive compensation'. Alongside this, it identifies the shortfalls of the Wii as it is an 'off-the shelf' technology designed for use by able-bodied people, therefore the feedback for patients is negative such as being 'unbalanced; or having a high 'Wii Fit age' [26].

In many cases, patients are unable to get meaningful feedback from the Wii. This shows the importance of designing equipment that provides feedback that is specific to the individual patient and related to the patients previous exercise results.

6   Design Guidelines

These five design guidelines that resulted from this research can be used to design equipment to help patients with motivation when completing their rehabilitation.

DG1 - Allow for ease of setup - Interactive equipment should be simple and easy for physiotherapists and patients to set up. The interviews discussed how technology that is difficult to setup does not get used, as physiotherapists don't have the time and in some cases the technical knowledge to do so. Therefore the equipment needs to be 'plug and play' with no complex technical setup.

DG2 - Provide immediate and longer term feedback - Interactive equipment needs to provide immediate and longer term feedback. Initially a baseline needs to be created from which to measure improvement. Following this, patients need to receive immediate feedback about their movements when they are completing their exercises. This should be in the form of knowledge of performance, where the patient is getting consistent information about how to complete the exercise correctly as well as knowledge of results informing the patient of how many successful repetitions they did in a session. Alongside the immediate feedback, the equipment should track the patient's performance over time to allow the patient to understand if they have improved or not. It was found that this is an important factor for motivating patients.

DG3 - Allow for goal setting - The equipment should allow for patients to set both short and long term goals to help with motivation. The short term goals could be the number of repetitions which a patient will aim to complete in one day, whereas the long term goals are those which the patient wants to achieve over a longer period of time such as being able to walk. Breaking patient's long term goals into a number of short term goals helps with motivation.

DG4 - Design to be multilingual and multimodal- Patients come from a range of different language backgrounds and have varying levels of English. Therefore it is important that feedback is both multimodal and understandable by patients from a range of different backgrounds. An example is the use of a more universal language, such as icons.

DG5 - Allow for personalisation - A patient needs to be able to personalize their feedback depending on what works best for them. Factors such as age, severity of stroke and cognitive issues affect the types of feedback that are most useful for individual patients. For example, physiotherapists commented that older patients often do not relate the game based nature of the Nintendo Wii. Therefore it is important to allow patients or physiotherapists to personalize the type and frequency of the feedback provided, to suit the individual patient.

7   Conclusion

This study focused on understanding the motivation of stroke patients and the factors that affect motivation. Through observing physiotherapists doing their daily work, as well as interviewing six therapists, we gained an understanding of the physiotherapists' perspective of patient motivation as well as the types of feedback which are most suitable for patients. Our findings have resulted in a set of guidelines for researchers and designers who are designing equipment for stroke rehabilitation.

Acknowledgements. We would like to thank all the physiotherapists who participated in the study. The study was completed under national ethics approval (HREC/12/CRGH/185).

References

1. Gollwitzer, P.M., Oettingen, G.: Motivation, History of the concept. In: Wright, J. (ed.) International Encyclopaedia of Social and Behavioural Sciences, vol. 15, pp. 10109–10112. Elseview, Oxford (2001)
2. Maclean, N., Pound, P., Wolfe, C., Rudd, A.: The concept of patient motivation: a qualitative analysis of stroke professionals' attitudes. Stroke 33, 444–448 (2002)
3. Furnham, A.: The Psychology of Behaviour at Work, pp. 248–251. Psychology Press, East Sussex (1997)
4. Sugavanam, T., Mead, G., Bulley, C., Donaghy, M., van Wijck, F.: The effects and experiences of goal setting in stroke rehabilitation – a systematic review. Disability and Rehabilitation (3), 177–190 (2013)
5. Rosewilliam, S., Roskell, C., Pandyan, A.D.: A systematic review and synthesis of the quantitative and qualitative evidence behind patient-centered goal setting in stroke rehabilitation. Clinical Rehabilitation 25, 501–514 (2011)
6. Hartigan, I.: Goal setting in stroke rehabilitation: part 1. British Journal of Neuroscience and Nursing 8, 123–128 (2012)
7. Siegert, R.J., Taylor, W.J.: Theoretical aspects of goal-setting and motivation in rehabilitation. Disability and Rehabilitation 26, 1–8 (2004)
8. Fogg, B.: Creating Persuasive Technologies: An Eight-Step Design Process. In: Proceedings of the 4th International Conference on Persuasive Technology, pp. 1–6. ACM, California (2009)
9. IJsselsteijn, W.: deKort, Y., Midden, C., Eggen, B., van den Hoven, E.: Persuasive Technology for Human Well-Being: Setting the Scene. In: First International Conference on Persuasive Technology for Human Well-Being, pp. 1–5. Springer Link, Heidelberg (2006)
10. Caplan, L.: Stroke. Demost Medical Publishing, New York (2006)
11. Fasoli, S., Krebs, H., Hogan, N.: Robotic technology and stroke rehabilitation: Translating Research into Practice. Topics in Stroke Rehabilitation 11, 11–19 (2004)
12. Maclean, N., Pound, P., Wolfe, C., Rudd, A.: Qualitative analysis of stroke patients' in rehabilitation. British Medical Journal 321, 1051–1054 (2000)
13. Bongers, A.J., Smith, S.: Interactivating Rehabilitation through Active Multimodal Feedback and Guidance. In: Rocker, C., Ziefle, M. (eds.) Smart Healthcare Applications and Services: Developments and Practices, pp. 236–260. IGI-Global, Pennsylvania (2010)
14. Balaam, M., Rennick-Egglestone, S., Hughes, A., Nind, T., Wilkinson, A., Harris, E., Axelrod, L., Fitzpatrick, G.: Rehabilitation Centered Design. In: CHI 2010 Extended Abstracts on Human Factors in Computing Systems, pp. 4583–4586. ACM, New York (2010)
15. Blake, P., Chen, Y., Duff, M., Lehrer, N.: A novel adaptive mixed reality system for stroke rehabilitation: principles, proof of concept, and preliminary application in 2 patients. Topics in Stroke Rehabilitation 18, 212–231 (2011)
16. Harvey, N., Ada, L.: Suitability of Nintendo Wii Balance Board for rehabilitation of standing after stroke. Physical Therapy Reviews 17, 311–321 (2012)

17. Lange, B., Flynn, S., Rizzo, A.: Initial usability assessment of off-the shelf video game consoles for clinical game-based motor rehabilitation. Physical Therapy Reviews 14, 355–363 (2009)

18. Alankus, G., Lazar, A., May, M., Kelleher, C.: Towards Customizable Games for Stroke Rehabilitation. In: CHI 2010 Proceedings of the SIGCHI Conference on Human Factors in Computing Systems, pp. 2113–2122. ACM, New York (2010)

19. Bongers, A.J., Smith, S.T., Donker, V., Pickrell, M., Hall, R.: Interactive infrastructures – physical rehabilitation modules for pervasive healthcare technology. In: Holzinger, A., Ziefle, M., Röcker, C. (eds.) Pervasive Health – State of the art and Beyond, pp. 229–254. Springer, London (2014)

20. Braun, V., Clarke, V.: Using thematic analysis in psychology. Qualitative Research in Psychology 3, 77–101 (2006)

21. Pérez-Quiñones, M., Sibert, J.: A collaborative model of feedback in human-computer interaction. In: Proceedings of the SIGCHI Conference on Human Factors in Computing Systems (CHI 1996), pp. 316–323. ACM, New York (1996)

22. Orji, R., Vassileva, J., Mandryk, R.: LunchTime: a slow-casual game for long-term dietary behaviour change. Personal and Ubiquitous Computing 17, 1211–1221 (2013)

23. Consolvo, S., Klasnja, P., McDonald, D.W., Landay, J.A.: Goal-setting considerations for persuasive technologies that encourage physical activity. In: Proceedings of the 4th International Conference on Persuasive Technology (Persuasive 2009), pp. 1–8. ACM, New York (2009)

24. Holmqvist, L.W., Koch, L.: Environmental factors in stroke rehabilitation: Being in hospital itself demotivates patients. British Medical Journal 322, 1501 (2001)

25. Van Vliet, P., Wulf, G.: Extrinsic feedback for motor learning after Stroke: What is the evidence? Disability and Rehabilitation 28, 831–840 (2006)

26. Hilland, T., Murphy, R., Stratton, G.: The Feasibility and Appropriateness of Utilising the Nintendo Wii during Stroke Rehabilitation to Promote Physical Activity. A report by the Liverpool John Moores University (2011)

Formalizing Customization in Persuasive Technologies

M.C. Kaptein[✉]

Radboud University, Nijmegen
Assistant Professor, Artificial Intelligence, Nijmegen, The Netherlands
m.kaptein@donders.ru.nl

Abstract. Many authors have noted that customization increases the effectiveness of persuasive technologies. Also, many empirical demonstrations of successful customization efforts exist in the persuasive technology literature. However, a clear formal framework to describe and evaluate customization is lacking. This leads to the worrisome conclusion that statements like: "customization is beneficial" are often ill-defined given the empirical demonstration at hand. In this paper we forward a formalization of customization to prevent such problems. We derive a number of assumptions regarding the data-generating model that need to be met for customization to be fruitful, and we provide several examples of customization criteria. This paper serves as a discussion piece for the persuasive technology conference to evaluate the use and value of (mathematical) formalizations of customization.

Keywords: Persuasive technology · Customization · Personalization

1 Introduction

In many fields of the social sciences (e.g., marketing, psychology, health-care, education, etc.) scholars are examining the effects of customized treatments (see, e.g., 2; 4; 8; 19; 14; 10). This is known under a multitude of headings (personalization, customization, etc. etc. (15; 1; 24)), and many studies can be found ostensibly showing the positive effects of customization (e.g., 21). However, the interpretation of statements like "customization of advertisements is beneficial" (2) or "personalization of medical information is more persuasive than non-personalized information" (9) is often ambiguous. This paper introduces a formal mathematical notation to describe the effects of personalization. This formalization clearly *defines* customization attempts and serves to *derive assumptions* regarding the data generating model and the customization process that are of use in experimental evaluations of customized persuasive technologies.

This paper is organized as follows: First, we briefly review customization and personalization efforts in the persuasive technology field. This review does not aim to provide a complete overview of earlier attempts, but merely serves to highlight the importance of customization to our field. Second, we provide a formalized view on customization attempts and introduce the (mathematical)

© Springer International Publishing Switzerland 2015
T. MacTavish and S. Basapur (Eds.): PERSUASIVE 2015, LNCS 9072, pp. 27–38, 2015.
DOI: 10.1007/978-3-319-20306-5_3

formalization we use throughout. In the third section of this paper we analyze the simplest customization attempt possible using the proposed formalization and derive a number of results regarding the data generating process involved in such a simple customization effort. Subsequently, we introduce a numerical example of the use of our framework to guide customization efforts for a more elaborate customization attempt. Finally, we discuss the limitations of our proposed framework and discuss possible future work.

2   Customization and Personalization in Persuasive Technologies

The persuasive technology field has witnessed a number of attempts to understand customization in persuasive technologies. Much of the work on on customization in persuasive technology is theoretically based on dual-process models—the Elaboration Likelihood Model (ELM) (7) in particular—to work out how new or established psychological traits moderate persuasion. This is warranted by experimental studies in psychology which demonstrate that trait differences in motivations, such as need for cognition (NfC, 7) exists, and that these differences influence the peripheral and central processing of persuasive messages. Traits like NfC predict (e.g.,) differences in the effects of argument strength on attitudes, the degree to which individuals rely on product characteristics versus source liking (e.g., 13), attitude strength resulting from processing a persuasive message (e.g., 12), and metacognition in persuasion (e.g., 26). Hence, using trait differences in information processing is a fruitful approach for the design of persuasive technologies.

Taking a more applied approach, persuasive technology researchers have also worked on applications of individual differences in the design of persuasive technologies directly. (18) developed a customized persuasive systems in which persuasive messages were customized based on questionnaire measures of user susceptibility, while (16) developed a customized persuasive system in which persuasive messages were tailored to users based on observed user responses. (6) developed a scale to measure persuadability of users for use in the customization process, and in a CHI 2014 workshop on *Personalizing Behavior Change Technologies* personalization was actively discussed.[1] Customization was examined in the context of persuasive technologies designed to improve sleeping behaviors (5), and authors have discussed general architectures for personalized persuasive systems (22) and persuasive system design. Also, under the heading of computer tailored health interventions, customization is heavily researched (see, e.g., 24; 20).

To summarize, customization, or personalization, is heavily researched within the persuasive technology community. However, a formal language to evaluate and compare customization efforts is lacking: while many studies conclude that

---

[1] http://personalizedchange.weebly.com/1/post/2014/03/the-crowd-and-persuasion-a-necessity-for-individualized-persuasive-technologies.html

customization is "beneficial" in one way or another, there is no consensus in the methods that demonstrate such statements. Hence, it is unclear what exactly customization means, what beneficial means, and compared to what type of non-customized system the statement holds. In the next sections we develop a formalization of customization that, we hope, reduces some of these problems.

3 A Formalization of Customization

In this section we introduce a mathematical formalization of customization (or personalization) efforts that are undertaken in the design of persuasive systems and in other fields. We then provide a simple application of the proposed formalization based on an existing customization study (17).

We start with a number of definitions useful to formalize the customization problem. Abstractly, each customization effort can be described according to the following terms:

Definition 1. *Treatments (or actions)* $\boldsymbol{a}_i$. *Here,* $\boldsymbol{a}_i$ *specifies the treatments (or messages, or feedback) that a user i receives.* $\boldsymbol{a}$ *is possibly a vector describing treatment values in a high dimensional treatment space.*

Definition 2. *User features* $\boldsymbol{x}_i$. *Here,* $\boldsymbol{x}_i$ *denotes all relevant characteristics of the user that are used in the customization process. Also x is possibly a vector.*[2]

Definition 3. *The (assumed) data generating function* $y_i = \mathcal{M}_g(\boldsymbol{a}_i, \boldsymbol{x}_i)$. *Here,* y_i *denotes some outcome measure of the customization attempt (e.g., compliance), and* $\mathcal{M}_g(\boldsymbol{a}_i, \boldsymbol{x}_i)$ *denotes the function that maps the treatments given to a user i to the observed outcome given the user's features.*

Definition 4. *A criterion* $\mathcal{C}$. *The criterion is a statement regarding the observed outcomes,* y_i, *of the customization process which formalizes the* goal *of the customization attempt. In the remainder of this paper we assume that we choose the criterion such that effective customization* maximizes *the criterion.*

The above formalization does not yet specify what is intended with statements like "customization is effective". We propose to formalize such a statement using what we coin a *customization function*:

Definition 5. *The customization function* $\boldsymbol{a}_i = \eta_c(\boldsymbol{a}_i^B, \boldsymbol{x}_i)$. *This function describes how a certain* baseline *treatment,* $\boldsymbol{a}_i^B$, *interacts with the user features,* $\boldsymbol{x}_i$, *to produce a* customized *treatment.*

Note that if the function $\eta()$ does *not* depend on $\boldsymbol{x}_i$, then the treatments are *not customized*. The simplest case of such a non-customized treatment is denoted by $\boldsymbol{a}_i = \eta_{nc}(\boldsymbol{a}_i^B) = 1\boldsymbol{a}_i^B$ which we denote by the *nc* (non-customized) subscript.

---

[2] Note that this definition of user features also combines the notion of segmentation – adapting treatments to subgroups of users – and personalization: only if a each user has a unique combination of feature values then the term "personalization" would be distinct from "segmentation".

To state that "customization is effective" is thus the same as stating that for *some* customization function $\eta_c(a, x) \neq \eta_{nc}(a)$, that is selected by the researcher, the value of the criterion $\mathcal{C}$ is higher than for *any possible choice* of $\eta_{nc}(a)$.

3.1   Operationalization of the Definitions

To explain how the above definitions describe a concrete customization attempt consider the customization attempt described by (17): in this paper the authors measure, using a survey, whether or not users are "persuadable" (e.g., receptive to persuasive messages). The authors identify both "high" and "low" persuadables. Subsequently, the authors send email messages that either contain persuasive arguments (such as *"Both physicians and general practitioners recommend at least 30 minutes of moderate activity, such as walking, during a day."*) or not to motivate users to participate in a health related activity. The authors (amongst other things) measure the interest in the health related activity using a click on the (email) message.

In this specific case the treatment a_i is a scalar denoting either the persuasive message or the non-persuasive message (e.g., $a \in \{0, 1\}$). The user features for each user i can also be represented by a scalar x_i denoting high or low persuadable users (thus, also $x \in \{0, 1\}$). The data generating model $\mathcal{M}_g$ describes the assumed relationship between the treatments and the user features. In (17) this model is not described explicitly, but a flexible model mapping the four (2×2) possible treatment-feature combinations to possible observed outcomes y is given by:

$$y_i = \mathcal{M}_g(a_i, x_i) = \beta_0 + \beta_1 a_i + \beta_2 x_i + \beta_3 a_i x_i + \epsilon_i \tag{1}$$

where ϵ_i denotes the noise in the measurements and $\theta = \{\beta_0, \ldots, \beta_3\}$ is a set of model coefficients that need to be estimated from empirical data.[3]

The customization function in this experiment is simple, and merely "flips" the treatment for the two possible user features:

$$a_i = \eta_c(a_i^B, x_i) = (1 - a_i^B)^{(1-x_i)}(a_i^B)^{x_i}$$

resulting in the fact that for a specific baseline treatment $a_i^B = 0$, the users with a feature value $x_i = 0$ receive the treatment 0, while users with a feature value $x = 1$ receive treatment 1 and vice versa.

Finally, the authors examine the percentage of users showing interest in each of the four treatment-feature combinations. This can be formalized into the criterion $\mathcal{C}_{perc} = 100 * \frac{\sum_{i=1}^{N} y_i}{N}$. Note however, that since N is a constant *given* the experiment, maximizing the criterion $\mathcal{C}_{perc}$ is equivalent to maximizing $\mathcal{C}_{sum} = \sum_{i=1}^{N} y_i$ which we regard quite a common criterion and denote "$\mathcal{C}_1$" from now on.

---

[3] Note that in this paper we do not discuss estimation methods and from now on for simplicity assuming that θ can be estimated without error.

4 Analysis of the 2 × 2 Customization Case

In this section we analyze the 2 × 2 customization study as presented in (17), and derive a number of general results regarding the data generating model $\mathcal{M}_g(a_i, x_i)$ which are general for the 2 × 2 setting and can thus be used to evaluate other customization attempts with the same formalization.

For "customization" to be effective — given the criterion $\mathcal{C}_1$, the customization function $\eta_c(a_i^B, x_i) = (1 - a_i^B)^{(1-x_i)}(a_i^B)^{x_i}$, and the non-customized assignment function $\eta_{nc}(a_i^B, x_i) = 1a_i^B$, and furthermore using the assumed data generating model specified in Equation 1 — the following must hold:

$$\underset{a^B}{\mathrm{argmax}} \sum_{i=1}^{N} \mathcal{M}_g(\eta_c(a_i^B, x_i), x_i)) > \underset{a^B}{\mathrm{argmax}} \sum_{i=1}^{N} \mathcal{M}_g(\eta_{nc}(a_i^B), x_i) \qquad (2)$$

Using this mathematical formalization, we can derive the following facts in the 2 × 2 case:

Theorem 1. *Treating x as a random variable, personalization will not be effective (thus, the inequality presented in Equation 2 will not hold) if $V[x] = 0$ where $V[]$ denotes the variance of the random variable.*

The proof is omitted but intuitively obvious: if each user has the exact same features x, then $\eta_c()$ reduces to $\eta_{nc}()$ for all users i and hence $\mathcal{M}_g(\eta_c()) = \mathcal{M}_g(\eta_{nc}())$.

Theorem 2. *Given the data generating model defined in Equation 1 personalization can only be effective if $\beta_3 \neq 0$.*

Here again the proof is trivial: if there is no interaction between user features and treatments, then $\underset{a^b}{\mathrm{argmax}} \sum_{i=1}^{N} \mathcal{M}_g(\eta_c()) = \underset{a^b}{\mathrm{argmax}} \sum_{i=1}^{N} \mathcal{M}_g(\eta_{nc}())$ since, irrespective of the user features, there is a optimal choice for the treatment which will be optimal *for all users*.

Since Theorem 2 is intuitively obvious, one often finds empirical demonstrations of the benefits of personalization which show, using null-hypothesis significance tests, that $\beta_3 \neq 0$ by rejecting $H_0 : \beta_3 = 0$. However, even in the simple 2 × 2 case such a demonstration is, while necessary, not *sufficient* for the statement in Equation 2 to hold. This is true since:

Theorem 3. *With criterion $\mathcal{C}_1$ personalization is effective (in the sense specified in Equation 2 and with data generating model specified in Equation 1) if and only if*

$$\beta_1 + \beta_3 > 0 \text{ when } \beta_1 < 0 \text{ or} \qquad \beta_1 + \beta_3 < 0 \text{ when } \beta_1 > 0$$

or, in words, the interaction term is larger, and of opposite sign, then the main effect of the treatment.

The proof is simple and can be given by enumerating the different options of user features and treatment combinations for this simple setup. However, a more general method for deriving the proof is to differentiate $\sum_{i=1}^{N} \mathcal{M}_g()$ with respect to a for both η_{nc} and η_c, setting to zero to find its maximum, and comparing $\mathcal{C}_1$ evaluated at that point for both the cases of η. Note that in applied cases x will be *given* by the population distribution of the user features and is thus a *constant* when determining properties of $\mathcal{M}_g()$.

Using the data presented in Table 1 of (17) and focussing on the first dependent measure ("Interest") we obtain – using a logit link function – $\beta_1 = 1.0116$ and $\beta_3 = -1.1163$ and thus, if we take theses point estimates as *true* values of $\mathcal{M}_g()$, the authors have indeed shown that personalization was effective in their experiment (although not very convincingly).

5   Continuous Treatment Personalization

To demonstrate the versatility of the formalization of customization that we present here, we explore another case in which both the treatment a is continuous, and the feature x is continuous (but again both are one-dimensional). Here we focus on the use of the introduced formalization to determine a customization function $\eta()$.

The following scenario describes a case in which this setting realistically occurs: suppose we are designing a persuasive technology that aims to motivate knowledge workers to lead a healthy lifestyle (See, e.g., 11). The system could send messages with suggestions for walks of different lengths (in kilometers), and the system could measure, using GPS, the number of kilometers a user actually walks. The suggested number of kilometers by the systems possibly interacts with the age of the user. Thus we have:

- Actions $a_i \in \{0, \dots\}$, the suggested number of kilometers for the walk.
- User features $x_i \in \{0, 99\}$, the age of the user.
- Outcomes y_i: the number of kilometers that the user ends up walking after receiving the suggestion.

Let us further suppose that we have carried out a large randomized experiment testing different messages, for a large set of users, with diverse ages (and thus with variance in the features in the dataset), and that we have measured their respective responses. We (ostensibly) find that a model that fits the data well is the following:

$$y_i = \mathcal{M}_g(a_i, x_i) = -\frac{1}{4}\left(a_i - (15 - \frac{1}{4}x_i)\right)^2 + 10 + \epsilon_i \tag{3}$$

where ϵ is some random noise with $E[\epsilon] = 0$ which is plotted (discarding ϵ) for users of different ages, $x \in \{20, 30, 40, 50\}$, in Figure 1. Basically the model describes that for suggestions that are either too low or too high, users fail to comply with the suggestion. In between a "best" suggestion can be found leading to the largest observed outcome. However, older users are more likely to regard a suggestion as too high: thus, the same suggestion has a different effect for users of different ages (hence, there is an interaction between user features and assigned treatments).

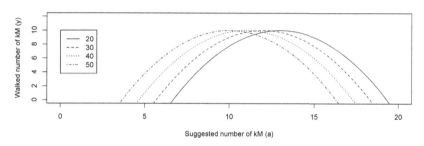

Fig. 1. Relationship between the suggested number of kilometers a, and the observed number of walked kilometers y, for users of different ages as described by the model specified in Equation 3.

5.1 Evaluating Customization for $\mathcal{C}_1$

Now that we have a formulation of the actions, features, and outcomes, and furthermore have specified the data generating model, we can use our formalization to find a customization function which maximizes an outcome criterion such as the sum of the outcomes over all users, $\mathcal{C}_1$.

Suppose we aim to treat a population of 1000 users, with ages distributed uniformly random between 20 and 50. We can then explore whether a specific customization function $\eta_c()$ "outperforms" a non-customized version of treatment selection (formalized by $\eta_{nc}(a_i^B, x_i) = 1a_i$). Figure 2 presents the value of $\mathcal{C}_1$ for a group of 1000 users as a function of a_i^B for the non-customized version (solid line), and various customization functions (dashed lines) given by:

$$\eta_c(a_i^B, x_i, \beta) = a_i^B - \left(\frac{1}{\beta} * (x_i - 20) \right) \tag{4}$$

where $\beta \in \{1, 5, 10, 15\}$. This customization function formalizes the idea that users with a high age (x value) should receive lower suggestions. As is clear from Figure 2, with the appropriate choice of β, customization can outperform non-customized messaging in this specif case.[4] The maximum value of $\mathcal{C}_1$ for the non customized version is (on average, dependent on the simulation run) about 9819 (averaged over 100 simulation runs), while for the customized version, with $\beta = 10$, a maximum value of 10000 can be obtained (regardless of the simulated ages).

5.2 Evaluating Customization for Alternative Criteria

In the previous section we examined the customization function defined in Equation 4 using criterion $\mathcal{C}_1$. However the proposed formalization of customization allows for the investigation of different types of objectives of customization at-

---

[4] And, obviously, given this particular choice of customization function.

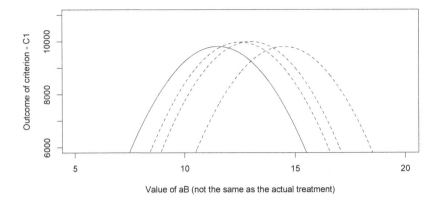

Fig. 2. Values of $\mathcal{C}_1$ as a function of a_i^B for different values of β in Equation 4. Note that several customization functions outperform the non-customized version (solid line), and that the highest value of $\mathcal{C}_1$ can be obtained using $\beta = 10$.

tempts. For example, we could also specify as a criterion:

$$\mathcal{C}_2 = -1 \times \sum_{i=1}^{N} (y_i - k)^2$$

where k is a constant denoting the optimal value of the outcome for individuals (which, in this case, is the same for all individuals). Setting $k = 10$ — and thus denoting that the *optimal* walk length is 10 kM, and both longer and shorter walks are infeasible — we can again numerically examine the criterion as a function of a^B. Figure 3 shows, for $\beta \in \{1, 5, 10, 15\}$ the possible outcomes. Here again, given the appropriate choice of β, customization clearly outperforms non-customized messaging. Note that in each case 2 distinct values for a^B maximize the criterion, hence two different baseline treatments would lead to the same outcome(s) in this specific setting.

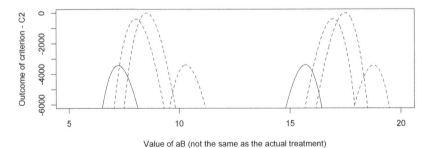

Fig. 3. Values of $\mathcal{C}_2$ as a function of a_i^B for different values of β in Equation 4. Note that several customization functions outperform the non-customized version (solid line), and that the highest value of $\mathcal{C}_1$ can again be obtained using $\beta = 10$. Also note that there are two possible maxima for each customization method.

6   Discussion

In this paper we presented a possible formalization of customization attempts consisting of a description of:

- Actions (or treatments) $\boldsymbol{a}$.
- Features of the user, $\boldsymbol{x}$.
- Observed outcomes y provided by the data generating function $\mathcal{M}_g(\boldsymbol{a}, \boldsymbol{x})$.
- The customization function $a_i = \eta_c(a_i^B, x_i)$.
- A criterion $\mathcal{C}$.

We have demonstrated that using this formalization seemingly distinct customization efforts can be formally described, and that the formalization can be of use to disambiguate statements regarding customization. Furthermore, the introduced formalism can be used to a) derive features of the assumed data-generating model $\mathcal{M}_g$, and b) determine optimal customization functions $\eta()$. However, we consider the current article merely a starting point: the value of methods to (mathematically) formalize customization attempts for the persuasive technology field remains to be seen. Notably, relationships between the currently proposed formalization, and those proposed in surrounding fields (see, e.g., 3; 25; 23) need further discussion. In the remainder of this discussion section we introduce a number of possible extensions to the formalization and some practical problems that can be foreseen.

6.1   Criteria

In this article we introduced two possible criteria to evaluate customization: $\mathcal{C}_1$ denoted the summed overall outcome y, while $\mathcal{C}_2$ denoted the squared distance from some objective for each user. The formalization presented in this paper however gives rise to alternative specifications of customization criteria. For example, one could consider:

$$\mathcal{C} = \sum \mathbb{1}\{y_i > k\}$$

as a personalization criterion where $\mathbb{1}$ denotes the indicator function and thus the criterion states to maximize the number of users that have at least outcome k. Contrary to $\mathcal{C}_1$ this customization function does not consider the absolute size of y_i, but rather only the passing of a certain threshold.

6.2   Estimation

In this paper we have not discussed the role of empirical data in the estimation of $\mathcal{M}_g$. In most practical situations $\mathcal{M}_g$ will be unknown and both model selection as well as parameter estimation need to be undertaken to find a suitable form. In practice the estimated coefficients (e.g., β's in Equation 3) will contain error that need to be considered when examining different customization functions.

6.3   Analytical Solutions

In this paper, and primarily in Section 5, we have presented a number of numerical (based on simulations) results of customization functions. However, there is a clear analytical procedure available once the customization function is selected: one merely plugs in the customization function into the data generating model, and evaluates its maximum (given the chosen criteria and possible population estimates of x) by differentiating with respect to a^B. In practice this might be cumbersome for a high dimensional set of features and possible treatments, however, theoretically this provides a clear method to evaluate different customization functions. This needs further demonstration.

6.4   Dynamic (over-time) Customization

The current paper introduced a formalization of customization in which fixed features x, and a single treatment a per user are considered. In practice, we observe more and more customization efforts which are dynamic over time (e.g., 16). In these cases the action $a_{(i,t+1)}$ selected for user i at timepjoint $t+1$ depends on $y_{(i,t)}$, the observed outcome at time t. We currently think that such attempts can easily be reconciled with our formalization by using $y_{(i,t)}$ as a feature when customizing for $y_{(i,t+1)}$. However, the applicability of our framework for dynamic customization attempts needs future work.

6.5   Conclusions

In this paper we forwarded an initial attempt to formalize customization efforts in persuasive technology. Based on this formalization we derived a number of assumptions of the (assumed) data-generating model that need to be met for customization to be fruitful, and we provided several examples of definitions of customization and their implications. This paper should serve as a discussion piece for the persuasive technology conference to evaluate the use and value of (mathematical) formalizations of the customization process for the design of persuasive systems.

References

[1] Adomavicius, G., Tuzhilin, A.: Personalization technologies. Communications of the ACM 48(10), 83–90 (2005),
    http://dl.acm.org/ft_gateway.cfm?id=1089109\&type=html
[2] Ansari, A., Mela, C.F.: E-Customization. Journal of Marketing Research 40(2), 131–145 (2003)
[3] Armentano, M.G., Amandi, A.A.: Recognition of user intentions for interface agents with variable order markov models. In: Houben, G.-J., McCalla, G., Pianesi, F., Zancanaro, M. (eds.) UMAP 2009. LNCS, vol. 5535, pp. 173–184. Springer, Heidelberg (2009)

[4] Arora, N., Dreze, X., Ghose, A., Hess, J.D., Iyengar, R., Jing, B., Joshi, Y., Kumar, V., Lurie, N., Neslin, S.: Putting one-to-one marketing to work: Personalization, customization, and choice. Marketing Letters 19(3), 305–321 (2008)

[5] Beun, R.J.: Persuasive strategies in mobile insomnia therapy: alignment, adaptation, and motivational support. Personal and Ubiquitous Computing 17(6), 1187–1195 (2013)

[6] Busch, M., Schrammel, J., Tscheligi, M.: Personalized persuasive technology–development and validation of scales for measuring persuadability. In: Berkovsky, S., Freyne, J. (eds.) PERSUASIVE 2013. LNCS, vol. 7822, pp. 33–38. Springer, Heidelberg (2013)

[7] Cacioppo, J.T., Petty, R.E., Kao, C.F., Rodriguez, R.: Central and peripheral routes to persuasion: An individual difference perspective. Journal of Personality and Social Psychology 51(5), 1032–1043 (1986)

[8] Churchill, E.F.: Putting the person back into personalization. Interactions 20(5), 12–15 (2013), http://dl.acm.org/ft_gateway.cfm?id=2504847\&type=html

[9] Dijkstra, A., De Vries, H.: The development of computer-generated tailored interventions. Patient Education and Counseling 36(2), 193–203 (1999), http://www.ncbi.nlm.nih.gov/pubmed/10223023

[10] Dijkstra, A.: Working mechanisms of computer-tailored health education: evidence from smoking cessation. Health Education Research 20(5), 527–539 (2005), http://her.oxfordjournals.org/cgi/content/abstract/20/5/527

[11] Halko, S., Kientz, J.A.: Personality and persuasive technology: An exploratory study on health-promoting mobile applications. In: Ploug, T., Hasle, P., Oinas-Kukkonen, H. (eds.) PERSUASIVE 2010. LNCS, vol. 6137, pp. 150–161. Springer, Heidelberg (2010)

[12] Haugtvedt, C.P., Petty, R.E.: Personality and persuasion: Need for cognition moderates the persistence and resistance of attitude changes. Journal of Personality and Social Psychology 63(2), 308–319 (1992)

[13] Haugtvedt, C.P., Petty, R.E., Cacioppo, J.T.: Need for cognition and advertising: Understanding the role of personality variables in consumer behavior. Journal of Consumer Psychology 1(3), 239–260 (1992)

[14] Hirsh, J.B., Kang, S.K., Bodenhausen, G.V.: Personalized Persuasion: Tailoring Persuasive Appeals to Recipients' Personality Traits. Psychological Science (April 2012), http://www.ncbi.nlm.nih.gov/pubmed/22547658

[15] Ho, S.Y., Bodoff, D., Tam, K.Y.: Timing of Adaptive Web Personalization and Its Effects on Online Consumer Behavior. Information Systems Research 22(3), 660–679 (2010), http://isr.journal.informs.org/cgi/doi/10.1287/isre.1090.0262

[16] Kaptein, M.C., van Halteren, A.: Adaptive Persuasive Messaging to Increase Service Retention. Journal of Personal and Ubiquitous Computing 17(6), 1173–1185 (2012)

[17] Kaptein, M., Lacroix, J., Saini, P.: Individual Differences in Persuadability in the Health Promotion Domain. In: Ploug, T., Hasle, P., Oinas-Kukkonen, H. (eds.) PERSUASIVE 2010. LNCS, vol. 6137, pp. 94–105. Springer, Heidelberg (2010)

[18] Kaptein, M.C., de Ruyter, B., Markopoulos, P., Aarts, E.: Tailored Persuasive Text Messages to Reduce Snacking. Transactions on Interactive Intelligent Systems 2(2), 10–35 (2012)

[19] Moon, Y.: Personalization and Personality: Some Effects of Customizing Message Style Based on Consumer Personality. Journal of Consumer Psychology 12(4), 313–325 (2002), http://ezproxy.stanford.edu:2197/stable/1480285

[20] Neville, L.M., O'Hara, B., Milat, A.J.: Computer-tailored dietary behaviour change interventions: a systematic review. Health Education Research 24, 699–720 (2009)

[21] Noar, S.M., Benac, C.N., Harris, M.S.: Does tailoring matter? Meta-analytic review of tailored print health behavior change interventions. Psychological Bulletin 133(4), 673–693 (2007), http://www.ncbi.nlm.nih.gov/pubmed/17592961

[22] Oinas-Kukkonen, H., Harjumaa, M.: Persuasive Systems Design: Key Issues, Process Model, and System Features. Communications of the Association for Information Systems 24(1), 485–500 (2009), http://aisel.aisnet.org/cais/vol24/iss1/28/

[23] Pentland, A.: A computational model of social signalin. In: 18th International Conference on Pattern Recognition, ICPR 2006, vol. 1, pp. 1080–1083. IEEE (2006)

[24] Smeets, T., Brug, J., de Vries, H.: Effects of tailoring health messages on physical activity. Health Education Research 23(3), 402–413 (2008), http://her.oxfordjournals.org/content/23/3/402.short

[25] Sollenberger, D.J., Singh, M.P.: Methodology for engineering affective social applications. In: Gomez-Sanz, J.J. (ed.) AOSE 2009. LNCS, vol. 6038, pp. 97–109. Springer, Heidelberg (2011)

[26] Tormala, Z.L., DeSensi, V.L.: The Effects of Minority/Majority Source Status on Attitude Certainty: A Matching Perspective. Personality and Social Psychology Bulletin 35(1), 114–125 (2009)

Understanding How Message Receivers' Communication Goals are Applied in Online Persuasion

E. Vance Wilson[(✉)]

Worcester Polytechnic Institute, 100 Institute Road,
Worcester, MA, USA
vancewilson@gmail.com

Abstract. Prior research demonstrated that message receivers' primary and secondary communication goals are important predictors of their evaluation of online persuasive messages. The present study was undertaken to illuminate the process by which these communication goals are applied in response to received messages. The findings demonstrate that communication goals are applied immediately upon viewing even a simple message directory listing containing subject, sender, and date information. Once activated, communication goals significantly predict intention to comply with a message request, although predictiveness increases substantially when the complete message is read. Further analysis suggests that message receivers' communication goals can offer rich explanations of the cognitive processes that are used to evaluate online persuasive messages.

Keywords: Influence · Compliance · Computer-mediated communication (CMC) · Email · Goals-planning-action model

1 Introduction

This paper extends the work of Wilson and Lu [1], who propose that receivers of online persuasive messages[1] evaluate them using a two-tiered goal structure. Goals are "internal representations of desired states, where states are broadly construed as outcomes, events or processes" ([2] p. 338). Goals are characterized by several properties that provide important background to the study of online persuasion.

- *Goals are motivational as well as aspirational*—where gaps are encountered between the current state and the desired goal state, individuals tend to act to achieve their goals rather than to simply internalize them [3]. This property implies that where individuals have unmet goals, e.g., related to online persuasive messages, these goals will tend to motivate behavior.

---

[1] In this paper the phrase *online persuasive messages* is used to describe messages that urge receivers to comply with one or more requests and are delivered via a computer-mediated communication (CMC) medium, such as email, and *online persuasion* is used to describe the processes by which these messages are created by senders and evaluated by receivers.

© Springer International Publishing Switzerland 2015
T. MacTavish and S. Basapur (Eds.): PERSUASIVE 2015, LNCS 9072, pp. 39–50, 2015.
DOI: 10.1007/978-3-319-20306-5_4

- *Goals demonstrate equifinality*—goals can be achieved through multiple means that are not necessarily dependent on the current state [2]. This makes it possible for individuals to maintain stable goal structures while applying diverse methods to achieve their goals.
- *Goals provide standards against which outcomes may be measured* [4]—this property implies that goals are readily available for individuals to reference and also incentivizes individuals to maintain stable goal structures.
- *Goals are interrelated and hierarchical*—individuals commonly prioritize goals and subgoals. Thus it is essential to identify and understand interrelations that occur within overall goal structures in order to explain goal-based behaviors [2]. This property suggests that goals research should focus on reconciling comprehensive effects of goal structures rather than emphasizing individual goals.
- *Different goals predominate under different circumstances* [5]—this property reinforces the need to study goal structures vs. individual goals in order to develop explanations of online persuasion that are generalizable across diverse contexts.

Dillard, Segrin, and Harden [6] present a goal structure of interpersonal influence that responds to these properties in the context of individuals producing persuasive messages (referenced hereafter as *message senders*). They propose that such attempts to persuade are instigated by the primary goal of influencing others and that four secondary goals act in concert to determine the form of the message.

- *Identity goals* relate to the individual's self-concept, including moral standards, principles, and other internal standards.
- *Interaction goals* relate to social appropriateness, including the desire to manage others' impressions of oneself, to avoid threatening or embarrassing others, and to appear relevant and coherent.
- *Relational resource goals* include intrinsic, gratificational rewards that the individual desires from participating in a relationship with others, such as attention, emotional support, and social comparison.
- *Arousal management goals* refer to the individual's desire to maintain his or her state of arousal and apprehension concerning the interaction within tolerable limits by avoiding conditions that cause anxiety or discomfort.

Empirical tests of this goal structure have confirmed that it is capable of predicting numerous behaviors of message senders, including the level of planning, effort, directness, positivity, and logic they incorporate into persuasive messages [6] and the system features they utilize in creating online persuasive messages, including use of graphics and text formatting [7][8].

Wilson and Lu [9] proposed that the secondary goal components of identity, interaction, and arousal management are applicable to *receivers* of online persuasive messages as well as message senders. (Relational resource goals were not included in their analysis, as receivers of online persuasive messages frequently do not have any existing relationship with the message sender.) They further proposed that message receivers apply dual primary goals of *obtaining benefits* and *avoiding costs* to evaluate online persuasive messages (see Figure 1).

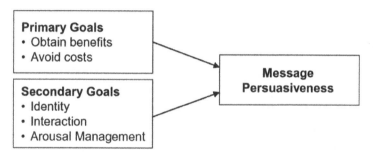

Fig. 1. Communication goals model of online message persuasiveness [1]

Initial empirical testing demonstrated that the goal structure presented in Figure 1 is predictive of numerous aspects of message persuasiveness, including message receivers' involvement with the message, attitude toward the message contents, perception of sender credibility, perceived information quality, and behavioral intention to comply with requests made in the message [1].

One question that initial testing of the communication goals model did not address, however, is the process by which these communication goals are applied in response to online persuasive messages. The authors write,

"Our findings do not tell us whether goals vary substantially based on perceived characteristics of the message and its sender or the extent to which goals are applied as 'preformatted' scripts or templates. It is not clear from the prior literature or from our findings whether communication goals are stable characteristics of the individual . . . or occupy a more ephemeral tier within a goals hierarchy." ([1] p. 2571)

The present study was designed to shed light on the processes by which message receivers' communication goals are applied in response to different levels of message exposure and sender characteristics.

2   Research Method

This research was conducted through use of a custom-developed online experimental simulation and survey application. Subjects were presented with a simulated online persuasive message (see Table 1) and were then asked to rate their goals and other perceptions in response to one of four treatments in a 2 x 2 fully factorial design.

The first dimension addressed by the research design assesses communication goals at multiple stages. Prior research indicates that goals become salient in response to stimuli in the individual's environment [5]. In the case of online persuasive messages, two stages of stimuli are commonly encountered: an initial directory listing stage containing the message subject, identity of the message sender, and date followed by a complete message stage containing message text in addition to the directory listing information. Two corresponding message exposure treatments were used: a *Directory View* treatment in which subjects were asked to rate goal scale items immediately after viewing the directory listing, and a *Complete View* treatment in which subjects rated goal scale items after viewing the complete message.

The second dimension of the research design responds to a limitation acknowledged in the Wilson and Lu [1] study, which addressed only online persuasive messages received from an unknown sender. Two sender characteristic treatments were implemented: an *Unknown Sender* treatment in which the sender was identified only through a fictitious email address following the design of [1] and a *Known Sender* treatment in which subjects were told that they had received the message from an existing acquaintance.

2.1   Subjects

Subjects were 495 undergraduate students at a large urban Midwest U.S. University enrolled in business communications and information systems courses who earned extra course credit by voluntarily participating in the study or completing an alternative assignment. The average subject was 20 years old, 56% were male, and 44% were female. Subjects were notified via an email message containing participation instructions and a hyperlink to access the online application, which was available for completion during a period of one week following notification. Subjects who had not completed the survey after five days were sent a follow-up reminder via email.

2.2   Research Measures

This study tested direct effects of communication goals on message involvement and direct effects and indirect effects (mediated by message involvement) on intention to comply, a measure of message persuasiveness studied previously by [1]. Measurement scale items used in the research are presented in Table 2. Communication goals used items from [1], message involvement used the personal involvement inventory developed by Zaichkowsky [9], and intention to comply used new items developed for the research context based on a seminal definition of behavioral intention [10].

2.3   Administration Procedure

On entry into the application, subjects were informed regarding their rights and the research process and were then randomly assigned to one of the research treatments presented in Table 1. Subjects assigned to either of the Directory View treatments were notified that they had received an online message with the subject title "Need your help" from either "bdayo@texts2africa.com" (unknown sender) or "Your Favorite Professor" (known sender). The known sender treatment was selected to emphasize key principles of influence, including reciprocity, social proof, liking, and authority [11]. At this point they were instructed to rate their communication goals toward the message. Subsequently, they were asked to read the entire message, as presented in the Complete View version of the applicable Known Sender or Unknown Sender treatment, to rate their message involvement and intention to comply with the request, and to respond to demographic questions. Subjects then exited the application.

Table 1. Explanation of research treatments

Treatment	Viewed by Subjects Prior to Rating Communication Goals
Directory View- Unknown Sender	You have received the following message: Received: 10/2/2014 8:23:19 AM From: bdayo@texts2africa.com Subject: Need your help
Complete View- Unknown Sender	You have received the following message: Received: 10/2/2014 8:23:19 AM From: bdayo@texts2africa.com Subject: Need your help African students need your used textbooks. Students in African countries like Zambia and Nigeria have little money to pay for college textbooks, and they need your help. When you finish your coursework this semester you can make a big difference in their lives by donating your used textbooks to deserving African students instead of reselling them to book buyers. Textbooks are needed in all subject areas. Here's how to donate. First, reply to this message to pledge a donation of one, two, or all your used textbooks. When you are finished using your textbooks for the semester, carefully package them and ship them to: Texts2Africa P.O. Box 43502 Brooklyn, NY 10024 Our volunteers will be waiting to accept your donation in fulfillment of your pledge. I look forward to receiving your reply, and really appreciate your help in this good cause.
Directory View- Known Sender	You have received the following message: Received: 10/2/2014 8:23:19 AM From: Your Favorite Professor Subject: Need your help
Complete View- Known Sender	You have received the following message: Received: 10/2/2014 8:23:19 AM From: Your Favorite Professor Subject: Need your help African students need your used textbooks . . . [*same message text as in Complete View/Unknown Sender treatment*] . . . I look forward to receiving your reply, and really appreciate your help in this good cause.

Table 2. Measurement items and CFA loading (combined treatments)

Construct		Measurement Items	Loading
Benefit Goals	B1	I feel complying with this request would actually be good for me.	0.835
	B2	I am looking forward to positive things resulting from this message.	0.832
	B3	I am interested in benefits the message might have for me.	0.779
Cost Goals	C1	I am concerned about personal costs of complying with this request.	0.738
	C2	I am concerned that complying with this request might be bad for me.	0.843
	C3	I worry about the downsides for me that this message might produce.	0.867
Identity Goals	ID1	I am concerned about being true to my values and myself.	0.850
	ID2	I am concerned with not violating my own ethical standards.	0.740
	ID3	It is important to me that I represent myself honestly.	0.780
Interaction Goals	IX1	I don't want to look stupid to the message sender.	0.794
	IX2	I will be careful to avoid interacting in a way that is socially inappropriate.	0.717
	IX3	I am concerned with putting myself in a bad light in this situation.	0.831
Arousal Management Goals	AM1	The potential of this message for making me nervous and uncomfortable worries me.	0.876
	AM2	I am afraid of being uncomfortable or nervous.	0.833
	AM3	I worry that this message could make me anxious.	0.795
Message Involvement	Inv1	My feeling is that this message is: (Important / Unimportant	0.838
	Inv2	My feeling is that this message is: (Boring / Interesting)	0.844
	Inv3	My feeling is that this message is: (Relevant / Irrelevant)	0.808
	Inv4	My feeling is that this message is: (Unexciting / Exciting)	0.822
	Inv5	My feeling is that this message: (Means Nothing to Me / Means a Lot to Me)	0.832
	Inv6	My feeling is that this message is: (Appealing / Unappealing)	0.867
	Inv7	My feeling is that this message is: (Fascinating / Mundane)	0.815
	Inv8	My feeling is that this message is: (Worthless / Valuable)	0.812
	Inv9	My feeling is that this message is: (Involving / Uninvolving)	0.648
	Inv10	My feeling is that this message is: (Not Needed / Needed)	0.803
Intention to Comply	IC1	How likely is it you would comply with the request made in the 'Need your help' message? (Very Unlikely / Very Likely)	0.891
	IC2	If I actually received the 'Need your help' email message, I would do what it requests.	0.892
	IC3	I would pledge to donate at least one book if I actually received the 'Need your help' message.	0.886
	IC4.	I would not pledge to donate any books if I received the 'Need your help' message. *(Reverse coded)*	0.849

* All responses used 7-point scales end-marked as 1 = Strongly Disagree and 7 = Strongly Agree or as shown in parentheses; loadings are produced through Promax rotation.

For subjects in one of the Complete View treatments, after being notified that they had received an online message they viewed the entire message prior to responding to all survey items, i.e., combined ratings of communication goals, message involvement, intention to comply, and response to demographic measures. Subjects then exited the application. For all subjects, administration ordering of survey items was individually randomized as recommended by [12].

3   Results

Descriptive statistics and results of between-groups mean differences tests are shown in Table 3. In order to account both for the presence of significant skewness in several constructs [13] and non-linear relationships which often are encountered in cognitive and behavioral research [14] WarpPLS version 4.0 [15] was used to perform confirmatory factor analysis (CFA) and structural model analysis.

CFA conducted on the overall subject pool indicates that measurement items load primarily on the theorized construct (see Table 2) and demonstrates satisfactory convergent and discriminant validity of the measurement model (see Table 4).

Separate structural models were created for the Directory View and Complete View datasets (see Table 5). In both datasets, communication goals significantly predict message involvement and intention to comply, however, communication goals are substantially more predictive of message involvement and intention to comply in the Complete View treatment. Each communication goal was found to be significantly associated with message involvement and/or intention to comply in at least one of the view treatments.

4   Discussion

The results suggest that communication goals play a front-stage role in receivers' evaluation of online persuasive messages and that the communication goals model can provide a rich explanation of message persuasiveness, assessed in this study by measures of receivers' message involvement and intention to comply with message requests. Several implications of the results are discussed in the remaining sections.

4.1   Communication Goals as Predictors of Message Persuasiveness

Prior research showed that communication goals can be important predictors of message persuasiveness where receivers have read a complete message [1]. The findings of the present study demonstrate that this effect extends to reading a Directory Listing of the message that contains only subject, sender, and date information and to situations where the message receiver knows the message sender in addition to the Unknown Sender treatment previously assessed by [1]. These extended findings imply that the communication goals model is robust and generalizable across research contexts.

Table 3. Descriptive statistics and results of between-groups mean differences tests

Measure	Group Mean* (Standard Deviation)			
	Known Sender (n = 247)	Unknown Sender (n = 248)	Directory View (n = 249)	Complete View (n = 246)
Benefit Goals	**5.37** (1.27)	**3.83** (1.70)	4.56 (1.84)	4.64 (1.51)
Cost Goals	**3.81** (1.56)	**4.63** (1.56)	**4.53** (1.60)	**3.91** (1.67)
Identity Goals	**4.92** (1.37)	**4.60** (1.48)	4.85 (1.44)	4.67 (1.43)
Interaction Goals	**4.60** (1.57)	**3.73** (1.41)	**4.56** (1.49)	**3.75** (1.51)
Arousal Mgmt. Goals	3.47 (1.66)	3.42 (1.66)	**3.97** (1.57)	**2.92** (1.57)
Message Involvement**	**4.20** (1.19)	**3.53** (1.33)	3.88 (1.31)	3.85 (1.30)
Intention to Comply**	**4.49** (1.66)	**3.32** (1.67)	3.93 (1.79)	3.88 (1.75)

*   Bolding indicates significant difference ($p < .05$, two-tailed t-test) between group means of Known Sender vs. Unknown Sender or Viewed Sender and Subject vs. Viewed Complete Message

** All subjects viewed the complete message prior to responding to items measuring message involvement and intention to comply

Table 4. Relationships among latent variables and construct validation statistics

	AVE	Alpha	CR	B	C	ID	IX	AM	MI	IC
Benefit Goals (B)	0.67	0.75	0.86	**0.82**						
Cost Goals (C)	0.67	0.75	0.86	-0.14	**0.82**					
Identity Goals (ID)	0.62	0.70	0.83	0.42	0.19	**0.79**				
Interaction Goals (IX)	0.61	0.68	0.83	0.26	0.11	0.23	**0.78**			
Arousal Mgmt. Goals (AM)	0.71	0.78	0.87	0.28	0.09	0.14	0.68	**0.84**		
Message Involvement (MI)	0.66	0.94	0.95	0.64	-0.37	0.34	0.49	0.05	**0.81**	
Intention to Comply (IC)	0.77	0.77	0.90	0.57	0.11	0.35	0.16	0.16	0.79	**0.88**

*   Means and standard deviations (SD) are calculated as averaged summations of the raw data; Cronbach's alpha (Alpha), and composite reliability (CR) are shown as reported by WarpPLS; the square root of average variance extracted (AVE) for each latent factor as reported by WarpPLS is shown as a bolded entry in the diagonal.

Table 5. Output of structural models run with Directory View and Complete View datasets*

Antecedent	Directory View				Complete View			
	Path Weight to MI	Path Weight to IC	Indirect Effects on IC	Total Effects on IC	Path Weight to MI	Path Weight to IC	Indirect Effects on IC	Total Effects on IC
Benefit Goals	**0.25**	**0.17**	**0.19**	**0.36**	**0.49**	0.09	**0.31**	**0.40**
Cost Goals	-0.01	0.07	-0.01	0.07	**-0.33**	**-0.15**	**-0.21**	**-0.36**
Identity Goals	0.02	-0.05	-0.01	-0.06	**0.18**	**0.12**	**0.11**	**0.23**
Interaction Goals	**0.15**	0.05	**0.12**	**0.17**	**0.10**	0.03	**0.06**	**0.09**
Arousal Mgmt. Goals	0.07	0.05	0.05	**0.10**	**0.11**	**0.12**	**0.07**	**0.19**
Message Involvement	—	**0.78**	—	—	—	**0.63**	—	—
Explained Variance (R^2)	0.11	0.72	—	—	0.53	0.68	—	—

* MI = Message Involvement, IC = Intention to Comply; bolded path weights and indirect and total effects statistics indicate statistical significance ($p < 0.05$); indirect and total effects on intention to comply as reported by WarpPLS 4.0.

4.2   Communication Goals Structure

The original GPA model of message senders' communication goals [5] and the extension of the model to message receivers by [1] postulate that these goals form a hierarchy in which actions are initiated principally by primary goals of influence among message senders and benefits/costs among receivers. Secondary goals relating to factors such as maintaining one's identity, interacting with others, and managing arousal and apprehension principally determine the form of the message.

Both primary and secondary goals are theorized to be ubiquitously applicable to human interactions [16]. As a test to distinguish the two goal categories and demonstrate the instrumentality of primary goals in initiating action, Wilson and Lu [1] proposed that primary goals should meet the dual criteria of *universality* (applying in all test cases) and *prominence* (showing higher level of association than secondary goals with dependent factors). Findings of the present study confirm that benefit goals are universal and prominent predictors of message involvement and intention to comply across treatments (see Table 5). Cost goals also meet these criteria in the Complete View treatment, where subjects read all message contents prior to rating their communication goals, but not in the Directory View treatment. Similar equivocal findings regarding cost goals were reported by [1], suggesting that targeted research is needed to more clearly delineate the conditions that make cost goals salient to message persuasiveness. Overall, however, the results support the communication goals hierarchy used in the present study.

4.3   View Stages and Application of Communication Goals

The results demonstrate that communication goals are immediately activated on exposure to online persuasive messages. Goal ratings are significantly higher for cost, interaction, and arousal management goals in the Directory View treatment vs. the Complete View treatment (see Table 3). It seems likely that these heightened goal ratings result at least in part from uncertainty arising from the limited information that is available in the Directory Treatment. Those subjects were aware only of the subject, sender, and date of the message at the time they rated their communication goals. Previous research has showed that uncertainty can affect individual performance goals [17] and strategic management goals [18]. One implication of this finding is that communication goals may be important antecedents to the decision whether to read online persuasive messages or to discard them based on subject and sender information in the directory listing [19], however, this issue will require new research to address. In any case, findings of the present study demonstrate that individuals' communication goals are readily accessible to them and that these goals are applied to evaluate even limited message stimuli.

4.4   Communication Goals and Sender Characteristics

Ratings of most communication goals vary significantly between Known and Unknown Sender treatments (see Table 3). The distinctive goal ratings patterns that are illustrated in Figure 5 provide a further, unique perspective on the cognitive processes that receivers apply to evaluate online persuasive messages.

- Benefit goals diverge strongly between Known and Unknown Senders in the Directory View treatment but move toward convergence in the Complete View, indicating that message contents can substantially mitigate negative responses to a message from Unknown Senders and can also subdue overenthusiastic initial responses to messages from Known Senders. Interestingly, predictiveness of benefit goals does not improve substantially across view treatments, as measured by total effects on intention to comply (see Table 5).
- Cost goals are higher for Unknown Senders, reinforcing the interpretation that uncertainty tends to heighten goal ratings. Unlike benefit goals, cost goals developed in the Directory View treatment have no predictive association with intention to comply, a rating which is made after those subjects read the remainder of message text. This finding suggests that receivers evaluate online persuasive messages holistically rather than by applying situational stereotypes [20].
- Interaction goals are greater overall for Known Senders, suggesting message receivers place higher priority on how existing acquaintances view them. Unlike other goals, the total effects of interaction goals on intention to comply were reduced in the Complete View treatment, suggesting that concerns for social appropriateness and image management are subordinated by message contents.
- Identity and arousal management goals show only small differences between Known and Unknown Sender treatments, suggesting that these goals are primarily internal to individuals rather than responsive to the sender, however, both goals significantly predict intention to comply in the Complete View treatment.

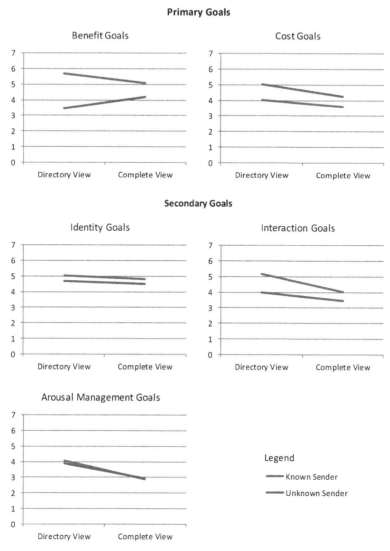

Fig. 3. Communication goals ratings across treatments

The findings answer some questions regarding the process by which communication goals are applied. Goal strength does vary substantially based on sender characteristics as well as message content. And although goals may be applied as a script, e.g., when reading a directory listing, these effects can be overcome by subsequent information.

4.5   Conclusion

This study reinforces the proposition put forward by [1] that communication goals are useful predictors of message persuasiveness. In addition, it extends prior research by demonstrating how a communication goals structure can enrich explanations of the process by which message receivers evaluate online persuasive messages.

References

1. Wilson, E.V., Lu, Y.: Communication Goals and Online Persuasion: An Empirical Examination. Comput. Hum. Behav. 24(6), 2554–2577 (2008)
2. Austin, J.T., Vancouver, J.B.: Goal Constructs in Psychology: Structure, Process, and Content. Psychol. Bull. 120(3), 338–375 (1996)
3. Ryan, T.A.: Intentional Behavior. Ronald Press, New York (1970)
4. Hacker, W.: On some fundamentals of action regulation. In: Ginsberg, G.P., Brenner, M., von Cranach, M. (eds.) Seeking Compliance, pp. 63–84. Academic Press, London (1985)
5. Dillard, J.P.: A Goal-driven Model of Interpersonal Influence. In: Dillard, J.P. (ed.) Seeking Compliance: The Production of Interpersonal Influence Messages, pp. 41–56. Gorsuch Scarisbrick, Scottsdale (1990)
6. Dillard, J.P., Segrin, C., Harden, J.M.: Primary and Secondary Goals in the Production of Interpersonal Influence Messages. Commun. Monogr. 56(1), 19–38 (1989)
7. Wilson, E.V.: Persuasive Effects of System Features in Computer-mediated Communication. J. Org. Comp. Elect. Com. 15(2), 161–184 (2005)
8. Wilson, E.V., Zigurs, I.: Interpersonal Influence Goals and Computer-mediated Communication. J. Org. Comp. Elect. Com. 11(1), 59–76 (2001)
9. Zaichkowsky, J.L.: The Personal Involvement Inventory: Reduction, Revision, and Application to Advertising. J. Advertising 23(4), 59–70 (1994)
10. Warshaw, P.R., Davis, F.D.: Disentangling Behavioral Intention and Behavioral Expectation. J. Experimental Soc. Psychol. 21(3), 213–228 (1985)
11. Cialdini, R.B.: Influence: Science and practice. Allyn & Bacon, Boston (2001)
12. Wilson, E.V., Lankton, N.K.: Some Unfortunate Consequences of Non-randomized, Grouped-item Survey Administration in IS Research. In: Proceedings of the 2012 International Conference on Information Systems, Orlando, FL (2012)
13. Chin, W.W.: The Partial Least Squares Approach to Structural Equation Modeling. In: Marcoulides, G.A. (ed.) Modern Methods for Business Research, pp. 1295–1336. Lawrence Erlbaum Associates, Mahwah (1998)
14. Kock, N.: WarpPLS 4.0 User Manual, ScriptWarp Systems, Laredo, TX (2013)
15. Kock, N.: WarpPLS (2014), http://www.scriptwarp.com/warppls/
16. Schrader, D.C., Dillard, J.P.: Goal structures and interpersonal influence. Commun. Stud. 49(4), 276–293 (1998)
17. Darnon, C., Harackiewicz, J.M., Butera, F., Mugny, G., Quiamzade, A.: Performance-approach and Performance-avoidance Goals: When Uncertainty Makes a Difference. Pers. Soc. Psychol. B 33(6), 813–827 (2007)
18. Bourgeois, L.J.: Strategic Goals, Perceived Uncertainty, and Economic Performance in Volatile Environments. Acad. Manage. J 28(3), 548–573 (1985)
19. Andersson, M., Fredriksson, M., Berndt, A.: Open or Delete: Decision-makers' Attitudes Towards E-mail Marketing Messages. Adv. Soc. Sci. Res. J. 1(3), 133–144 (2014)
20. West, P., Wilson, E.V.: A simulation of strategic decision making in situational stereotype conditions for entrepreneurial companies. Simulat. Gaming 26(3), 307–327 (1995)

Empowering Individuals

What Makes You Bike? Exploring Persuasive Strategies to Encourage Low-Energy Mobility

Matthias Wunsch[1,3(✉)], Agnis Stibe[2], Alexandra Millonig[1], Stefan Seer[1],
Chengzhen Dai[2], Katja Schechtner[2], and Ryan C.C. Chin[2]

[1]Austrian Institute of Technology, Vienna, Austria
{Matthias.Wunsch.fl,Alexandra.Millonig,Stefan.Seer}@ait.ac.at
[2]MIT Media Lab, Cambridge, MA, USA
{agnis,chengdai,katjas,rchin}@mit.edu
[3]Human Computer Interaction, Vienna University of Technology, Vienna, Austria

Abstract. This paper explores three persuasive strategies and their capacity to encourage biking as a low-energy mode of transportation. The strategies were designed based on: (I) triggering messages that harness social influence to facilitate more frequent biking, (II) a virtual bike tutorial to increase biker's self-efficacy for urban biking, and (III) an arranged bike ride to help less experienced bikers overcome initial barriers towards biking. The potential of these strategies was examined based on self-reported trip data from 44 participants over a period of four weeks, questionnaires, and qualitative interviews. Strategy I showed a significant increase of 13.5 percentage points in share of biking during the intervention, strategy II indicated an increase of perceived self-efficacy for non-routine bikers, and strategy III provided participants with a positive experience of urban biking. The explored strategies contribute to further research on the design and implementation of persuasive technologies in the field of mobility.

Keywords: Low-energy mobility · Persuasion · Biking · Cycling · Behavior change · Transportation · Sustainability · Socially influencing systems

1   Introduction

Cities around the world are growing at an unprecedented pace, creating a manifold of new opportunities to meet and exchange ideas and goods. At the same time, however, they generate more traffic. Creating a transport system that supports high-quality life in urban areas requires shifting from high-energy modes of transportation, such as private cars or even public transport, to sustainable low-energy urban mobility, such as walking and biking [21]. Doing so reduces emissions of greenhouse gases, provides health benefits, and enhances the quality of urban life. However, an adoption of new modes of transportation requires a substantial behavior change [11]. Beyond hard policy measures, persuasive strategies embedded in technologies can be useful in facilitating such behavioral change [8],[12],[19]. The aim of this work is to explore such strategies and suitable technologies to promote sustainable low-energy mobility.

© Springer International Publishing Switzerland 2015
T. MacTavish and S. Basapur (Eds.): PERSUASIVE 2015, LNCS 9072, pp. 53–64, 2015.
DOI: 10.1007/978-3-319-20306-5_5

A promising low-energy mode for urban mobility is biking, as it is easily accessible, fast, low-cost, and uses less space than most other modes of transportation. Although previous work has covered mode choices and bike use, little attention has been paid to a change of choice from high-energy modes to biking as a low-energy mode and how this can be supported by persuasive technologies. Heinen et al. [14] classified five groups of determinants for bike commuting. Amongst them are psychological factors; these are attitudes, perceived social norms and habits, which can be at the center of persuasive strategies. Gatterslaben & Appleton [13] applied the transtheoretical model of behavior change [18] to bike commuting. Their findings suggest that different strategies are needed depending on current attitudes and behavior of individuals. Froehlich et al. [9] developed a mobile phone application that semi-automatically sensed and revealed information about transportation behavior. In combination with a personal ambient display, the app engaged users with the goal of increasing green transportation choices (e.g. walking, biking, public transport). Although some statements from qualitative interviews indicated the willingness for such change, no evaluation of actual change in mobility behavior was conducted. A similar but more recent study by Gabrielli and Maimome [10] examined the effect of a mobile app on supporting eco transport choices by citizens of an urban area. The transport choices and habits of the participants were influenced with several persuasion strategies and an overall increase of sustainable transport choices of 14%, as well as a higher environmental awareness among participants, was observed. However, the study design did not include a control group to better attribute behavior change to the experimental intervention. Even more recently, Flüchter et al. [7] found a positive impact of social normative feedback on e-bike commuting.

In accordance with the literature [14], a preliminary survey conducted at the beginning of this research showed that safety concerns are one of the main barriers for adapting biking as a regular mode of transportation. Therefore, the strategies in this study were designed with a focus on perceived safety of biking. All study participants were given access to bikes in order to prevent issues with bike availability and to concentrate research on motivational aspects.

The research question tackled in this paper is: What types of persuasive strategies can lead to a modal shift towards low-energy mobility by increasing bike use? Three different strategies were designed and evaluated in a pretest-posttest control group experimental design.

Section 2 presents the developed persuasive strategies. Section 3 describes the data collection and data analysis. Results are shown in section 4 and discussed in section 5. The paper ends with a conclusion and an outlook towards future research in section 6.

2   Deployed Persuasive Strategies

We designed and developed three strategies for this study.

Strategy I: Frequent Biking Challenge

In this strategy, the following principles of persuasion (see also [6], [8], [20]) have been combined: triggering, recognition, competition, cooperation, and comparison. The overall hypothesis is that this strategy increases bike use.

Triggering. Participants received emails (Fig. 1) between 3 to 5 times a week, providing them with information about their performance in the challenge and acting as a trigger for biking [8]. Emails were chosen as they are likely to be regularly read as opposed to a webpage or a mobile app providing the same information. They were sent in the evening to influence mobility planning for the next day. The regular email updates also contained a set of notifications tailored to each participant, such as daily weather forecasts and entertaining elements. The purpose of these notifications was to keep the sent emails useful and engaging for the participants. Additionally, the emails provided motivational facts about biking and suggestions on when to use a bike.

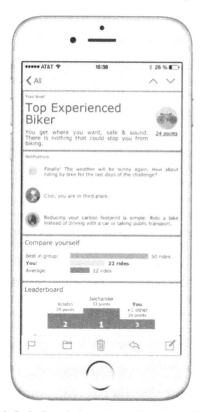 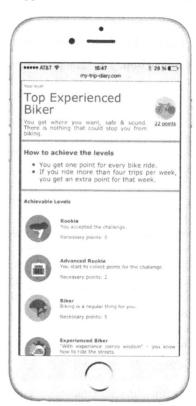

Fig. 1. Left: Regularly sent email updates: Notifications, comparison chart and leaderboard. Right: Explanation of the point scheme and achievable levels within the Frequent Biking Challenge.

Recognition. Based on the number of reported bike trips, participants received points and were awarded different statuses depending on the total number of points. These status levels had titles, were visualized with images and had an exploratory slogan. For example, participants achieving 5 points were recognized with the status "Experienced Biker" and the slogan: "With experience comes wisdom. You know how to ride the streets." Such recognition typically increases enjoyment [4] and influences future behavior [15].

Competition. The email updates furthermore included a leaderboard, showing one's own rank based on the achieved points in comparison to the other participants of the group. It was visualized with a podium for places 1, 2 and 3, followed by a list of the other ranks. Such salient metrics for people to observe their performances among other participants typically promotes competition, which consequently influences their thoughts and behavior [15].

Cooperation. At start, a collective goal (achieving 100 points collectively) was included in the email to facilitate cooperation among participants [15]. This was visualized with a bar graph that showed the sum of points from all participants and how much more were needed to reach the collective goal. The collective goal was reached in the second week of the challenge. Four days later it was replaced with the "compare yourself" comparison chart.

Social Comparison. The "compare yourself" design element allowed participants to compare their number of their bike rides to the average of bike rides and the best participant within the group. This possibly influences motivation as people tend to look for self-enhancement [22] and self-improvement [6],[23].

Strategy II: Virtual Bike Tutorial
The concept of perceived self-efficacy "is concerned with judgments of how well one can execute courses of action required to deal with prospective situations" [3]. Prior studies, such as Chittaro [5], used a persuasive game to increase the perceived self-efficacy[1] of passengers in the situation of an aircraft accident. In this study, the concept of perceived self-efficacy was used in relation to perceived risk and safety, thereby assessing how users perceive their control over their own safety in a biking context. The related assumption is that an increased self-efficacy towards biking will help to overcome safety barriers and hence encourage more biking.

Participants were provided with a short video tutorial on safe urban biking. The safety related information is based on safety guidelines from city officials from New York City, Boston and Vienna. The core concept of the training session is based on the content of a city biking school program. An expert-interview with an experienced biking instructor was conducted in order to gain knowledge on how biking in the city can be taught most effectively to novice bikers.

After the tutorial, a participant should experience the effects of different biking-related decisions in an interactive video training session. The procedure started with a first-person-view video where the participant saw a typical biking scene. The video was then stopped and the participants had to decide on how to continue the ride. (Fig. 2) The consequences of each possible decision were shown in a subsequent video. Different real-life scenarios (e.g. conflict with pedestrian) were tested and partici-

---

[1]   Chittaro referred to it as "safety locus of control". See Ajzen [1] for a discussion on the difference between these concepts.

pants could learn about the consequences of their decisions. An increase of perceived self-efficacy due to that intervention was expected. To measure that, a self-efficacy in biking questionnaire[2] had to be completed by the participant before and after the video training session. The same questionnaire was also included in the survey at the end of the experimental period.

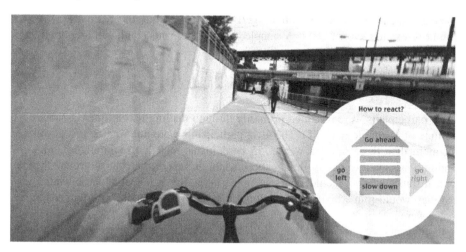

Fig. 2. Screenshot of the Virtual Bike Tutorial showing a conflict situation with a pedestrian

Strategy III: Bike Buddy Program

The start of a new physical exercise is often supported by an experienced person such that guidance and training is provided. In order to apply this kind of learning to the biking context, participants received a one time "bike buddy experience". The hypothesis in this regard is that for novice bikers, the experience of biking in an urban environment will change the perceived safety and risk of doing so. It was expected that this would lead to more positive attitudes towards biking and an overall increase of biking within the participants.

Bike buddies were recruited out of the potential participants for this study who were regular bikers and comfortable biking with new bikers. Bike buddies and participants were matched based on where they live and what routes they usually take. The bike buddies furthermore received instructions for the ride, covering safety aspects and clarifying the goal of showing the participant a safe and enjoyable biking route. They therefore were asked to find a safe and easy route for the planned bike ride and preferable inspect this route prior to the ride. They were also requested to set up a meeting point (ideally at the participant's home) for conducting the ride.

Several persuasive principles were implemented [6],[8]. *Authority*, by having the bike buddy as a guide for the bike ride. *Reduction*, by reducing the effort of the user to find a safe route (complex behavior) in the city to a simple behavior (follow the bike buddy). *Tunneling*, by guiding participants along the route and allowing them to

---

[2] Items were adapted from a self-efficacy in driving questionnaire. [2]

experience the potential benefits of biking. Finally, ***tailoring***, by providing tailored information and personalized support to the user.

3   Data Collection and Analysis

The experiment took place in Cambridge/Boston, Massachusetts area over the period of four weeks in October 2014. A sample of 44 participants continually reported their trip data on a daily basis.

3.1   Sample

Study participants were recruited primarily through mailing lists at the Massachusetts Institute of Technology (MIT). The ideal participants were non-routine bikers (biking not more than three times a week). 55 participants met that requirement and were randomly assigned to one of three experimental groups or the control group. Typical route distance was not included as selection criteria, but as potential participants knew that they would join a biking related study it is likely that people with longer routine routes were less prone to join.

Participants were primarily part of the MIT community. Students made up a large portion of the sample. Therefore, the study sample is not representative of a broader population. Furthermore, the sample most likely exhibits self-selection bias. The process by which participants were recruited encourages those who want to bike, but do not have the means to do so, to join.

44 participants reported their trip data continuously over the period of four weeks. Group sizes were n=12 for (I) Frequent Biking Challenge, n=11 for (II) Virtual Bike Tutorial, n=11 for (III) Bike Buddy Program and n=10 for the control group. Out of all participants, 33 had no access to a bike and were provided with a one-month local bike sharing scheme subscription. 24 participants were provided with a helmet. As prior research shows that there are significant gender differences regarding utilitarian bike use [14], the sample should be balanced in terms of gender. The 44 participants that continually reported their trip data consisted of 22 women and 22 men.

3.2   Data Collection

Participants reported their trips on a daily basis. The collected mobility data included trip purpose and used mode(s). Participants were provided with a web-application that sent the data to a webserver with a relational database. To get continuous trip data, participants were automatically reminded via email in case they forgot to input their trips for the day. The trip diary included a calendar to navigate through the days, a help section, and a statistics graphic where users could see the amount of reported trips and how they were distributed among different modes of transportation. A settings section allowed the users to set a time for the daily reminders, put in custom trip purposes and to set their time zone.

Online questionnaires were used to measure perceived risk and perceived safety in biking at the beginning and end of the experimental period. Open questions were also included at the final questionnaire to ask for perceived behavior change. Interviews were conducted in order to gain further insight on the effect of the strategies. Six participants and six bike buddies from the Bike Buddy Program, two participants of each the Frequent Biking Challenge, the Virtual Bike Tutorial and the control group agreed to be interviewed after the experimental period.

3.3   Data Analysis

Analysis of Quantitative Trip Data. Based on the self-reported mobility data the modal split between modes was computed per person per day. To correct for bad weather, all days with precipitation above average were excluded from the analysis.[3] As can be seen in (1), the difference between the daily bike share of each participant of an experimental group $y_{g,d}$ and the mean of daily bike share within the control group $\bar{y}_{c,d}$ was computed for each day. The sum of these daily differences was divided by the number of days N_{pre} before or N_{post} after the (start of the) intervention.

$$z_{g,pre} = \frac{1}{N_{pre}} \sum_{d=1}^{N_{pre}} \left(y_{g,d} - \bar{y}_{c,d} \right) , \; z_{g,post} = \frac{1}{N_{post}} \sum_{d=1}^{N_{post}} \left(y_{g,d} - \bar{y}_{c,d} \right) \quad (1)$$

As can be seen in (1), the result is a value for average bike-share above control per participant before the intervention $z_{g,pre}$ and after the (start of the) intervention $z_{g,post}$. This approach provides a per-day correction of data which is more accurate than just comparing uncorrected per participant pre- and post-intervention mean values between experimental and control group.[4] Based on the computed values a one-sided paired sample t-test[5] was used to test the hypothesis of an increase in bike-share above the control group value.

As an indicator for the dependence between the share of biking and the share of high-energy modes Pearson r correlations have been computed at per participant level. To test for a difference in the means of perceived risk and perceived safety scores, a paired sample t-test was conducted.

Analysis of Qualitative Interview and Questionnaire Data. Qualitative content analysis [16] was used to analyze data obtained through ex-post-interviews and open question surveys. Category application was carried out in a deductive way, with aspects of analysis based on existing theoretical and empirical work.

4   Results

The effect of the presented strategies on actual bike use has to be viewed in light of many other factors with influence in this regard. The analysis of the gathered qualita-

---

[3]   Weather data from NOAA [0] was used for that. Average precipitation was 4.8 mm.

[4]   For that reason, the common method for pre post control designs of ANCOVA (analysis of covariance) was not applied.

[5]   Shapiro-Wilk tests were conducted prior to all t-tests to check for normal distribution.

tive data showed that good biking infrastructure, such as protected bike lanes, makes biking more attractive and is perceived as safe. Knowing a route with good cycling infrastructure or otherwise comfortable interaction with motorized traffic helped participants to bike. Travel distance and difference in travel time compared to other possible modes of transportation played another crucial role. The analysis of the interviews suggests, that participants who could gain significant time savings by taking a bike instead of walking or using public transportation were more motivated to bike. Financial aspects like the upfront costs of buying a bike or the cost of using a bike sharing scheme were also taken into consideration, especially by the financially constrained study participants. For actual day to day bike use, situational factors such as weather, having to wear elegant clothing or having a lot to carry was reported as influential for the decision on whether or not to bike.

The reported mobility data showed an overall increase of bike trips that was mainly fueled by the participants that were provided with access to bikes. Participants with positive experiences while trying out biking subsequently considered buying a bike in the future. The study-participation and especially the use of the trip diary raised general awareness of biking and the experimental period was described as a time of personal reflection on mobility. One participant mentioned: "I also now consider what form or transportation I take before I take it because the trip diary made me consider the different forms of transportation." Another one reported that she wanted to show that she is able to bike more. A self-monitoring effect was also reported by other participants. One told that he was regularly checking the provided statistics in the trip diary out of curiosity to see his personal statistics. But thinking actively about possible modes of transportation made participants also more aware of problems associated with urban biking: "I watched people get checked by car doors all the time and other bikers not obey lights or pedestrians".

As for perceived safety and risk, the hypothesis has been that for non-routine bikers the experience of biking in an urban environment will lead to an increase in perceived safety and decrease in perceived risk of doing so. However, comparing the scores of these two variables for the beginning and end of the experimental period did not show a change.

4.1   Mode Shifts

The analysis on an individual level provides an overview on how the share of modes shifted. A change in mobility patterns towards more biking could be rooted in a decrease in use of high-energy modes (car and public transportation), but could also stem from a decrease in walking. The former is of special interest for this research. Pearson r correlations have been calculated as a basic indicator for the dependence of mode share over the four weeks in which the mobility data was recorded. These correlations show a statistically significant ($p<.05$) negative dependency of bike use and use of high-energy modes for at least 16 out of 44 (36%) participants, ranging from $r=-.97$ to $r=-.40$. As can be expected there are also statistically significant ($p<.05$) negative correlations between bike use and walking for 13 out of 44 (30%) participants, ranging from $r=-.94$ to $r=-.41$.

4.2 Strategy I: Frequent Biking Challenge

As shown in Fig 3, an increase in bike share occurred. It rose from 2% in week one to 15% in week two to 33% in week three. Week four showed a decrease to 23%. The change from pre- to during-intervention values of bike share was 13.5 percentage points[6] above the control group at statistically significant levels (p=0.03). Results based on interviews show that the constant reminders of possible mobility choices and the trip diary, which separated mobility patterns into several smaller parts, helped a participant "break the prospect of biking to/from down into achievable goals for myself, e.g. bike from home to the train station or from the train to work [...]" The daily reminders were described as interesting and funny. The interviews also inform that cooperation and competition could have been more effective when involving social ties to other participants in the group.

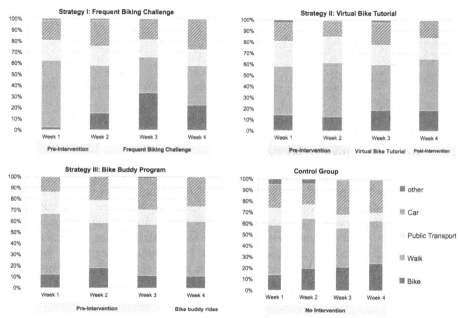

Fig. 3. Modal split during the experimental period

4.3 Strategy II: Virtual Bike Tutorial

The participants in the self-efficacy group conducted the tutorial in weeks two and three of this study. The results demonstrate an increase of biking share within all trips after the intervention from about 14% in week one and two to 19% in weeks three and four. When compared to control group shares, the change in bike use is not statistically significant for this strategy.

---

6   These values refer to percentage points within the modal split.

Self-efficacy of participants that reported lower levels at the beginning of the intervention showed a slight increase. (Fig. 4) However, on average, no clear rise in perceived biking self-efficacy emerged. In line with that, the conducted interviews suggest that the tutorial content was more suited for people without prior biking experience whereas regular bikers did not perceive the scenarios as challenging and could not learn from them. As for the design of the intervention, participants underlined the experience as realistic and immersive.

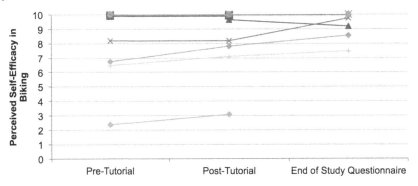

Fig. 4. Perceived self-efficacy in biking. Each line represents one participant.

4.4   Strategy III: Bike Buddy Program

Due to difficulties with scheduling, only six participants did the bike buddy rides in week 4 or after. Because the rides took place so late, no post-intervention trip data is available. The participants reported a positive experience with their "bike buddies" and perceived this strategy to be valuable for new bikers. In addition, they provided several suggestions on how this strategy could be improved. However, no clear rise in intention to bike more in the future emerged. The bike buddies were overall satisfied with helping less experienced bikers to overcome their fears and barriers. This indicates that voluntary work can be utilized in this matter.

5   Discussion

Strategy I (Frequent Biking Challenge) resulted in a significant increase in bike use above control group levels. To improve this strategy, the individual effect of the included principles should be studied. The gathered qualitative data at least suggests that competition and the collective goal elements should be designed in a way to allow social comparison also with familiar besides unknown participants. Notably, this strategy was the only one out of three that lasted for a long period of time (20 days), conveyed several main principles of socially influencing systems [20], and it used messages dependent on the actual behavior of participants, as recommended by Gatersleben & Appleton [13].

Although the design of strategy II (Virtual Bike Tutorial) was described as an immersive experience, it should be examined how to achieve a higher rise in perceived self-efficacy. Furthermore, it remains unclear if this change will actually lead to an increase in bike use. Due to scheduling issues and subsequent low actual participation the effect of strategy III (Bike Buddy Program) could not be examined by the quantitative trip data. The conducted interviews with the participants suggest that this one time biking experience did not change their intention to bike. Therefore it must be assumed, that this intervention design does not lead to a sufficient behavior change.

No change in perceived risk and perceived safety in biking could be identified. This indicates, that as most participants were already used to biking, they already had an estimate on the related safety and risk aspects. A change in actual bike use did not lead to a subsequent change of the individual evaluation of risk and safety associated with biking, at least not in the short term of this study. Our future research will therefore focus on more and other aspects that influence biking (e.g. bike availability, experience of biking or general attitudes). Furthermore, it will emphasize the use of qualitative methods to better assess why interventions show certain outcomes.

6   Conclusions and Future Research

This paper provides several contributions. Three persuasive strategies were designed for persuading people to bike as a low-energy mode of transportation and an evaluation of these were presented. The Frequent Biking Challenge showed an increase in bike use. Future research can focus on the individual principles applied as well as the analysis, for whom these are effective under which circumstances. The Virtual Bike Tutorial and Bike Buddy Program got promising feedbacks, but no clear conclusions about their outcomes can be drawn yet. Further evaluation of these strategies is needed and future research should focus more on novice bikers and evaluate the potential of these strategies to encourage them to bike. More elaborated technologies (e.g. immersive virtual environments) to simulate biking could improve the persuasive power of this design. This may be combined with a virtualized bike buddy experience, providing guidance to a user.

Overall, the presented study explored a set of strategies and features that shall act as a valuable base for future research on how to design and implement persuasive technologies [8] and socially influencing systems [20] in the field of mobility.

Acknowledgments. The authors gratefully acknowledge Kent Larson and Geraldine Fitzpatrick for their advice and support within this research project. We thank Bernhard Dorfmann for providing his expertise in tutoring novice bikers. Our special acknowledgement is due to Sandra Richter for her contributions to this research project and her help in performing the presented experiments.

References

1. Ajzen, I.: The Theory of Planned Behavior. Organizational Behavior and Human Decision Processes 50(2), 179–211 (1991)
2. Bandura, A.: Guide For Constructing Self-Efficacy Scales. In: Pajares, F., Urdan, T.C. (eds.) Self-Efficacy Beliefs of Adolescents, pp. 307–337. Information Age Publishing, Greenwich (2006)
3. Bandura, A.: Social Foundations of Thought and Action: A Social Cognitive Theory. Prentice-Hall, Englewood Cliffs (1986)

4. Baumeister, R.F.: The Self. In: Gilbert, D.T., Fiske, S.T., Lindzey, G. (eds.) The Handbook of Social Psychology, pp. 680–740. McGraw-Hill, New York (1998)

5. Chittaro, L.: Changing User's Safety Locus of Control through Persuasive Play: An Application to Aviation Safety. In: Spagnolli, A., Chittaro, L., Gamberini, L. (eds.) PERSUASIVE 2014. LNCS, vol. 8462, pp. 31–42. Springer, Heidelberg (2014)

6. Cialdini, R.B.: Influence: The Psychology of Persuasion. HarperCollins ebooks (2007)

7. Flüchter, K., Wortmann, F., Fleisch, E.: Digital Commuting: The Effect of Social Normative Feedback on E-Bike Commuting – Evidence From A Field Study. In: Proceedings of the European Conference on Information Systems ECIS, pp. 1–14. Tel Aviv (2014)

8. Fogg, B.J.: Persuasive Technology: Using Computers to Change What We Think and Do. Morgan Kaufmann, San Francisco (2003)

9. Froehlich, J., Dillahunt, T., Klasnja, P., Mankoff, J., Consolvo, S., Harrison, B., Landay, J.A.: UbiGreen: Investigating a Mobile Tool for Tracking and Supporting Green Transportation Habits. In: Proceedings of the SIGCHI Conference on Human Factors in Computing Systems, pp. 1043–1052. ACM, New York (2009)

10. Gabrielli, S., Maimone, R.: Are Change Strategies Affecting Users' Transportation Choices? In: Proceedings of the Biannual Conference of the Italian Chapter of SIGCHI, pp. 1–4. ACM, New York (2013)

11. Gärling, T., Fujii, S.: Travel behavior modification: Theories, Methods, and Programs. In: The Expanding Sphere of Travel Behaviour Research, pp. 97–128. Emerald Group (2009)

12. Gass, J.S., Seiter, R.H.: Persuasion, Social Influence, and Compliance Gaining. Allyn & Bacon, Boston (2010)

13. Gatersleben, B., Appleton, K.M.: Contemplating Cycling to Work: Attitudes and Perceptions in Different Stages of Change. Transportation Research Part A: Policy and Practice 41(4), 302–312 (2007)

14. Heinen, E., van Wee, B., Maat, K.: Commuting by Bicycle: An Overview of the Literature. Transport Reviews 30(1), 59–96 (2010)

15. Malone, T.W., Lepper, M.: Making Learning Fun: A Taxonomy of Intrinsic Motivations for Learning. In: Snow, R.E., Farr, M.J. (eds.) Aptitude, Learning and Instruction: III. Conative and Affective Process Analyses, pp. 223–253. Erlbaum, Hillsdale (1987)

16. Mayring, P.: Qualitative Content Analysis. Forum Qualitative Sozialforschung / Forum: Qualitative Social Research 1(2), Art. 20 (2000), http://nbn-resolving.de/urn:nbn:de:0114-fqs0002204

17. NOAA (2014), http://www1.ncdc.noaa.gov/pub/orders/cdo/435898.csv

18. Prochaska, J.O., DiClemente, C.C.: The Transtheoretical Approach: Crossing Traditional Boundaries of Change. Dow Jones/Irwin, Homewood IL (1984)

19. Stibe, A.: Socially Influencing Systems: Persuading People to Engage with Publicly Displayed Twitter-based Systems. Acta Universitatis Ouluensis (2014)

20. Stibe, A.: Towards a Framework for Socially Influencing Systems: Meta-Analysis of Four PLS-SEM Based Studies. In: MacTavish, T., Basapur, S. (eds.) Persuasive Technology. LNCS, vol. 9072, pp. 171–182. Springer, Heidelberg (2015)

21. United Nations, Department of Economic and Social Affairs, Population Division. World Urbanization Prospects: The 2014 Revision Highlights (2014)

22. Wills, T.A.: Downward Comparison Principles in Social Psychology. Psychological Bulletin 90(2), 245–271 (1981)

23. Wilson, S.R., Benner, L.A.: The Effects of Self-Esteem and Situation upon Comparison Choices During Ability Evaluation. Sociometry 34(2), 381–397 (1971)

Preliminary Evaluation of Virtual Cycling System Using Google Street View

Shota Hirose and Yasuhiko Kitamura[✉]

Department of Informatics,
School of Science and Technology,
Kwansei Gakuin University,
2-1 Gakuen, Sanda 669-1337, Japan
{eav00014,ykitamura}@kwansei.ac.jp
http://ist.ksc.kwansei.ac.jp/~kitamura/index.htm

Abstract. Overweight and obesity due to lack of physical activities incur a serious social problem. Recently, a large number of people have interest in physical exercise to keep themselves well, but it is not easy to continue to do it. Persuasive technology can provide solutions to encourage them to continue physical activities. Exercise bikes are one of indoor exercise tools, but the users easily get tired of the bikes because they just only pedal at the same spot. Several virtual cycling systems have been developed, which encourage exercise by showing scenery videos or virtual reality CG movies in accordance with the pedaling speed, but the choices of the cycling routes are limited. We are developing a new virtual cycling system with Google Street View to provide almost unlimited route choices to the users. It reproduces scenery along a cycling route by showing Street View images one after another in accordance with the pedaling speed. This paper shows how our system promotes physical exercise as a preliminary evaluation.

Keywords: Virtual cycling · Promoting physical activities · Google street view

1 Introduction

Overweight and obesity due to lack of physical activities incur a serious social problem. Recently, a large number of people have interest in physical exercise to keep themselves well, but it is not easy to continue to do it. Persuasive technology can provide solutions to encourage them to continue physical activities [1,2].

Cycling is one of popular and casual physical activities. People ride a bicycle not only for commuting and traveling but also for diet, fitness, and training. The physical load of cycling on legs is lighter than that of running or jogging and can be adjusted to the exercise intensity. Moreover, it motivates the riders to continue the physical exercise because they can go anywhere they like enjoying the scenery and feeling the wind. In contrast, exercise bikes are an indoor exercise tool. They do not motivate the riders as much as bicycles, because the riders just pedal at the same place.

© Springer International Publishing Switzerland 2015
T. MacTavish and S. Basapur (Eds.): PERSUASIVE 2015, LNCS 9072, pp. 65–70, 2015.
DOI: 10.1007/978-3-319-20306-5_6

To deal with the drawback, a number of virtual cycling systems have been developed. Atari Corp. released an interactive cycling game Puffer [3] in 1982, as a precursor of virtual cycling systems. The users ride an exercise bike and play the game operating the control stick and pedaling the bike. Mokka [4] developed a fitness game "Virku" with an exercise bike in a 3D virtual space. The users play mini games pedaling the bike to move in the virtual space. The study shows that the users immersed themselves in playing games rather than in doing exercise. "Tacx Trainer software 4 Advanced" of Tacx Corp. is a sport bike training system [5]. The users can compete virtually with each other in a well known race course or in a 3D virtual space. Ijesselsteijn et al. [6] also have developed a virtual cycling system and they show that the reality of virtual space heighten an effect on promoting physical exercise.

These systems have positive effects to promote physical exercise, but they show only scenery videos along cycling routes prepared in advance. The users may soon get tired of the systems and it is difficult for them to keep exercise fun continuously. Lee et al. [7] have developed a new system that shows scenery images from Google Street View one after another along the route. Google Street View is a Web service provided by Google Inc., which provides a huge number of scenery images along streets taken all over the world. "Tour de France PRO" is a commercial product developed by PROForm Corp., which employs Google Street View images [8].

We have interest in how virtual cycling systems with Google Street View promote physical exercise. We have developed a virtual cycling system using Google Street View as mentioned in Section 2, and show how the system promote physical exercise through an experiment as a preliminary evaluation in Section 3. We conclude this paper with our future work in Section 4.

2   Virtual Cycling System Using Street View

We developed a virtual cycling system consisting of a bicycle, a computer and a display as shown in Fig. 1. When a user bikes the bicycle, the computer calculates the pedaling speed from the sensor information and shows a sequence of scenery images retrieved from Google Street View on the display in accordance with the pedaling speed.

Google Street View is a Web service featured in Google Maps and provides panoramic images taken at about 10 meter intervals by mostly car-mounted cameras along streets all over the world . This system shows Street View images one after another along the route to the user and makes him/her feel like cycling outdoors.

Fig. 2 shows the system components of the virtual cycling system. Initially, a user chooses a cycling route on the computer by using the Route Setting Module. He/She searches for a preferred cycling location and designates the start and goal points on Google Maps by using a mouse. The cycling route is automatically created by the Google Maps API route service. The user can add prefered via points by drag-and-drop operations. After creating the route, he/she starts cycling.

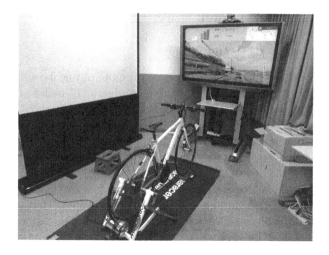

Fig. 1. Virual Cycling System using Google Street View

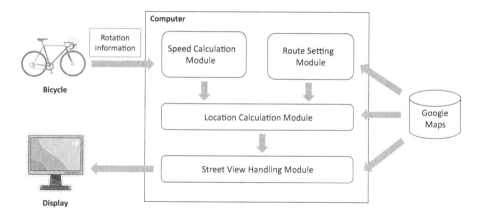

Fig. 2. System components

The number of wheel rotations is counted by a sensor (MINOURA speed sensor) attached to the bicycle and is transmitted to the computer through the ANT wireless communication interface. The Speed Calculation Module transforms the number of wheel rotations into the speed of the virtual bicycle, and the Location Calculation Module locates it on the route. The virtual bicycle is indicated by an icon on a Google map, and moves along the route in accordance with the pedaling speed. The Street View Handling Module retrieves a Street View image within 10 meters from the virtual bicycle, and shows it on the display.

As shown in Fig. 1, the display shows a Street View image with a route map and cycling information such as current speed, cycling distance, elapsed time, and so on.

3   Evaluation Experiment

3.1   Participants and Method

We evaluated how our virtual cycling system promote physical exercise. The participants of this experiment are 23 university students (17 males and 6 females) from 20 to 24 years old. We assigned the participants into three groups. The Normal group (5 males and 2 females) is the baseline of this experiment and just pedals the bicycle without any information on the display. The Map group (6 males and 2 females) pedals the bicycle watching an icon moving on the map in accordance with the pedaling speed, but no Street View images are given. The Street View group (6 males and 2 females) pedals the bicycle watching Street View images changing in accordance with the pedaling speed, but no map information is given. Participants of each group ride the bicycle twice. At first, we ask them to just ride it for 5 minutes without any information on the display to measure their average pedaling speed. Then, they take a rest about 5 minutes for recovery. Finally, we ask them to ride the bicycle again for 5 minutes with the information depending on the assigned group to measure their average pedaling speed. No information about the pedaling speed is given to the participants.

We compared the difference of the average speed between two rides depending on the group. We also asked the participants to answer questions about their impression of the virtual cycling system as shown in Table 1. The route of virtual cycling is fixed to our university campus from the nearest train station. The distance of the route is about 5 km, and it is long enough for no participant to reach the goal in 5 minutes.

3.2   Results

Fig. 3 shows the differences of the average speed between two rides according to each group. We performed statistical testing on every pair of the groups. There is a significant difference between the Normal group and the Street View group ($t(13) = 3.02, p = .013$), and a significant trend between the Normal group and

Table 1. Answers to the questionnaire. N, M, and SV mean Normal, Map, and Street View respectively.

Question	N-M	N-SV	M-SV
Was it fun?	2.75-4.25 **	2.75-4.13 **	4.25-4.13
Did you feel like cycling outdoors?	2.38-3.00	2.38-3.88 **	3.00-3.88
Were you tired?	3.38-3.75	3.38-3.75	3.75-3.75
Did you feel like a training?	3.00-3.88 *	3.00-4.00 *	3.88-4.00
Was it boring?	3.25-2.13 **	3.25-2.63	2.13-2.63
Did you want to ride again?	2.63-3.50	2.63-3.13	3.50-3.13
Did you recognize where you were?	2.88-4.38 *	2.88-4.50 ***	4.38-4.50

$^*p < 0.1,$ ** $p < 0.05,$ *** $p < 0.01$

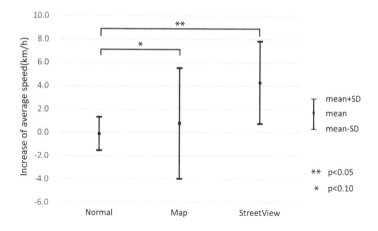

Fig. 3. Difference of the average speed between two rides

the Map group ($t(13) = 0.47, p = .064$), but no significant difference between the Map group and the Street View group ($t(14) = 1.56, p = .139$).

Table 1 summarizes answers to the questionnaire. Participants answer to each question by using the Likert scale; 1 (strongly disagree), 2 (disagree), 3 (neither agree nor disagree), 4 (agree), and 5 (strongly agree). The table shows the average score to each question.

3.3   Discussion

The difference of the average speed between the Normal group and the Street View group shows the virtual cycling system with Street View promotes physical exercise more than the one without it, even a sequence of scenery images is shown in a discrete manner. Table 1 shows the system with Street View makes the users have fun ($p < 0.05$) and feel like cycling outdoors ($p < 0.05$) more than the one without it.

Since there is a significant trend between the Normal group and the Map group, even the system with Map has an effect to promote exercise to some extent. We have no significant difference between the Map group and the Street View group. The answers to the questionnaire also look similar between the two groups. The result may come from the fact that 94% of the participants knew the route chosen in the experiment and they may be able to imagine the scenery even when they watch an icon on the map. To show the superiority of the system with Street View images over the one with Google Maps, we need to make an experiment with the route that the participants do no know.

4   Summary and Future Work

We developed a virtual cycling system with Google Street View and evaluated how the system promotes physical exercise by measuring the average pedaling speed of the users in an experiment. We show there is a significant difference between the system with Street View and the one without it. To further clarify the results, we need to evaluate the systems in detail using more participants.

Comparing the conventional virtual cycling system with scenery videos, we have more choices of cycling route because the system utilizes Google Street View that contains almost unlimited number of scenery images. We need to evaluate how much and how long the freedom of route choice affects users to promote physical exercise in our future work.

References

1. Fogg, B.: Persuasive Technology: Using Computers to Change What We Think and Do (Interactive Technologies). Morgan Kaufmann (2002)
2. Fogg, B., Eckles, D.: Mobile persuasion: 20 perspectives on the future of behavior change, vol. 1. Stanford Captology Media Standford, CA (2007)
3. Atari: Atari gaming headquarters - atari project puffer page (1982), http://atarihq.com/othersec/puffer/index.html
4. Mokka, S., Väätänen, A., Heinilä, J., Välkkynen, P.: Fitness computer game with a bodily user interface. In: ICEC 2003 Proceedings of the Second International Conference on Entertainment Computing, pp. 1–3. Carnegie Mellon University (2003)
5. Tacx: Tacx trainer software 4 advanced (2014), http://www.tacx.com/en/products/software/tacx-trainer-software-4-advanced
6. IJsselsteijn, W., de Kort, Y., Bonants, R., de Jager, M., Westerink, J.: Virtual cycling: Effects of immersion and a virtual coach on motivation and presence in a home fitness application. In: Proceedings Virtual Reality Design and Evaluation Workshop, pp. 22–23 (2004)
7. Lee, H.C., Kange, K.H., Joo, J.H., Kim, E.S., Hur, G.T.: Development of fitness cycle system using google streetview. IJCSNS 11(2), 121 (2011)
8. ProForm: Tour de france (2013), http://www.proform.com/fitness/en/ProForm/Exercise-Bikes/tour-de-france

Bet4EcoDrive:

Betting for Economical Driving

Caroline Atzl[1]([✉]), Alexander Meschtscherjakov[2], Stefan Vikoler[3],
and Manfred Tscheligi[2]

[1]Research Studios Austria iSPACE, Salzburg, Austria
`caroline.atzl@researchstudio.at`
[2]Christian-Doppler-Laboratory "Contextual Interfaces",
Center for HCI, University of Salzburg, Salzburg, Austria
`{alexander.meschtscherjakov,manfred.tscheligi}@sbg.ac.at`
[3]University of Salzburg, Salzburg, Austria
`stefan.vikoler@stud.sbg.ac.at`

Abstract. We present *Bet4EcoDrive*, an in-car app, which intends to persuade drivers to change their driving behavior towards an economical driving style. This is achieved by suggesting the driver to bet that (s)he can reach a predefined goal. In our study scenario, the driver can bet to stay within a certain RPM range to avoid driving at high revs and, thus, to reduce fuel consumption. We have implemented Bet4EcoDrive as an Android-based smartphone app, which can be connected to the vehicle via ODB-II over Bluetooth, in order to read car data (e.g., RPM). It provides feedback of the actual state while driving through different visualizations. An exploratory in-situ study with five participants proves the feasibility of our approach. The results show that participants were persuaded to reduce average RPM values while driving by the desire to win the bet.

Keywords: Economic driving · OBD-II · Betting app

1   Introduction

Both automotive industry and smartphone industry are part of fast and permanent growing markets. Vehicles are equipped with many sensors and have become a place for information access, communication, media consumption, and entertainment [1]. The same holds true for smartphones. The combination of these two components with a suitable interface enables novel features and services for car drivers and passengers [2]. In literature, many applications integrate, analyze, and visualize automotive sensor data with the aim of making car driving more secure or economic. The reduction of the fuel consumption is a topic that is often addressed. Aside from technical improvements, driving behavior influences fuel consumption up to 50% [3]. A smart and adapted way of driving can lead to a reduction of the average fuel consumption up to 20% [4]. This can only be achieved through changes in the driving behavior and requires a special motivation to take on new ways of driving [5]. Persuasive technologies are aiming at such behavioral changes and increase the motivation of the user [5].

© Springer International Publishing Switzerland 2015
T. MacTavish and S. Basapur (Eds.): PERSUASIVE 2015, LNCS 9072, pp. 71–82, 2015.
DOI: 10.1007/978-3-319-20306-5_7

In this paper, we present *Bet4EcoDrive* (i.e., betting for an economical driving behavior), which is a persuasive application that aims to motivate drivers to perform an economical driving style through making bets. The basic idea is to allow drivers to bet that they are able to drive in a certain way for a predefined distance. For example, the driver could bet that (s)he is able to drive so that the average fuel consumption for the next 100 kilometers is below a certain value. Another example is that the driver bets (s)he can stay within a certain RPM (revolutions per minute) range for the next two hours of driving. Since one of the golden rules of eco-driving is that low RPM values lead to an increased reduction of fuel consumption, this can lead to an economical driving style (cf. www.ecodrive.org). The driver should be able to set his/her own competition goals (i.e., to bet against him/herself) or, alternatively, (s)he could accept bets from others (e.g., friends). Gamification elements, such as high scores or the loss of virtual lives, could be used as an incentive to win the bet. For example, a virtual wager in form of coins could be passed to the account of the winner. Bet4EcoDrive should be implemented as a smartphone app, which provides an interface to make the bet, as well as a visualization of the ongoing bet. It should be connected to the vehicle in order to access car data and provide feedback in an appropriate way to the driver during a ride (i.e., simplified to avoid distracting the driver).

To show the feasibility of this approach, we have implemented a prototypical version of Bet4EcoDrive as an app for Android smartphones, which allows the driver to bet to stay within a certain RPM range for a chosen distance. The app combines GPS data collected by the smartphone itself with the RPM of the vehicle. The RPM is read using the standard on-board diagnostic interface of the vehicle (OBD-II) and transmitted to the smartphone via Bluetooth. This data is used to inform the driver about the status of ongoing bets in real-time and to monitor, analyze, and ensure the accuracy and compliance of completed bets. We have implemented three different types of visualizations (i.e., gamification in form of remaining lives, current RPM, and a map showing the actual route). Chapter 3 introduces the implementation of our prototype, including the software used and screenshots of Bet4EcoDrive.

In order to explore the persuasive potentials of our approach, we have conducted an initial user study with five participants using Bet4EcoDrive in-situ (see Chapter 4). The main objective of the study was to find out if the bet has the potential to persuade the driver to change his/her driving behavior. In our case, the driver bets that (s)he is able to stay below a certain RPM threshold for a predefined route. Additionally, we collected feedback on the information visualization and general attitude of participants towards the application.

2   Related Work

People love to play, win, and compare, and many games use the entertainment factor to train, educate, and inform their users [6]. The term "gamification" is often used to describe such applications and is defined by Deterding et al. as "the use of game design elements in non-game contexts" [7]. Especially the interaction with such apps while driving can have negative effects on the driving behavior, since these activities affect the driving performance and the attention of the driver (e.g., [1] [5] [6]). But gamification approaches have potentials in the automotive realm. Bihler et al. [8] conducted a study with 276 participants about the general acceptance of games while driving. Overall, 51% of the participants could imagine using context-based games in the car. They also show that getting hints from a technical system for an economic driving style is well accepted (86%). Ecker et al. [5] show that users are only pressured and distracted a little by a game contest within the car. Their results show that participants experience a lot of joy, motivation, and fun during using a gaming app while driving. Miranda et al. [9] have examined the efficacy of a persuasive technology package in reducing texting and driving behavior.

In the automotive domain, persuasion and gamification have already been used to change driver behavior towards an eco-friendly driving style. The general acceptance of persuasive in-car interfaces towards an economic driving behavior has been explored by Meschtscherjakov et al. [10]. Lee et al. [11] present a critical view on the long term persuasive effect of an ambient dashboard feedback system in an automobile called Eco-driving System. Another example is EcoChallenge, a persuasive and location-based in-car game with the goal of motivating the driver to develop a fuel-saving driving style in a multiplayer fuel-saving competition [5]. Eco-Driver is a prototypical game that aims to reduce the fuel consumption based on car data read from the ODB-II interface [8]. The user can compare current fuel consumption with the past and is ranked.

Car manufacturers have developed similar applications for their users. Fiat's Eco-Drive[1] provides a statistical analysis of recorded routes within an online community. Users receive hints for improving their fuel consumption and can compare their last routes. Ford's SmartGauge with EcoGuide[2] has been developed for hybrid vehicles and informs the driver about the current efficiency level of driving. Once the driver has reached the highest level of efficiency, so-called "efficiency leaves" grow on the dashboard.

The difference between these approaches and Bet4EcoDrive is the combination of economical driving with a playful betting principle. Current available betting apps allow mainly betting on sporting events or creating a bet against friends, such as AnteUp[3] and Youbetme[4]. None of these betting apps use vehicle data or aim at economical and safe driving. Based on our literature review, no prototype comparable with Bet4EcoDrive could be discovered.

3   Implementation

In this chapter, we present the current prototype of Bet4EcoDrive and the software used for its implementation. In the current version, only the functions needed for conducting an initial field study are implemented.

---

[1] http://www.fiat.com/ecodrive
[2] http://smartdesignworldwide.com/work/ford-smart-gauge/
[3] https://www.facebook.com/goanteup
[4] http://youbetme.com/

3.1   Software

The Android-based Bet4EcoDrive prototype was implemented using the Eclipse IDE for EE Java Developers (Eclipse Luna 4.4.1). Using the Google Android Development Tools (Android SDK and ADT Plugin v22.6.2 for Eclipse) allowed us to access the API libraries and tools that are necessary to develop, test, and debug Android apps. The Android platform was chosen because of the widespread use on the smartphone market and its open-source nature. In addition, we have used PhoneGap/Cordova in version 2.9.1 to develop the graphical user interface (GUI) of Bet4EcoDrive with JavaSript, HTML5, and CSS3 instead of Java.

For the communication between the smartphone and the vehicle or more specifically for the verification of the bet and display of vehicle data in real-time, an OBD-II connector with Bluetooth function was used (Wireless Bluetooth OBD2 CAN BUS Diagnose Interface V1.5). The OBD-II standard includes several elements such as the connector for the diagnosis, protocols, and the message format. In addition, there is a list of parameters that can be monitored by means of assigned codes. Hence, ODB-II provides access to various vehicle data such as RPM.

3.2   Bet4EcoDrive Prototype

As recommended by Ecker et al. [5], the driver receives direct feedback on the state of the bet while driving and gets statistical analysis of past trips after driving. Apart from the creation of new bets, additional information about the vehicle type can be stored and technical settings can be done. The home page of Bet4EcoDrive is the starting point to enter these four areas (see Fig. 1 A):

- **New Bet**: Creation and monitoring of new bets (see Fig. 1 B)
- **My Car**: Input of car data that can be used to create new bets (see Fig. 1 C)
- **Statistics**: Statistical analysis and graphical evaluations in the form of a dashboard
- **Settings**: Technical settings such as acoustic feedback (e.g., sound on/off, volume and different tones) and selection of a theme (e.g., light or dark design)

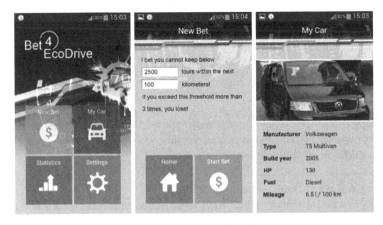

Fig. 1. Home page (A), "New Bet" area (B) and "My Car" area (C) of Bet4EcoDrive

The focus of the Bet4EcoDrive prototype is on the "New Bet" area, because we want to find out whether the fact that a bet is running has a positive influence on the driving behavior. The functionality behind "My Car", "Statistics", and "Settings" is not implemented yet.

After clicking on the "New Bet" button, a page opens where the parameters for the creation of a new bet can be set. Currently, it is only possible to set the maximum RPM value that is not allowed to be exceeded more than 3 times and the distance in kilometers for which the bet is valid. For future development, more adjustment parameters and other bet types, such as fuel consumption, are planned. In Fig. 1 B, we illustrate that the driver is challenged to keep below 2,500 RPM within the next 100 kilometers. If (s)he exceeds this threshold more than three times for three seconds each, (s)he loses the bet. We have chosen a value of three seconds in order not to punish very short accelerations.

In a further development stage, a virtual coin concept should be implemented. This enables friends to set a certain amount of coins for, or against, the bet and the profit is shared between the winners.

After starting the bet, a connection to the OBD-II connector is created via Bluetooth to query the RPM values in real-time while driving. If the internal GPS of the smartphone is not enabled, it is turned on to retrieve the actual GPS position that corresponds to the recorded RPM value. This data is the foundation for the three visualization types that provide feedback for the users while driving (see Fig. 2).

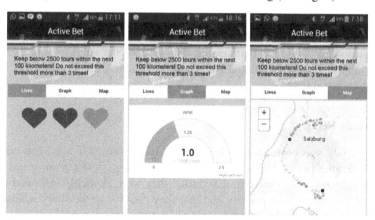

Fig. 2. Three visualizations for the driver: lives (A), RPM (B), and GPS data on a map (C)

The first visualization uses a gamification approach by showing three lives represented by three red hearts, corresponding to the three times the driver may exceed the upper RPM limit. The driver receives feedback of how many of the three lives are still available. In Fig. 2 A, the driver can see that (s)he has two lives left (two red hearts) and one life already lost (one grey heart). If the driver exceeds the maximum allowed RPM value, the driver is alerted by a beep. After that, the driver has three seconds to reduce the speed, otherwise (s)he loses a life. For losing a life, another acoustic signal is used as feedback and one of the three red heart icons changes to gray. If the user has lost all three lives, the bet is lost and a "Game Over" appears on the screen.

Another indicator is the visualization of the current RPM value (see Fig. 2 B). For the display of the RPM value, the "solid gauge" of the Highcharts API is used. This representation resembles the rev-counter in the car. The current RPM value is displayed with consideration of the value defined as maximum. In other words, the color in the chart will change from green to yellow or from yellow to red depending on how close the actual RPM value is to the maximum. Thus, the user can quickly realize how well the driving style is at the moment.

The third visualization is a map (see Fig. 2 C) showing the GPS positions of the route driven. The dots on the map are colored according to the height of the RPM value at this location with regard to the limit in green, yellow, or red. This means, if the user drives at a certain location with a very high RPM and exceeds the maximum allowed value, the specific dot on the map is highlighted in red. Hence, the user can see exactly on which part of the road it was more difficult to drive with an appropriate RPM and where a life has been lost.

The users can switch between these three visualization types while driving by means of a swiping gesture. In all three visualizations, we tried to keep a minimalistic design in order not to distract the driver with too much information.

4   User Study

In order to evaluate the feasibility of our approach, we have conducted an exploratory in-situ user study with five participants. The goal of the study was to evaluate the persuasive potentials of Bet4EcoDrive and to get feedback on the prototype, including potential improvements.

4.1   Study Setup

The field study was conducted with five participants (4m, 1f), aged between 22 and 33 years. Participation was voluntary and participants signed a informed consent. Since participants had to drive in real traffic, they were explicitly informed that driving safely had the highest priority and that they could stop the study whenever they wanted. Participants could choose to drive with their own car or a car provided by us (VW Polo 6N2 1998). The technical preparation of the study included the plug-in of the OBD-II Bluetooth dongle and the mounting of the Android smartphone, on which Bet4EcoDrive was installed in the car console so it was easily visible for the driver while driving. During the study RPM values (from the OBD-II dongle), GPS data (from the smartphone) and a time stamp were written automatically into a log file using Bet4EcoDrive. During the drives, two researchers were sitting in the car. One researcher was controlling the technical setup and functioning of the prototype, another researcher was taking notes.

Participants were asked to drive a preselected route twice. The first drive was used as a baseline for typical RPM values of the participant without any intervention (i.e., the Bet4EcoDrive visualization was turned off). Before the first test drive, participants were not introduced to the goals of the study. The reason for this was that we wanted participants to drive as usual without being influenced in advance. After the first drive, a brief introduction to the use and purpose of Bet4EcoDrive was given. Thereafter, a bet, which participants should try to comply to, was created in the Bet4EcoDrive app. To win the bet, the participant must not exceed a certain threshold more than three times during the second drive. The threshold was individually calculated for each participant based on the RPM data from the first baseline drive. For the calculation of the individual thresholds, we used 70% of the maximum RPM value of each participant. By comparing the average RPM values of both drives, we could evaluate if driver behavior has changed.

The selected route was a section of a street in Salzburg, Austria. The test drive took between 7 and 15 minutes, depending on the traffic situation. Two of the participants preferred to drive in their own cars (VW T5 Multivan 2003, Opel Corsa 2014); three participants drove with the provided vehicle. After each drive, participants were interviewed. The first interview included demographics and questions regarding the participants attitude towards eco-driving. In the second interview, we asked for subjective persuasiveness and potential improvements of Bet4EcoDrive.

4.2   Results

After the study, we analyzed the logged data and the two interviews after each of the two drives. The first interview was conducted to find out if the participants thought about ecological driving. Two of the participants have noted that they do not care about an ecological driving style because they want to have "fun" when driving their cars. "Driving fun" means for them to "drive in the upper RPM range", "race", "speed up fast", and "suddenly decelerate." The other three participants claimed to drive in an economic manner. They do so by "driving with low RPM", "avoiding sudden deceleration", "avoiding speeding and unnecessary acceleration", "turning off the engine during long waiting times", and "avoiding unnecessary routes."

The second round of interviews was conducted immediately after the second drive, in which the Bet4EcoDrive app was used. All participants stated that their driving behavior had changed due to Bet4EcoDrive. All participants noticed that they paid more attention to the RPM display and drove with less RPM. Two participants reported that they drove more attentive and shifted to the next gear earlier. One participant stated (s)he started slower at traffic lights. The reason for the change in driving behavior for all participants was the fact that "a bet is running" and they "want to win" the bet. This indicates that betting has the potential to change driving behavior.

Above that, we asked participants about their attitude towards the Bet4EcoDrive idea. Four of the five participants were willing to use the app while driving. One of those four stated that he would only use it when integrated into the dashboard. Another one stated that he would bet, but did not like the visualizations of the app while driving. The reason for not using the app in the future for another participant was that it would be too laborious to plug-in the OBD-II dongle every time.

When asked if they would accept bets from others, four participants agreed and one participant would only accept a bet if many of his friends would also bet. Four of the five participants stated that they would like to bet against family members and friends; one wanted to bet against firms. None of the participants wanted the bets to be integrated in their social networks. Four participants could imagine that the bets are public (e.g., worldwide rankings). Regarding the type of bets, three participants stated that a bet to stay below a certain fuel consumption would be interesting. Additionally, one participant suggested that winning a bet should lead to actual prizes (e.g., a gas voucher).

None of the participants stated that they were distracted from driving when using the app. One participant stated that the audio signal was somehow annoying. Another participant stated to prefer only the audio feedback during the drive and the visualization at the end of the trip.

Another question of the second interview focused on the three visualization types of the app (see Fig. 2) and the preference of participants. Four participants found the "RPM visualization" the most useful (see Fig. 2 B), whereas one of them would prefer a combination with the "lives visualization" (see Fig. 2 A). Two participants mentioned that "the display of the lives available is only interesting if you are at risk to lose the bet." For one participant, the "map visualization" is the most useful one while driving (see Fig. 2 C). The others stated that "the map is only interesting if you want to see the route again after driving."

In order to investigate design alternatives for the "RPM visualization" (see Fig. 2 B), we presented three alternative paper prototypes (see Fig. 3) to each participant during the second interview. They included a bar chart of the current RPM value (see Fig. 3 A), a graph showing RPM values throughout the trip (see Fig. 3 B), and the RPM value in form of a number (see Fig. 3 C). Three participants favored the default Bet4EcoDrive RPM visualization most (see Fig. 2 B). One of these participants also liked the digit visualization (see Fig. 3 C). The display in the form of a bar chart (see Fig. 3 A) is preferred by one participant and named by two of the participants as their second choice. One participant favored the graph visualization (see Fig. 3 B), although this display type was perceived as the least appealing by the others.

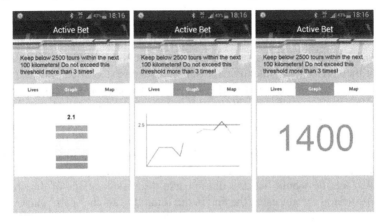

Fig. 3. Alternative visualization types: bar chart (A), diagram (B), and digit (C)

In addition to the two interviews, we compared the RPM values recorded during both drives for each of the participants. Since the number of participants is low, we have concentrated on an analysis of the data using only descriptive statistics. First, we have calculated the average RPM values of the two test drives of each participant and compared those values. For the first drive (i.e., baseline), RPM values ranged between 662 and 5,164 revs with an average RPM value of 1,710 revs. For the second drive (i.e., bet running), RPM values ranged between 635 and 2,756 revs with an average RPM value of 1,315 revs. Thus, the highest logged RPM value dropped from 5,164 revs to 2,756 revs and the overall average RPM value decreased by 395 revs (23%).

When comparing the first and second drive for each participant, we found that participants have lowered their average RPM values to between 160 and 569 revs, which means an improvement of between 13% and 30% (see Fig. 4). In particular, the participants who mentioned to pay little attention to economical driving in the first interview (participant 1 and 5) have improved their average RPM. The participant with the least change in the mean RPM value (participant 2) was the only driver with a diesel vehicle. The reason, therefore, could be the fact that diesel engine cars are driven at a lower RPM in general.

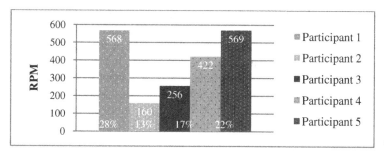

Fig. 4. Average improvement of the RPM values between the first and second drive

In addition, we have compared the two drives of all participants. Fig. 5 and Fig. 6 exemplary visualize the RPM values over time of two drives from two participants. It shows that there are nearly no high peaks in the RPM values of the second drive. This was also true for the other participants. Additionally, we discovered that the second drives (M=10.8 minutes) took, on average, 10% longer than the first drives (M=9.8 minutes). One reason for this is that all participants were leaving traffic lights and intersections with more care.

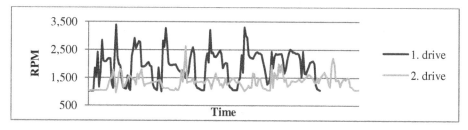

Fig. 5. Comparison of the RPM values during the first and second drive of participant 1

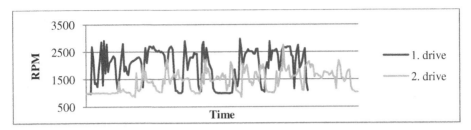

Fig. 6. Comparison of the RPM values during the first and second drive of participant 5

Overall, we can conclude that the logged RPM data supports the subjective statements of participants in the interviews that the Bet4EcoDrive app led to lower RPM values on average. This again would lead to an eco-friendly driving behavior and lower fuel consumption.

5   Discussion

The results of the study show the persuasive potentials of the Bet4EcoDrive approach. Both subjective, as well as objective, results indicate that betting to stay below a certain RPM threshold is feasible and leads with the help of the right feedback to decreased average RPM values. Participants agreed that the Bet4EcoDrive app leads to a change in driving behavior, which was supported by logged RPM data. Not surprisingly, the highest improvements were achieved by participants who did not drive eco-friendly beforehand. Winning the bet was a major motivational aspect to change the behavior. Overall, we can assume that betting to reduce fuel consumption by including gamification elements is an appropriate method to change short-term behavior.

Additionally, we have shown that the Bet4EcoDrive prototype works in a real world scenario. Both the general approach and the idea to use bets as a motivation to change behavior were approved by our participants. Overall, participants could image using the app in the future. In order to be successful, the app should be integrated in the car's eco system to avoid cumbersome installation processes. Feedback should be minimal during driving to avoid distraction. Since we only implemented one type of bet (i.e., not to exceed an RPM threshold), the type of visualization should be selected carefully for each type of bet. In general, the visualization of typical game elements (in our case, heart symbols to represent lives) worked well. The visualization of the actual RPM value in the form of a solid gauge is perceived as the most appropriate while driving. Even after showing further alternatives for the RPM presentation, the solid gauge was still the favored one, closely followed by the bar chart visualization. Some of the participants would prefer a combination of specific visualizations for a future version of Bet4EcoDrive.

Nonetheless, our findings also have some shortcomings. First, we critically annotate that the number of five participants for the field study is too small to get an expressive result. It was not our purpose to provide generalizable results, but to show the initial feasibility of betting as means for driving behavior change, as well as an in-situ study for the Bet4EcoDrive prototype. In order to validate our findings, studies with more participants would be needed. Additionally, we have to acknowledge that we only evaluated the first time usage of the Bet4EcoDrive app and it cannot be guaranteed that the betting app is persuasive when used more often. Another aspect, which we did not target in the current version of Bet4EcoDrive, is how to balance between rewards and punishments for winning or losing a bet.

Another shortcoming is that we only evaluated short-term behavior changes. This is due to the nature of the user study and due to the nature of the betting idea in general. Bets are made for a specific period of time or distance. We have shown that the behavior may be changed using bets for this period, but it is not clear if this would persuade drivers to drive more eco-friendly in general. Thus, the sustainability of the learning effect needs to be proven. Will the driving behavior remain changed when no bet is running? Will the behavior rebound when the app is removed or is not present because one drives in another car? Do personality traits have an influence on the susceptibility of the user? How does the social environment influence individual behavior if we include competition elements? In order to answer these questions, field studies over a longer period of time are needed.

The availability and accuracy of the smartphone's internal GPS is another deficit that was identified during the study. Due to the tall buildings and narrow streets within the city of Salzburg, the GPS signal was lost frequently and led to gaps in the map visualization. In addition, some of the points on the map were far apart from the actual road, because of the poor position accuracy of the smartphone devices. This deficit could be overcome by the use of an external GPS module.

6   Conclusion

With Bet4EcoDrive, we have introduced betting as a persuasive method to change driver behavior to reduce fuel consumption. An initial user study has shown that betting not to exceed a certain RPM threshold led to a change in driving behavior. The presented study results show an improvement in the average RPM values and a reduction of extreme values by using Bet4EcoDrive. In summary, we have found out that the fact that a bet is running leads to a positive change in the driving behavior with focus on the RPM.

In a next steps we plan to the implementation of a scoring, friend, and ranking system, further betting types (e.g., reducing of the fuel consumption), the programming of GUI extensions (e.g., statistics and setting areas), and the architecture of the underlying data management. Further studies will target at long-term persuasive effects.

Acknowledgements. The financial support by the Austrian Federal Ministry of Science, Research and Economy and the National Foundation for Research, Technology and Development and AUDIO MOBIL Elektronik GmbH is gratefully acknowledged (Christian Doppler Laboratory for "Contextual Interfaces").

References

1. Schmidt, A., Dey, A.K., Kun, A.L., Spiessl, W.: Automotive User Interfaces: Human Computer Interaction in the Car. In: CHI 2010 Extended Abstracts on Human Factors in Computing Systems, pp. 3177–3180. ACM, Atlanta (2010)
2. Zaldivar, J., Calafate, C.T., Cano, J.C., Manzoni, P.: Providing Accident Detection in Vehicular Networks Through OBD-II Devices and Android-based Smartphones. In: Proceedings of the 2011 IEEE 36th Conference on Local Computer Networks, pp. 813–819. IEEE Computer Society, Bonn (2011)
3. Dorrer, C.: Effizienzbestimmung von Fahrweisen und Fahrerassistenz zur Reduzierung des Kraftstoffverbrauchs unter Nutzung telematischer Informationen. Expert Verlag, Germany (2004)
4. ADAC, http://www.adac.de/infotestrat/tanken-kraftstoffe-und-antrieb/spritsparen/
5. Ecker, R., Holzer, P., Broy, V., Butz, A.: EcoChallenge: a race for efficiency. In: Proceedings of the 13th International Conference on Human Computer Interaction with Mobile Devices and Services, pp. 91–94. ACM, Stockholm (2011)
6. Diewald, S., Möller, A., Roalter, L., Stockinger, T., Kranz, M.: Gameful Design in the Automotive Domain: Review, Outlook and Challenges. In: Proceedings of the 5th International Conference on Automotive User Interfaces and Interactive Vehicular Applications, pp. 262–265. ACM, Eindhoven (2013)
7. Deterding, S., Dixon, D., Khaled, R., Nacke, L.: From Game Design Elements to Gamefulness: Defining "Gamification". In: Proceedings of the 15th International Academic MindTrek Conference: Envisioning Future Media Environments, pp. 9–15. ACM, Tampere (2011)
8. Bihler, P., Blumenau, D., Bendel, S., Pilger, S.: Eco-Driver: Using Automotive Sensor Data to Control Mobile Driving Games. In: Proceedings of the IADIS International Conference on Game and Entertainment Technologies, pp. 111–115. IADIS Press, Rome (2010)
9. Miranda, B., Jere, C., Alharbi, O., Lakshmi, S., Khouja, Y., Chatterjee, S.: Examining the Efficacy of a Persuasive Technology Package in Reducing Texting and Driving Behavior. In: Berkovsky, S., Freyne, J. (eds.) PERSUASIVE 2013. LNCS, vol. 7822, pp. 137–148. Springer, Heidelberg (2013)
10. Meschtscherjakov, A., Wilfinger, D., Scherndl, T., Tscheligi, M.: Acceptance of Future Persuasive In-Car Interfaces Towards a More Economic Driving Behaviour. In: Proceedings of the 1st International Conference on Automotive User Interfaces and Interactive Vehicular Applications, pp. 81–88. ACM, Essen (2009)
11. Lee, S.-S., Lim, Y.-K., Lee, K.-P.: A long-term study of user experience towards interaction designs that support behavior change. In: CHI 2011 Extended Abstracts on Human Factors in Computing Systems, pp. 2065–2070. ACM, Vancouver (2011)

Persuasive Technology Based on Bodily Comfort Experiences: The Effect of Color Temperature of Room Lighting on User Motivation to Change Room Temperature

Shengnan Lu[✉], Jaap Ham, and Cees Midden

Human-Technology Interaction, Eindhoven University of Technology, P.O. Box 513, 5600 MB, Eindhoven, The Netherlands
{s.lu,j.r.c.ham,c.j.h.midden}@tue.nl

Abstract. In this paper we propose a new perspective on persuasive technology: *Comfort-Experience-Based Persuasive Technology*. We argue that comfort experiences have a dominant influence on people's (energy consumption) behavior. In the current research, we argue that room lighting can influence heating-related comfort experiences (by emitting a 'warm' versus 'cold' lighting color temperature). Two studies were conducted to investigate the effect of lighting color temperature on participants' perceptions of room lighting temperature and their estimations of room temperature, their experiences of the comfort related to room lighting temperature and related to room temperature, and also their motivation to change room temperature settings and participants' temperature-setting behavior. Results indicated that lighting color temperature can influence a user's perception of the temperature in the room, and can also motivate the user to change room temperature. This research revealed that using persuasive strategies that targets user comfort experiences could help users decrease their energy consumption.

Keywords: Ambient persuasive technology · Sustainability · Comfort experiences · Lighting · Color temperature

1 Introduction

According to the U.S. Department of Energy (2014), room heating is the largest energy expense in the average U.S. home, accounting for about 45 percent of energy bills. In the Netherlands, around 333 million m^3 gas could be saved each year when the home heating thermostat would be turned down by only one degree.

Next to purely technological solutions such as efficient systems and the development of renewable energy sources, behavior change is also crucial if not a necessity and Persuasive Technology [1] incorporated into the interfaces of the devices that are used to consume energy with (e.g., the house heating thermostat) might be optimally suited to motivate users to change their behavior. Previous research indicated that persuasive interventions aimed at stimulating energy conservation have been employed

© Springer International Publishing Switzerland 2015
T. MacTavish and S. Basapur (Eds.): PERSUASIVE 2015, LNCS 9072, pp. 83–94, 2015.
DOI: 10.1007/978-3-319-20306-5_8

with varying degrees of success [2]. For example, McCalley and Midden [3] found evidence that by adding an energy bar to the user interface of a washing machine, 18% energy could be saved both in lab and field studies. Different from this kind of factual feedback (presenting the user with a number indicating the amount of kWh used), another form of persuasive feedback, social feedback, provided by an embodied robotic agent (e.g., when the robot says "your energy consumption is bad") had even stronger persuasive effects on energy-saving behavior [4].

More recently, lighting, as a medium of *Ambient Persuasive Technology* (e.g., [5], [6]), was employed as successful feedback about energy consumption (e.g., [7], [8]). For example, a device called HeatSink consisted of a lighting source illuminating the water stream from the tap while changing lighting color according to water temperature and thereby providing feedback information about the temperature of the water without altering the function of the sink [7]. Recent research [9] suggested that ambient lighting feedback might be effective because it is relatively easier to process, and therefore still effective in various situations in which more focal persuasive technology might lose its effectiveness. That is, Maan [9] tested the effect of feedback provided by a lamp that could gradually change color dependent on the amount of energy consumption of the participant in a certain task, and compared these effects to more widely used factual feedback. Results showed feedback through ambient lighting was more effective than numerical feedback. An important reason for the ease of processing and the effectiveness of ambient lighting feedback was proposed in follow-up studies by Lu [10], which indicated that only when people have strong preexisting associations between ambient lighting colors (i.e., red vs. green) and energy consumption (i.e., high vs. low), such feedback systems can be effective.

However, the basic persuasive strategies employed by these forms of ambient persuasive technology that use lighting are persuasive interventions that necessitate *information processing*. In other words, these forms of ambient persuasive technology use *interactive forms of feedback* that can effectively change (energy consumption) behavior only when users make cognitive efforts to understand the information that the feedback carries.

In the current paper we argue that (at least with respect to saving energy by decreasing room temperature) another important guiding factor in people's environment is their comfort experiences. We argue that comfort experience may often have a dominant influence on people's (energy consumption) behavior. Indeed, earlier studies showed that people mentioned comfort as a cause or as the main cause to not save natural resources [e.g., 11, 12]. For example, research on thermal comfort as experienced when taking a shower [see 13] showed a negative correlation between water flow and water temperature. That is, when participants were asked to use less water, they increased the temperature of the water to compensate for the decrease of thermal comfort. Moreover, Merkus [14] provided energy consumption (and water consumption) feedback to people taking a shower in a field experiment, but could not find evidence for energy-saving effects of such feedback. In sum, these findings suggested that the influence of energy feedback (at least in temperature-related context) is limited because of comfort issues. We argue that more attention is needed for comfort experience in persuasive strategies.

Therefore, we propose an additional, new perspective on persuasive technology: ***Comfort-Experience-Based (CEB) persuasive technology.*** Persuasive technology that is based on comfort experience can be distinguished from persuasive technology that uses other kinds of persuasive strategies by (at least) the following characteristics: **1**. Instead of information-based strategies (e.g., directly indicating the amount of kWh), *CEB persuasive technologies* use persuasive strategies that are more experience-based (e.g., feeling of the current environment); **2**. *Information-based persuasive strategies* involve mostly cognitive processes, while *CEB persuasive strategies* involve mainly bodily and perceptual processes; **3**. *Information-based persuasive strategies* influence people's behavior consciously (or at least partly consciously), and *CEB persuasive strategies* mainly have an unconscious influence on people's behavior; and **4**. *Information-based persuasive strategies* have an impact on people's thinking, whereas *CEB persuasive strategies* have a relatively intrusive (and direct) impact on people's comfort experiences.

In the current research, we assessed the effectiveness of the comfort-experience-based forms of persuasive technology we proposed. Therefore, the current research investigated the effect of color temperature of room lighting (as a *CEB persuasive technology*) on bodily comfort perceptions, and on user motivation to save energy and energy-saving behavior. In other words, we wanted to investigate whether the lighting color temperature (e.g., 'warm' lighting) could increase perceived bodily comfort experiences, in order to influence the user's motivation to decrease room temperature and save more energy. In line with this proposal, previous research indicated that people prefer low color temperature (i.e., 'warm' lighting) in winter [15]. Also, based on several studies, Ishikawa [16] estimated that household energy consumption for heating systems could be reduced by 5% to 8% by using 'warm' lighting in winter and 'cold' lighting in summer, while maintain the same thermal comfort level.

To investigate the effectiveness of *CEB persuasive technology*, in the current paper we describe two experiments in which we tested the effectiveness of persuasive technology that manipulated bodily comfort perceptions with the goal of influencing user motivation for changing energy consumption behavior. That is, we performed two studies in which we changed lighting settings in a room by manipulating room lighting color temperature ('warm' vs. 'cold' lighting). Based on the research findings as described earlier we expected to find evidence that room lighting color temperature influences participants' perceptions of room temperature, and most importantly, their motivation to change room temperature. More specifically, in Experiment 1, we hypothesized that participants in the 'warm' lighting condition would perceive the room temperature to be higher than participants in the 'cold' lighting condition (H1.1). Also, we hypothesized that participants in the 'warm' lighting condition would perceive the lighting in the room to be warmer than participants in the 'cold' lighting condition (H1.2). And finally, we hypothesized that participants in the 'warm' lighting condition would express a stronger motivation to decrease the room temperature than participants in the 'cold' lighting condition (H1.3).

2   Experiment 1

2.1   Method

2.1.1   Participants and Design

Sixty-six visitors of Eindhoven University of Technology participated in this study. Of these, thirty-eight participants were high school students (average age 17.2 years old, $SD = 1.87$) and twenty-eight were their parents (average age 50.1 years old, $SD = 3.86$). All participants were native Dutch speakers and participated during a visit of the lighting lab at the school of Innovation Sciences, Eindhoven University of Technology during the University Open Day 2014. Six groups (approximately ten visitors for each group) were randomly assigned to either 'warm' lighting condition or 'cold' lighting condition. In our lighting lab, the physical room temperature could not be controlled. We measured and continuously recorded room temperature (with an average of $22.9°C, SD = 0.70$) during this experiment, which was conducted in March 2014.

2.1.2   Experimental procedure

Before the groups entered the lab room, the lighting of the room was set to either a 'warm' (2700 Kelvin), or to a 'cold' lighting condition (5500 Kelvin). The lighting in the room was programmed to the specific settings ('warm' or 'cold') before the group entered the room, and stayed in those settings until the experiment finished.

After entering the lab room, the participants were given a short (verbal) general introduction to this lighting lab. In these explanations, neither the ceiling luminaries and their lighting settings nor potential influences of lighting on people were discussed. So no effect relative to the experiment was explained. After this introduction (of approximately 5 minutes), each participant was asked whether he or she wanted to participate in a short study, by filling out a one-page questionnaire (in Dutch, as described in the Materials section below). Answering the questions of the questionnaire took approximately 2 minutes. After this, the lighting lab demonstrations continued, and the confederate (lab tour guide) provided more extensive explanations including details on the ceiling lighting, how lighting might be used to influence users, and also debriefed all members of the group on the purpose of the study they had participated in, and thanked them for their participation. The whole visit to the lighting lab lasted approximately 20 minutes.

2.1.3   Materials

To assess perceived room temperature, perceived lighting temperature, and motivation to change room temperature, we asked participants to fill out a questionnaire. This questionnaire contained a variety of questions about the lab room, amongst them the three questions of focus. That is, this questionnaire asked participants first of all for their perceptions of the room temperature (using the question "What do you think about the temperature in this room?", to which they could answer on a 7-point rating scale ranging from 1 very cold to 7 very warm).

Also, the questionnaire asked participants for their perceptions of the lighting temperature in the room (using the question "What do you think about the lighting in this room?" to which they could answer by indicating whether "Warm" was applicable on a 7-point rating scale ranging from 1 absolutely not applicable to 7 very much applicable).

Also, the questionnaire asked participants for their motivation to change the temperature in the room (using the question "If you could adjust the temperature in this room, by how many degrees would you like to change it?" to which participants could answer on a 7-point rating scale ranging from -3°C to +3°C).

Finally, participants were asked to indicate their age, gender and the number of layers of clothing they were wearing.

2.2   Result and Discussion

Results showed that the distribution of all three of our dependent variables deviated from a comparable normal distribution (as indicated by a Kolmogorov-Smirnov test, for perceived room temperature, $D(64) = 0.18, p < .001$, for perceived lighting's temperature appearance, $D(64) = 0.15, p = .001$, and for motivation to change room temperature, $D(64) = 0.22, p < .001$). Therefore, all the three dependent variables were separately submitted to non-parametric Mann-Whitney test.

Another issue was that on our measure for motivation to change room temperature, three participants' scores were outliers, with a z-score of > 2.9. More specifically, these participants expressed the motivation to increase the room temperature by +3°C (which was maximum of the rating scale), even though these participants also expressed that they found the room temperature (on another question) to be relatively warm. Therefore, below, we report our analysis of the variable motivation to change room temperate with and without these participants.

Results provided no evidence in support of our first hypothesis (H1.1), that is, no evidence was found that participants in the 'warm' lighting condition perceived the room temperature to be higher or lower ($M = 5.11, SD = .96$) than participants in the 'cold' lighting condition ($M = 4.83, SD = 1.04$), $U = 421.50, z = -1.21, p = .23, r = -.15$. In line with our second hypothesis (H1.2), results showed that participants in the 'warm' lighting condition perceived the room lighting to be warmer ($M = 4.00, SD = 1.83$) than participants in the 'cold' lighting condition ($M = 5.48, SD = 1.21$), $U = 290.00, z = -3.30, p = .001, r = -.41$. Most interestingly, results also supported our third hypothesis (H1.3): Participants in the 'warm' lighting condition expressed a stronger motivation to decrease the room temperature by an average of 1.91°C, ($SD = .96$) than participants in the 'cold' lighting condition who wanted to decrease room temperature by an average of 1.13°C, ($SD = 1.45$), $U = 315.5, z = -2.57, p = .01, r = -.32$.[1]

---

[1] When including the three outliers on the measure for motivation to change temperature, results were comparable. That is, participants in the 'warm' lighting condition express a stronger motivation to decrease the room temperature (by an average of 1.49°C, $SD = 1.67$) than participants in the 'cold' lighting condition (who expressed to want to decrease room temperature by an average of 1.20°C, $SD = 1.20$, $U = 408.5, z = -1.78, p = .076, r = -.22$.

In sum, results indicated that participants in a room with lighting set to a low color temperature (i.e., 'warm' lighting) indeed perceived the lighting temperature to be warm, and importantly, expressed a stronger motivation to decrease the room temperature. Thereby, Experiment 1 presents evidence that the lighting of a room a person is in influences that person's motivation to change the room temperature.

However, the psychological mechanisms for stronger motivation to decrease the room temperature are still unclear. Crucially, earlier research [e.g., 11, 12] showed that comfort of a dwelling is one of the main reasons for conserving energy or not.

So, we conducted a follow-up study taking into account user comfort experience measure. Additionally, the psychological mechanisms for stronger motivation to decrease the room temperature might also be used to actually diminish energy consumption. Thus, in Experiment 2, we investigated whether a person in a room with 'warm' lighting diminish his or her energy consumption in a (virtual) energy consumption task (programming the heating thermostat for that room).

3   Experiment 2

For Experiment 2, we argued that room lighting temperature might influence the comfort experiences of a person in that room, and such experiences might influence that person's room temperature perception, his or her motivation to change the room temperature and even the person's energy consumption behavior in the room (i.e., actually taking measures to increase room temperature).

Therefore, in Experiment 2, we wanted to replicate Experiment 1, and we also included measures for perceived comfort of lighting temperature, perceived comfort of the room temperature and a behavioral energy consumption measure as additional dependent variables. We argue that 'warm' lighting also has positive effects on these three additional variables. More specifically, we expected that participants in the room with the 'warm' lighting indicate the lighting temperature in the room to be warmer (H2.1) and also more comfortable (H2.2) as compared to participants in the room with the 'cold' lighting. We also expected that participants in the room with 'warm' lighting would perceive the room temperature to be warmer (H2.3) and more comfortable (H2.4) as compared to participants in the room with the 'cold' lighting. Finally, we expected that participants in the room with the 'warm' lighting consume less energy (H2.5) in the thermostat programming tasks (i.e., setting lower temperature) than participants in the room with 'cold' lighting.

3.1   Method

3.1.1   Participants and Design

Forty-eight students (average age 22.1 years old, $SD = 2.76$) of Eindhoven University of Technology (29 male and 19 female) were recruited by using a local participant database. They participated in the current experiment in either the 'warm' lighting condition first and then the 'cold' lighting condition, or in the 'cold' lighting condition first and then the 'warm' lighting condition. Whether a participant received the 'warm' or the 'cold' lighting condition first, was strictly counterbalanced. All participants were native Dutch speakers. The experiments lasted approximately 45 minutes, and participants received 7 euros for their participation. In this lighting lab, the physical room temperature could not be controlled. We measured and continuously recorded room temperature (with an average of 24.6°C, $SD = 1.10$) during the experiment, which was conducted in June 2014.

3.1.2   Experimental procedure

Participants were welcomed in the central hall of the lab building. Each participant was asked to read and sign a consent form stating the general purpose of the research and their willingness to participant in this research. In the lab room, a thermometer was put on a table in the corner of the room to record the average room temperature during the experiment.

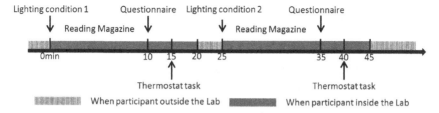

Fig. 1. Experimental procedure

Before participants entered the lab room (see Figure 1), for half of the participants the lighting of the room was set to 'warm' lighting in the first session (and to 'cold' lighting in the second session). For the other half of the participants, the lighting in the room was set to 'cold' lighting in the first session (and to 'warm' lighting in the second session). We used fluorescent ceiling lamps with a color temperature of 2500 Kelvin as 'warm' and 6100 Kelvin as 'cold' lighting conditions (see Figure 2).

For the first session, participants were asked to read a magazine for a period of ten minutes. For this, we supplied an issue of a Dutch popular science magazine (named "Quest") on the table right next to the laptop. After ten minutes, the computer indicated that the reading period was over and participants were asked to answer a set of fourteen questions that asked them to evaluate the lab room. This questionnaire consisted of fourteen questions (see the Material section below).

After answering these questions, we assessed energy consumption behavior by asking participants to perform a virtual thermostat task on the laptop. That is, participants received instructions on how to program a virtual room thermostat interface, and asked to program this thermostat for several scenarios. After two practice scenarios, participants completed programming the thermostat for six experimental scenarios. For each scenarios, the scenario itself was first described to the participants (e.g., "You and a friend are going to watch a television show for the next half hour.") and then the participant was asked to program the thermostat by setting the temperature for the room. For each scenario, participants were asked to strive for two goals: to consume as little energy as possible (for heating the room), and to maintain a temperature level that they deemed as comfortable as possible. After programming the room thermostat for the six scenarios, participants were told to leave the lab room, and to take a seat in the hall way outside of the lab room.

After a five-minute break, the second session of the experiment started. Participants were asked to retake their seats inside the lab room. The experimental procedure of the second session was completely identical to the first session, with the exception that lighting in the laboratory was manipulated to the other condition. After completion of the second session, participants were asked to answer demographic questions.

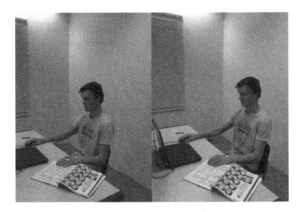

Fig. 2. Photographs of 'Warm' (left) and 'cold' (right) lighting condition

3.1.3   Materials

In each of the two sessions, participants were asked to fill out a set of fourteen questions (in Dutch). First of all, to assess a participant's perception of the lighting temperature in the room, participants were asked to answer four questions about the room lighting temperature ("What do you think about the lighting in this room?", "Do you think the lighting in this room is warm or cold?", "What feeling does the lighting in this room give you?", and "What do you think the light in this room looks like?") to which participants could answer by choosing an option on a 7-point rating scale ranging from 1 very cold to 7 very warm. We constructed a reliable (Cronbach's alpha = .86) measure of perceived lighting temperature by averaging participant's answers to these four questions.

Then, to assess a participants' evaluation of room and its lighting temperature, participants were asked to answer four questions about their evaluation of the room and its lighting temperature ("How comfortable do you think this room is?", "How comfortable to you think the lighting in this room is?", "Do you think the room lighting is comfortable?", "Do you think the room lighting is pleasant?"). Participants could answer these questions by choosing an option on a 7-point rating scale ranging from 1 very uncomfortable to 7 very comfortable. We constructed a reliable (Cronbach's alpha = .78) measure of room lighting comfort evaluation by averaging a participant's answers to these four questions.

Next, to assess a participants' perception of the room temperature, participants were asked to answer two questions about the room temperature ("How does the temperature of this room feel?", "Does the air in this room feel warm or cold?"). Participants could answer these questions by choosing an option on a 7-point rating scale ranging from 1 very cold to 7 very warm. We constructed a reliable (Cronbach's alpha = .83) measure of perceived lighting temperature by averaging participant's answers to these four questions.

Finally, to assess a participants' evaluation of the room temperature, participant were asked to answer four questions about their evaluation of the room temperature ("How comfortable do you experience the room temperature?", "How comfortable do you think the room temperature is?", "Do you think the room temperature is pleasant?", "Is the room temperature agreeable?"). Participants could answer these questions by choosing an option on a 7-point rating scale ranging from 1 very uncomfortable/very unpleasant/very disagreeable to 7 very comfortable/very pleasant/very agreeable. We constructed a reliable (Cronbach's alpha = .95) measure of evaluated room temperature by averaging a participant's answers to these four questions.

3.2   Result and Discussion

To analyze the effects of the room lighting color temperature on our various dependent variables, we used a one-way repeated measures analysis of variance (ANOVA), in which room lighting ('warm' vs. 'cold') was manipulated within participants.

Results supported our first hypothesis (H2.1). That is, when the room lighting was set to 'warm', participants indicated that they perceived the room lighting to be warmer ($M = 5.11, SD = .72$) than when the room lighting was set to 'cold' ($M = 3.15, SD = .84$), $F(1,47) = 175.5, p < .001, \eta^2 = .79$.

Confirming our second hypothesis (H2.2), results showed that when the lighting was set to 'warm', participants indicated the lighting temperature in the room to be more comfortable ($M = 5.05, SD = .86$) than when the lighting was set to 'cold' ($M = 4.15, SD = 1.00$), $F(1,47) = 34.8, p < .001, \eta^2 = .46$.

In addition to the perception of lighting temperature and perceived comfort of lighting temperature, we were especially interested in the effects on participant's perception of room temperature and perceived comfort of room temperature.

In line with our third hypothesis (H2.3), results indicated that when the room lighting was set to 'warm', participants perceived the room temperature to be warmer ($M = 4.72, SD = .81$) than when the lighting was set to 'cold' ($M = 5.05, SD = .86$), $F(1,47) = 9.9, p = .003, \eta^2 = .17$.

However, results provided no evidence in support of our fourth hypothesis (H2.4), that is, it presented no evidence that when room lighting was set to 'warm', participants perceived the room temperature to be more (or less) comfortable ($M = 5.01, SD = 1.03$) than when the room lighting was set to 'cold' ($M = 4.83, SD = .90$), $F(1,47) = 2.10, p = .16, \eta^2 = .04$.

Finally, results did not confirm our last hypothesis (H2.5). That is to say, participants in the room with the 'warm' lighting did not consume less (or more) energy in the thermostat programming tasks (i.e., setting lower temperature by an average of

19.68 °C, $(SD = 1.26)$ than participants in the room with 'cold' lighting (by an average of 19.75°C, $SD = 1.34$), $F(1,47) = .87, p = .36, \eta^2 = .02$. No effect of lighting color temperature on skin temperature was found.

4   General Conclusion and Discussion

In two studies, we explored the effectiveness of comfort-experience-based persuasive technology. More specifically, the current research investigated the effect of color temperature of room lighting (as a comfort-experience-based form of persuasive technology) on participants' perceptions of room lighting temperature and their estimations of the room temperature, their experiences of the comfort related to the room lighting temperature and related to the room temperature, and also their motivation to change room temperature settings and participant's temperature-setting behavior.

Results of both studies confirmed that our manipulation of room lighting was effective in showing that participants in the 'warm' lighting condition perceived the lighting in the room to be warmer than participants in the 'cold' lighting condition. More importantly, results of our second study confirmed that our manipulation of room lighting influenced participants' judgment of the temperature in the room. That is, in Experiment 2, participants in the room with the 'warm' lighting perceived the room temperature to be warmer than participants in the room with the 'cold' lighting.

However, this effect of lighting color temperature on participants' judgment of the temperature in the room was only found when the lighting conditions were manipulated within participants (as in Experiment 2), and was not found when these conditions were manipulated between participants (as in Experiment 1). Differences between participants (and their judgments of room temperature) may have caused more noise (in Experiment 1) on our dependent variable of room temperature perception making it more difficult to find effects of our manipulation of lighting color temperature on that variable in Experiment 1.

Interestingly, results of Experiment 1 also suggested that our manipulation of room lighting influenced participant's motivation to adjust the room temperature. That is, in Experiment 1, participants in the 'warm' lighting condition expressed a stronger motivation to decrease the room temperature than participants in the 'cold' lighting condition. This evidence indicated that user motivation for saving energy and related energy-saving behavior (e.g., setting a lower room temperature) could be enhanced when people were in a room with 'warm' lighting settings.

However, our second study provided no evidence that room lighting color temperature influenced actual energy saving behavior. That is, results of Experiment 2 provided no evidence that when participants were in a room with 'warm' lighting settings, they programmed the room thermostat differently from when they were in a room with 'cold' lighting settings. The lack of behavioral changes in our thermostat programming tasks may be due to a variety of reasons. Crucially, in our lighting lab, the actual room temperature could not be controlled and was relatively high (approximately 22.9°C in Experiment 1, which was conducted in March 2014; approximately 24.6°C in Experiment 2, which was conducted in June 2014). Indeed, all participants of Experiment 2 indicated the room temperature to be quite comfortable, in the both 'warm' and 'cold' lighting conditions. Thereby, participants may have lacked the motivation to change their behavior to attain a comfortable status (change the settings of the thermostat to a higher or lower temperature). In contrast, when people are in an uncomfortable status (e.g., feel slightly cold or hot), people might consume more energy (by increasing room temperature) in the 'cold' lighting condition than people in the 'warm' lighting condition (or vice-versa when they feel hot). Relatedly, earlier research [15] suggested that preference in the color temperature of general room lighting may vary depending on the previous experiences of air temperature before entering the room. So, future research might find the effect of room lighting color temperature on behavior change by diminishing the physical temperature in the experimental room.

Furthermore, results of our second study showed that when the room lighting was set to 'warm', participants indicated the lighting temperature in the room to be more comfortable than when the lighting was set to 'cold'. However, results (of Experiment 2) provided no evidence that our manipulation of room lighting influenced participant's comfort experience of the room itself. One reason might be that comfortable room temperature may vary considerably amongst individuals. Such differences between participants (caused by e.g., just having had a meal, taken a shower or wearing a sweater, see [12]) may have caused noise that made it more difficult to find effects of our manipulation of room lighting temperature. Future research investigating these effects could be conducted in real homes as a between subjects design, additionally increasing the external validity of the experiment by collecting the data over an extended period of time during normal usage of lights.

In sum, the current research shows that color temperature of the room lighting can influence on a user's perception of room temperature, and can motivate the user to change the room temperature. These findings contribute to the scientific literature crucial evidence that the effectiveness of persuasive technology could be also enhanced by targeting comfort experiences via mainly bodily and perceptual processes. This kind of persuasive technology can help users decrease their energy consumption, by using a category of persuasive strategies that targets user comfort experiences.

References

1. Fogg, B.J.: Persusaive Technology: Using Computers to Change What We Think and Do. Morgan Kaufmann, San Francisco (2003)
2. Abrahamse, W., Steg, L., Vlek, C., Rothengatter, T.: A review of intervention studies aimed at household energy conservation. Journal of Environmental Psychology 25, 273–291 (2005)
3. McCalley, L., Midden, C.: Energy conservation through product-integrated feedback: The roles of goal-setting and social orientation. Jounal of Economic Psychology 23, 589–603 (2002)
4. Ham, J., Midden, C.: A persuasive robotic agent to save energy: the influence of social feedback, feedback valence and task similarity on energy conservation behavior. In: Ge, S.S., Li, H., Cabibihan, J.-J., Tan, Y.K. (eds.) ICSR 2010. LNCS, vol. 6414, pp. 335–344. Springer, Heidelberg (2010)

5. Ham, J., Midden, C., Beute, F.: Can ambient persuasive technology persuade unconsciously?: using subliminal feedback to influence energy consumption ratings of household appliances. In: Proceedings of the 4th International Conference on Persuasive Technology, p. 29. ACM (2009)
6. Davis, J.: Towards participatory design of ambient persuasive technology. Presented at Persuasive Technology and Environmental Sustainability, Workshop at the 6th International Conference on Persuasive Computing (2008)
7. Arroyo, E., Bonanni, L., Selker, T.: Waterbot: exploring feedback and persuasive techniques at the sink. In: Proceedings of the SIGCHI Conference on Human Factors in Computing Systems, pp. 631–639. ACM (2005)
8. Wilson, G.T., Lilley, D., Bhamra, T.A.: Design feedback interventions for household energy consumption reduction (2013)
9. Maan, S., Merkus, B., Ham, J., Midden, C.: Making it not too obvious: the effect of ambient light feedback on space heating energy consumption. Energy Efficiency 4, 175–183 (2011)
10. Lu, S., Ham, J., Midden, C.J.H.: Using Ambient Lighting in Persuasive Communication: The Role of Pre-existing Color Associations. In: Spagnolli, A., Chittaro, L., Gamberini, L. (eds.) PERSUASIVE 2014. LNCS, vol. 8462, pp. 167–178. Springer, Heidelberg (2014)
11. Becker, L., Seligman, C., Fazio, R., Darley, J.: Relating attitudes to residential energy use. Environment and Behavior 13, 590–609 (1981)
12. Heijs, W., Stringer, P.: Research on residential thermal comfort: Some contributions from environmental psychology. Journal of Environmental Psychology 8, 235–247 (1988)
13. Ohnaka, T., Tochihara, Y., Watanabe, Y.: The effects of variation in body temperature on the preferred water temperature and flow rate during showering. Ergonomics 37, 541–546 (1994)
14. Merkus, B.: A shower meter to save water and energy: The influence of two feedback sources, goals, and the role of comfort on conservation behavior in a lab and Field experiment. Master's Thesis, Eindhoven University of Technology (2012)
15. Nakamura, H., Oki, M.: Influence of air temperature on preference for color temperature of general lighting in the room. Journal of the Human-Environmental System 4(1), 41–47 (2000)
16. Ishikawa, Y.: Energy-saving effect of heating/cooling system by illuminant color. J. Illum. Engng. Inst. Jpn 77(11), 690–692 (1993)

BrightDark: A Smartphone App Utilizing e-fotonovela and Text Messages to Increase Energy Conservation Awareness

Olayan Alharbi[✉] and Samir Chatterjee

School of Information Systems and Technology, Claremont Graduate University, 130 E.
9th Street, Claremont, CA, 91711, USA
{Olayan.alharbi,samir.chatterjee}@cgu.edu

Abstract. Global energy consumption is rapidly increasing, while natural energy resources are shrinking. Household energy consumption accounts for 22% of total energy consumption in U.S. Almost half of household energy consumption is electricity use. In the U.S., households spent on average $1,419 annually for electricity and it is accountable for over 70% of household CO_2 emissions. Households are looking to reduce their electricity consumption. In this paper, we present a novel persuasive approach, by using e-fotonovela (art-based research) and text messages to provide household with a customized motivation and awareness solution to reduce their electricity consumption based on either cost or environmental concern. Findings provide significant results for the efficacy of the customized e-fotonovela and text messages in motivating and raising households' awareness toward electricity conservation.

Keywords: Electricity conservation · Fotonovela · Text messages · Mobile apps · Persuasive technology

1 Introduction

Global energy consumption is rapidly increasing, while natural energy resources are shrinking [1]. Since the energy crisis of the 1970s and the current concerns about the role of energy consumption in environmental problems such as global warning, energy consumption has proven to have serious economic and environmental side effects. In 2011, energy production in the United States was less than the total consumption by 19 Quadrillion Btu [2]. Moreover, in 2013 the contribution of energy towards carbon dioxide emission increased by 2.5%. Those threats have encouraged scientists from different disciplines to find solutions that can lower consumer expenses and keep the environment safe. Energy efficiency and/or energy conservation have been marketed as main solutions to confront these threats [3, 4].

Household energy consumption accounts for 22% of total energy consumption in U.S. Almost half of that is electricity use, which accounts for about 4.39 Quadrillion Btu. In the U.S., households spent on average $1,419 annually for electricity in 2010. This amount is more than the average spent in 2006 by about $300 [5]. Regarding environmental concerns in the U.S., residential energy consumption is responsible for

© Springer International Publishing Switzerland 2015
T. MacTavish and S. Basapur (Eds.): PERSUASIVE 2015, LNCS 9072, pp. 95–106, 2015.
DOI: 10.1007/978-3-319-20306-5_9

about 5.7 billion metric tons of CO2 annually [6]. Specifically, electricity consumption is accountable for over 70% of household CO2 emissions. Thus, residential electricity consumption clearly has a primary share on increasing living costs and environmental threats. Electricity bills are affecting individual budgets and simultaneously increasing CO2 production rates globally.

According to Barreto et. al. [7], households believe energy conservation is important and has the potential to reduce expenses. Barreto [7] assert that *cost* is the first motivation to reduce electricity consumption. In addition to cost savings as an energy conservation driver, *environmental concerns* were considered a secondary driver for energy conservation. Thus, cost and environmental concerns are motivational factors for households to lower energy consumption.

While households are motivated and aware of the imperative needs to conserve energy, their energy consumption is growing. As mentioned above, both household spending on electricity and CO2 emissions rates are increasing. Thus, knowing the importance of energy conservation is not enough for sustainable energy reduction.

Fortunately, electricity consumption reduction is possible by changing consumers' behavior. According to [8], consumers are able to save up to 40% of their electricity consumption after following certain tips that reduce electricity wasting on a daily basis. In addition, [9] indicates that sustainable energy conservation actions for residents, such as reducing unnecessary standby mode for appliances, can improve energy conservation. On the other hand, [10] finds discomfort, forgetfulness, and lack of knowledge are important barriers to energy conservation. A total of 61% of the respondents in their study consider a lack of knowledge as being a barrier to achieve energy efficiency.

Technology-based solutions have been used in persuading households to reduce electric waste. Numerous studies use sensing technology to provide households with immediate feedback regarding their consumption rate [11–14]. On the other hand, social components and feedback solutions have been utilized to provide households with feedback and comparison solutions [15]. Those efforts regarding feedback solutions usually lack simple tips toward achieving energy conservation. Kjeldskov et al. [16] presents a study that combines feedback, comparison and saving tips. However, simple solutions and direct and attainable advices are imperative in designing a persuasive solution [17]. Moreover, households have different stimulus toward electricity conservation. Thus, customized awareness solutions and saving tips have better impacts toward changing recipient's behavior.

This paper presents BrightDark as a customized motivation and awareness solution. BrightDark is a smartphone application that adheres to the design science research guidelines [18, 19]. BrightDark application works in two stages. First, BrightDark determines household motivation toward electricity conversation. Then, based on household concerns, BrightDark utilizes fotonovela (comic book style storytelling) to increase motivation and awareness towards energy conservation. Second stage involves the use of text messages for daily tips to achieve the customized solution. The paper is organized as follows: Section 2 explains the adopted theoretical framework; Section 3 presents the build and design phase of BrightDark; Sections 4 provides an evaluation of BrightDark. Then, we provide insights on the effectiveness of e-fotonovela as a motivation and awareness tool, and the impact of the customized package (e-fotonovela and text messages) in electricity conservation. Finally, the paper concludes with limitations and future works.

2   Theoretical Framework

BrightDark aims to change human behavior for households to reduce their electricity consumption. Geller [20] suggests a behavioral change model that matches the intervention approach with the needs of the target individuals. There are four stages that a person goes through (unconscious incompetence, conscious incompetence, conscious competence, and unconscious competence), and there is a suitable intervention for each stage [20]. The model moves subjects who are not aware of the problem and the available solution (unconscious incompetence stage) into the successful stage, where they perform the desired behavior unconsciously (unconscious competence stage) through successive interventions (see Fig. 1). First, people with risk habits are in the "unconscious incompetence" stage where they are not aware of the threats of their habits. They usually perform automatically without any thinking about their habit. With instructional intervention, people become aware of the risks of their habit, and they understand the desired behavior. BrightDark through its use of e-fotonovela increases the awareness.

People with risk habits need to have instructions about the problem and about the available solutions. Instructional intervention is achieved by education. Awareness programs are required to help performers understand the desired behavior and ways to perform it. For better and effective results, instructional intervention needs to be specific and customized based on individual concerns. However, at this stage people may not continuously perform the desired behavior yet. Therefore, second intervention motivates conscious performers to achieve the desired behavior more often. Then people need support and motivation, to become more competent in the desired behavior. The motivation intervention requires external efforts such as incentives/rewards to increase the performers' abilities to perform the new behavior. The support intervention usually requires feedback about their progress and its positive consequences. It is more effective when the feedback comes from other performers.

Fotonovela has long been used to convey stories that can enhance awareness or educate people. BrightDark presents an e-fotonovela to encourage households to perform conservative behavior in consuming electricity. A traditional fotonovela is a small comic book that presents a dramatic story using photographs and bubble dialogs. It is mainly used for awareness purposes [21]. The fotonovela has been utilized as an awareness tool for raising knowledge about certain diseases such as depression and diabetes [21–24]. It is more readable than classic awareness tools such as pamphlets [23]. The success of the fotonovela in the context of healthcare encourages the research team to utilize it to reduce electricity consumption. This helps to improve education, as fotonovela is a much more digestible form of education than many of the traditional practices. For better accessibility and availability, BrightDark uses a mobile application platform to publish and disseminate the e-fotonovela.

By following the social cognitive theory, the fotonovela provides a model for electricity conservation behavior, which raises household self-efficacy toward electricity savings. The social cognitive theory points out that people could adopt new behaviors by direct experiences or observations [25]. The e-fotonovela acts as a model to educate households about available techniques in order to reduce electricity waste. It also presents the impacts of the desired behavior in decreasing costs and saving the environment. The e-fotonovela includes proven facts about the possible opportunities of saving money and reducing the rate of CO_2 emission by following the provided tips. The narrative is designed to help households observe the desired behavior and its financial and environmental impacts.

Thus, BrightDark follows Geller model and social cognitive theory for two purposes. First, Geller has been adopted to design and sort stages of the intervention (awareness and then motivation). Second, social cognitive theory is used in the first stage (awareness intervention) to provide household with a model for electricity conservation behavior (the e-fotonovela), which raises the household awareness regarding available tips to save electricity.

3   Designing the Smartphone Application

This design project includes designing and evaluating a smartphone app (BrightDark), implementing the fotonovela and a text messaging system. BrightDark is targeting households to promote electricity conservation behavior. It consists of two main components: an e-fotonovela as a motivation and awareness tool (mobile application), and a text messaging system as a daily awareness and reminder channel. To obtain better household engagement, the content in both of those components are customized based on individual consumer motivations. The entire project includes: 1) BrightDark mobile application, which has an embedded pre-survey, an e-fotonovela and subscription form, and 2) text messaging system.

3.1   BrightDark: Mobile Application Component

Households are typically driven by two factors to save electricity: cost or environmental concerns [7]. BrightDark starts by a pre-survey to uncover household concerns. The pre-survey helps BrightDark to customize the story according to person's interest. Consequently, the adaptable e-fotonovela focuses on electricity conservation within a context that matches the household motivation factor. Moreover, BrightDark stores pre-survey results in a cloud-based database. (These results are available for later analysis and discussion.) Based on their choices and after completing the pre-survey, the user can enjoy reading the e-fotonovela that matches his/her interests.

The e-fotonovela conversation script is written with three goals in mind, First, engage readers (households) in a scenario similar to their concerns. For instance, a user with a cost concern reads a customized version of the fotonovela that starts with a conversation about the continuous increase in monthly bills for electricity. Similarly, a reader with environmental concern is exposed to a different version of the fotonovela that introduces the discussion with CO_2 emission rates and individual roles to decrease it. Second, promote electricity conservation behavior by presenting valuable and attainable electricity saving tips (see Fig. 2). All these tips are simple and accessible to most households. Specifically, the e-fotonovela indicates three important electricity

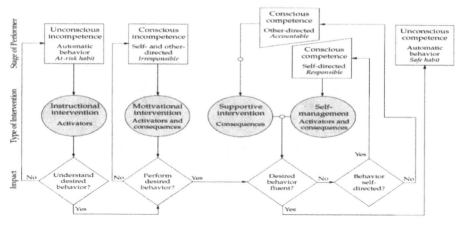

Fig. 1. Adopted Model: Geller behavioral change model

saving tips. For instance, appliances on standby mode waste almost 85% of the power that they use when they are working [26]. Moreover, there are 8 appliances on standby in the average house. The e-fotonovela points out the role of standby mode on several frames (see Fig. 2). These frames state the facts about standby mode threats. Then, they present a discussion about finding unnecessary working devices and calculating the waste amount in the average house. The other two advices are implied in the fotonovela content similarly. Third, the e-fotonovela motivates households to enroll in electricity conservation campaigns through a follow-up text message. Therefore, the final part of the e-fotonovela is designed to motivate households to subscribe to the text-messaging system. In both versions of the e-fotonovela, the end conversation invites households to subscribe to the text-messaging program. The invitation is part of the e-fotonovela dialog for a smooth transaction (see Fig. 3). Moreover, for simplicity the subscription form is embedded in the app similar to the pre-survey. BrightDark's users complete the pre-survey, the e-fotonovela, and the subscription form in one access. BrightDark's main task is to present a tailored e-fotonovela to households and invite them to daily text messaging campaigns.

3.2   BrightDark: Text Messaging System

The text-messaging system is used to maintain the new electricity conservation behavior of the household. The campaign where messages are sent lasts for four days. Each subscribed user receives a message daily at their preferred time based on the subscription form information. However, most subscribers are from one time zone, the messaging system is designed to serve different time zones. In addition, messages are personalized and short. Subscribers receive personalized messages that begin with their first name and a limit of 140 characters.

Messages are written to achieve three goals. First, messages serve as a trigger to remind the subscribers about their new behavior toward electricity conservation. Second, the messages continue to provide one of the e-fotonovela goals, which is "increasing awareness." According to [26], there are about one hundred simple

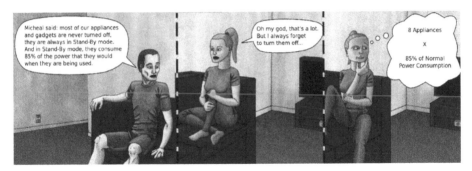

Fig. 2. Part of the conversation regarding stand-by mode (Cost concern version)

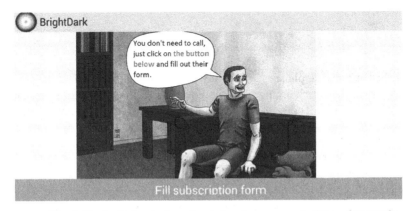

Fig. 3. The invitation to the subscription form as a part of the e-fotonovela

actions that almost anyone can apply without extra costs. BrightDark utilizes the text messages to raise household awareness regarding the available electricity reduction solutions. Third, messages aim to motivate the household to apply the received tips. Some of the messages end by asking about the household's actions toward earlier recommendations.

Finally, BulkSMS software is adopted for automating the text-messaging system tasks, such as scheduled messages, personalized messages, and group messages. BulkSMS software has several functions that empower the BrightDark system to send and receive group messages. Households are grouped based on their preferred time for receiving messages. The system sends messages for each group accordingly. In addition, BulkSMS is able to receive and categorize responses. For instance, some messages include follow-up questions. Then, BrightDark's users reply "Yes" or "No" to the questions, and the system adds the users to the appropriate groups. BulkSMS allows BrightDark messaging, scheduling and categorizing functions.

The entire BrightDark project (mobile application and text messaging system) is a collection of IT artifacts to provide households with a mobile application to find out their concerns, view the e-fotonovela and collect their contact information to subscribe in a follow-up awareness and motivation text-messaging program.

The BrightDark app can be downloaded from Google Play (Google's store for Android applications) at …..[http://goo.gl/fDVL3H]

3.3   Procedures

The BrightDark mobile application is applicable for smart phones with an Android operating system. The application is uploaded to Google Play Store. The research team promoted the application URL via their Facebook and Twitter accounts. Also, brochures were distributed in coffee shops and public places such as local libraries. Subjects who are interested in BrightDark download the application, and then complete the pre-survey and begin exploring the suitable version of the e-fotonovela based on their concerns. The last scene of the e-fotonovela, as mentioned above, asks subjects to subscribe to the text message campaign (Fig. 3). All subscriber information is saved in a cloud database that is accessible via Internet.

One week after distributing the mobile application, all subscribed users receive a text message to thank them for participating and to inform them that the second phase of BrightDark will start on the following day. At this point, the experiment moves to second stage, where households that downloaded the application and subscribed to the text-messaging campaign, start to receive a customized awareness message for four days (e.g. "Dear Frank, a typical household could save between $45.00 and $125.00 a year just by remembering to turn off appliances left on standby."). Also, in the following day, they receive a follow up message that asks them if she/he has completed the previous day's message (e.g. "Dear Frank, have you completed yesterday's tip [unplugging unnecessary plugged devices]? Reply Y/N'). The subscribers were grouped based on their preferred time of receiving messages.

4   Results and Discussion

We first present the results related to e-fotonovela's efficacy in motivating households to subscribe to the text-messaging campaign. We then present the impact of e-fotonovela in combination with the text-messaging campaign in order to reduce household electricity consumption. These results are presented by using a five-points Likert scale for questions on the level of agreement (i.e. The BrightDark motivated me to reduce my electricity consumption) and univariate analysis for direct questions (i.e. If you have access to your daily electricity consumption (e.g. SCE website), did you notice a decrease in the last four days?"). Table 1 shows participants' feedback about the e-fotonovela (the e-fotonovela and text messages) as a motivation and awareness tool in the context of electricity conservation.

BrightDark's mobile application was downloaded 50 times. A total of 92% (46) of the users who downloaded the application completed the pre-survey. Exactly 83% (35) of them considered cost concern as their main motivator for reducing electricity consumption. A third of the downloads are made by females. More than two thirds of the users are white. The e-fotonovela motivates more than 83% (41) of the users to subscribe in the text messaging campaign. This shows there is a major ability to motivate change among users of this project. Participants completed the pre-survey and were persuaded to subscribe in the text messages to receive a daily message for four days. Thus, a total of 41 subscribers are eligible to participate in the post survey because the post survey is built to collect participant feedback about the e-fotonovela and text-messaging campaign (Fig. 4).

A total of 82% of participants agreed to the effectiveness of the e-fotonovela in motivating them to reduce electricity consumption. The majority of participants (86%) agreed that the fotonovela was more enjoyable than regular awareness tools such as websites or pamphlets. As mentioned above, the e-fotonovela's content is customized based on participant motivation (cost or environmental). According to the post survey results, participants believe the e-fotonovela's content matches their concerns with 4.1 points on the Likert scale. One of the e-fotonovela objectives is to motivate participants to subscribe to the text-messaging campaign. As mentioned above, 84% of the users who downloaded the application are persuaded to subscribe to the text messages (Fig. 4). With similar results, Table 1 shows participant opinion about e-fotonovela's role in motivating them to subscribe to the text-messaging campaign.

BrightDark aims to increase household awareness about simple actions to reduce their electricity consumption. The e-fotonovela content includes three tips and a daily text message has an actionable tip. Leaving appliances on standby mode for a long time is a common wasting habit. On average, there are eight appliances unnecessarily on standby mode. Moreover, standby mode consumes 85% of the power that the appliances use when they are working. Therefore, the standby mode tip is included in both informants. Thus, the total awareness messages are six. The majority of participants were able to observe the imbedded messages regarding electricity conservation (86%). Even though the main objective for the e-fotonovela is to motivate households to subscribe to the text-messaging campaign, Table 1 shows the overall positive effectiveness of the e-fotonovela in raising household electricity conservation awareness.

The text messages are included in the last for four days. On the first day, only one awareness message was sent. During the rest of the days, subscribers received two customized messages. One was a regular awareness message similar to the first day message. The other message was a follow-up message that asks subscribers if she/he has completed the previous day's message (e.g. "Dear Frank, have you completed yesterday's tip [unplugging unnecessary plugged devices]? Reply Y/N'). On the fifth day, subscribers receive a follow-up text message and an invitation to the post survey. In total, BrightDark sends 164 awareness text messages in four days. More than half of the subscribers completed the tips and more than a third of them did not reply to the follow-up message (Fig. 5). On the other hand, most subscribers found the text messages to be a good reminder to maintain their new behavior toward electricity conservation (84).

Overall, most of the above analysis is based on household feedback regarding the e-fotonovela, daily text message and BrightDark. For further investigation about BrightDark's effectiveness, the research team asked participants to check their daily electricity consumption rate by accessing their accounts on their electricity provider's website. This question was optional. Interestingly, 34 of the participants have an access to their daily usage. A total of 64% of them noticed a reduction in their daily electricity consumption, while the remaining 36% had no significant reduction (see Fig. 6).

BrightDark has successfully motivated the majority of the participants toward electricity conservation. A total of 83% (41) of the users who have downloaded BrightDark's application were persuaded to subscribe in the text-messaging campaign. Moreover, 86% of the participants have become more aware of available

savings tips by reading the e-fotonovela. The messages were sent based on the participants' preferred time where they are usually at home and more able to follow the
tips. Therefore, the text messages are considered by the majority of the participants as
being an effective awareness and reminder tool. Although, given the time limit of the
experience, more than three quarters of the participants were able to obtain their daily
consumption rate by accessing the provider's website. Two-thirds of them have noticed a reduction in their daily consumption.

Table 1. Percentage of participants agreement on BrightDark effectivness

Measurement	Likert Scale	Strongly Agree	Agree	Neither Agree nor Disagree	Disagree	Strongly Disagree
The e-fotonovela as an awareness tool (n=41)	4.3	46%	44%	7%	0%	2%
The e-fotonovela as a motivation tool (n=41) To reduce electricity consumption	4.2	28%	58%	13%	0%	3%
To subscribe in text messages campaign		48%	34%	16%	2%	9%
The e-fotonovela overall effectiveness (n=41)	4.1	37%	51%	7%	2%	2%
BrightDark project (fotonovela and text messages) as a solution for reducing electricity consumption	4	37%	46%	12%	2%	2%
The text messages as a reminder	4.2	45%	39%	11%	0%	5%

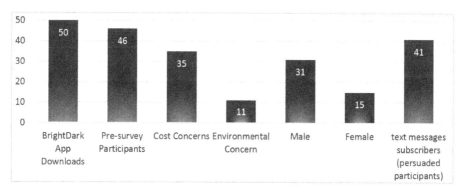

Fig. 4. Frequency Analysis: BrightDark application facts

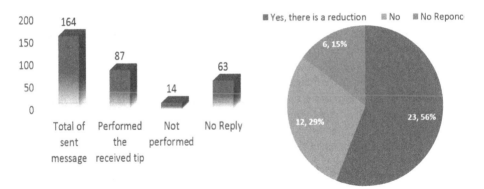

Fig. 5. Frequency analysis: follow up messages results

Fig. 6. Participant reports of electricity reduction rate

5   Future Study

This application is built by following Geller's behavioral change model. Geller's theory has four stages (Fig. 1) and our project addresses the first and second interventions: instructional and motivational interventions. The remaining stages of Geller's model help performers move from the conscious and competence stage, where performers maintain the new behavior consciously, to a desirable stage where performers maintain the new behavior unconsciously by applying it to interventions: supportive and self-management interventions. In future we will explore design solutions for other stages of Geller's model.

The majority of BrightDark's users believe e-fotonovela's content was customized to their concern regarding electricity conservation. The present project includes the top two concerns (cost and environment). Both choices are available under one platform, and by downloading one application. However, families specifically may have other concerns, such as a sense of control and security, and parents' self-perceived responsibility of their role as parents [7]. Thus, in the future we may include extra concerns to address segments of households that have different concerns.

The future study may overcome this project limitation by finding a simple solution that helps households easily figure out their daily electricity consumption and compare it to any other period of time. A total of 51% of the participants replied with positive feedback about finding out if there are savings in the daily consumption rate. Exactly 29% replied with a negative feedback, and 20% did not provide any responses. However, one limitation of this project is about discovering how much saving exactly was observed. In other words, measuring the differences in electricity consumption by the users is either difficult or time consuming. Thus, getting exact saving percentages to find the amount of reduction was not doable as opposed to measuring whether saving was observed or not. We were forced to make the question simple, in favor of receiving more positive or negative responses, instead of having no response because of the difficulties of calculating the daily consumption rate.

6   Conclusion

Although households are motivated and aware of the imperative need for energy conservation, their energy consumption is growing. Both household spending on electricity and the rate of CO_2 emissions are increasing. BrightDark is a novel persuasive technology that applies two innovations: a customized e-fotonovela and text messaging system. The use of e-fotonovela is very novel and has not been used in any persuasive solution to date. The e-fotonovela is effective in raising household awareness and motivation toward electricity conservation. More than three quarters of participants agreed about BrightDark's effectiveness in educating households about valuable and immutable tips to conserving electricity. BrightDark provides two interventions to move household with cost or environmental concerns from the "unconscious incompetence" stage of Geller's model to the "conscious competence" stage. BrightDark helps them build awareness about tips to reduce electricity waste and it motivates them to perform those tips. Interestingly, the combination of both enforcements helps reduce the electricity consumption for 64% of participants who have an access to their daily consumption rate. This is compared to their consumption before the experiment.

Besides the novel use of the fotonovela (art-based research) in the healthcare context, BrightDark's findings show significant results for art-based research in persuading households to improve electricity conservation behavior. Moreover, BrightDark presents an IT artifact that is capable of figuring out household concerns and providing them with a customized e-fotonovela that addresses those concerns. Two versions of the e-fotonovela dialog exist: a dialog for reducing the monthly bills, and the other for reducing CO_2 emission rates. A high level of agreement (82%) on the match between household concerns and the e-fotonovela scenario was obtained.

References

1. Energy Information Administration: International Energy Outlook (2014), http://www.eia.gov/forecasts/ieo/index.cfm
2. US EIA: Annual energy review 2011. Energy Inf. Adm. US Dep. Energy Wash. DC Www Eia Doe Govemeuaer (2011)
3. Steg, L., Gardner, G.T., Stern, P.C.: Environmental problems and human behavior, 2nd edn, p. 371. Pearson Custom Publishing, Boston (2002); ISBN 0-536-68633-5, $57.33; Nickerson, R.S.: Psychology and environmental change, p. 318. Lawrence Erlbaum Associates, Mahwah (2003), ISBN 0-8058-4096-6, $89.95(cloth), $37.50(paper); J. Environ. Psychol. 25, 120–123 (2005)
4. Abrahamse, W., Steg, L., Vlek, C., Rothengatter, T.: A review of intervention studies aimed at household energy conservation. J. Environ. Psychol. 25, 273–291 (2005)
5. Cauchon, D.: Household electricity bills skyrocket, http://www.usatoday.com/money/industries/energy/story/2011-12-13/electric-bills/51840042/1
6. Weber, C.L., Matthews, H.S.: Quantifying the global and distributional aspects of American household carbon footprint. Ecol. Econ. 66, 379–391 (2008)
7. Barreto, M.L., Szóstek, A., Karapanos, E., Nunes, N.J., Pereira, L., Quintal, F.: Understanding families' motivations for sustainable behaviors. Comput. Hum. Behav. 40, 6–15 (2014)

8. PIER: office plug loads: energy use and opportunities. public interest energy research (2012)

9. Gram-Hanssen, K., Kofod, C., Petersen, K.: Different everyday lives: Different patterns of electricity use. 2004 ACEEE Summer Study Energy Effic. Build., 1–13 (2004)

10. Stokes, L.C., Mildenberger, M., Savan, B., Kolenda, B.: Analyzing barriers to energy conservation in residences and offices: The Rewire program at the University of Toronto. Appl. Environ. Educ. Commun. 11, 88–98 (2012)

11. Petersen, D., Steele, J., Wilkerson, J.: WattBot: A Residential Electricity Moni-toring and Feedback System. In: CHI 2009 Extended Abstracts on Human Factors in Computing Systems, pp. 2847–2852. ACM, New York (2009)

12. Shiraishi, M., Washio, Y., Takayama, C., Lehdonvirta, V., Kimura, H., Nakajima, T.: Tracking Behavior in Persuasive Apps: Is Sensor-based Detection Always Better Than User Self-reporting? In: CHI 2009 Extended Abstracts on Human Factors in Computing Systems, pp. 4045–4050. ACM, New York (2009)

13. Kirman, B., Linehan, C., Lawson, S., Foster, D., Doughty, M.: There's a monster in my kitchen: using aversive feedback to motivate behaviour change. In: CHI 2010 Extended Abstracts on Human Factors in Computing Systems, pp. 2685–2694. ACM (2010)

14. Weiss, M., Mattern, F., Beckel, C.: Smart Energy Consumption feedback–Connecting Smartphones to Smart Meters. ERCIM NEWS 14 (2013)

15. Foster, D., Lawson, S., Blythe, M., Cairns, P.: Wattsup?: Motivating Reductions in Domestic Energy Consumption Using Social Networks. In: Proceedings of the 6th Nordic Conference on Human-Computer Interaction: Extending Boundaries, pp. 178–187. ACM, New York (2010)

16. Kjeldskov, J., Skov, M.B., Paay, J., Pathmanathan, R.: Using mobile phones to support sustainability: a field study of residential electricity consumption. In: Proceedings of the SIGCHI Conference on Human Factors in Computing Systems, pp. 2347–2356. ACM (2012)

17. Fogg, B.: A Behavior Model for Persuasive Design. In: Proceedings of the 4th International Conference on Persuasive Technology, pp. 40:1–40:7. ACM, New York (2009)

18. Hevner, A.R., March, S.T., Park, J., Ram, S.: Design Science in Information Systems Research. MIS Q. 28, 75–105 (2004)

19. Hevner, A., Chatterjee, S.: Design science research in information systems. Springer (2010)

20. Geller, E.S.: The challenge of increasing proenvironment behavior. Handb. Environ. Psychol. 525–540 (2002)

21. Unger, J.B., Cabassa, L.J., Molina, G.B., Contreras, S., Baron, M.: Evaluation of a Fotonovela to Increase Depression Knowledge and Reduce Stigma Among Hispanic Adults. J. Immigr. Minor. Health 15, 398–406 (2013)

22. Unger, J.B., Molina, G.B., Baron, M.: Evaluation of sweet temptations, a fotonovela for diabetes education. Hisp. Health Care Int. 7, 145–152 (2009)

23. Hernandez, M.Y., Organista, K.C.: Entertainment–education? A fotonovela? A new strategy to improve depression literacy and help-seeking behaviors in at-risk immigrant Latinas. Am. J. Community Psychol. 52, 224–235 (2013)

24. Valle, R., Yamada, A.-M., Matiella, A.C.: Fotonovelas: a health literacy tool for educating Latino older adults about dementia. Clin. Gerontol. 30, 71–88 (2006)

25. Bandura, A., McClelland, D.C.: Social learning theory (1977)

26. Clift, J.: Energy: Use Less-Save More: 100 Energy-Saving Tips for the Home. Chelsea Green Publishing (2009)

Designing and Analyzing Swing Compass: A Lively Interactive System Provoking Imagination and Affect for Persuasion

Kenny K.N. Chow[1(✉)], D. Fox Harrell[2], and Wong Ka Yan[3]

[1]School of Design, The Hong Kong Polytechnic University, Hong Kong, China
sdknchow@polyu.edu.hk
[2]CSAIL, Massachusetts Institute of Technology, USA
[3]School of Design, The Hong Kong Polytechnic University, Hong Kong, China

Abstract. Grounded in cognitive semantics in cognitive science, the psychology of emotion, and phenomenological approaches to interaction design, this paper first suggests a cognitive and interpretive approach to the imaginative and affective user experiences of "lively" interactive artifacts, which are reminiscent of everyday life experience. It then introduces Swing Compass, an interactive computing system that turns a tablet computer into a compass-like reflective device with artificial intelligence based on an analogy and moderation engine. With configurable analogy and moderation rules and changeable multimedia contents, the device can be instantiated differently, such as "daily activities advisors" or "app-launching guides", to help people from addiction or decidophobia in various contexts. User experience tests on the device have generated qualitative data showing how it provokes imagination and emotion via conceptual blends and emotional appraisals during different moments. This demonstrates the application of the proposed framework for interpreting users' meaning-making processes and informing possible orientations of the reflective design in hope of behavior change.

Keywords: Embodied cognition · Reflective design · Sensorimotor experience · Conceptual blending

1 Introduction

When a user of Mac OS X runs two fingers downward over a touchpad and sees pages scrolling upward in a window as a result, he or she might be provoked to imagine the scrolling process as reminiscent of panning a camera over the document. The action and perception are coupled up in a sensorimotor feedback loop, constituting conceptually meaningful interaction between the user and the system. Based upon this loop, some intriguingly designed interactive artifacts are able to provoke user imagination and emotion further at multiple cognitive levels. For example, the mobile phone NEC FOMA N702iS (designed by Oki Sato and Takaya Fukumoto) features a "water-level" battery meter, which is displayed on the phone's screen as an image looking like water. The subtle movement of the water in the interface prompts the

© Springer International Publishing Switzerland 2015
T. MacTavish and S. Basapur (Eds.): PERSUASIVE 2015, LNCS 9072, pp. 107–120, 2015.
DOI: 10.1007/978-3-319-20306-5_10

user to tilt the phone, resulting in animation of reactive water graphics (see Figure 1). The coupling of action and perception makes the user feel like holding a phone filled with water. Meanwhile, the water level descends gradually because it actually indicates the battery level. Noticing the descending water level, the user realizes the battery power consumption and starts to worry or becomes nervous. It is like he or she would not have enough drinking water for the following daily activities. This feeling emerges from metaphorical projection, which is a higher cognitive operation.

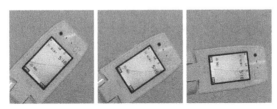

Fig. 1. The mobile phone N702iS whose battery level is indicated via the illusion of water inside the phone

Drawing upon insights from cognitive semantics in cognitive science, phenomenology in philosophy, and the psychology of emotion, the first author has articulated in length the phenomena of how a person perceives, acts upon, and responds affectively and imaginatively to "lively" interactive artifacts like the one mentioned above [1, 2]. Following the humanistic approaches, the previous work consisted of interpretive analyses, which offered possible meanings from the researcher's perspective about the phenomena, just like critiques in the humanities about a work of art, a film, or an event. Since the interpretations were based on cognitive models and phenomenological notions, the analyses were both cognitive and interpretive. In addition, we are currently working on a funded evaluation study of the user experiences of selected artifacts to collect empirical data in the laboratory environment as cross-references to the researcher's critiques. One lively interactive artifact involved in the study is Swing Compass, an interactive and generative computing system developed from the first author's another project. The system turns a tablet computer into a compass-like reflective device with artificial intelligence based on an analogy and moderation engine. With configurable analogy and moderation rules and changeable multimedia contents, variants of the compass can be instantiated, such as "daily activities advisors" or "app-launching guides", to help people from addiction or decidophobia in various contexts. User experience tests on the compass have been conducted in order to collect empirical data of how the interactions provoke one's imagination and emotion via conceptual blends, desires, and appraisals. The paper first introduces the above theoretical framework and the computational model employed in Swing Compass. It then articulates the research design of the user experience study, followed by interpretation of the cognitive processes based on the user's perspective.

2   Theoretical Framework

2.1   Lively Interactive Artifacts

By liveliness, we mean that the artifact enables interactions that are reminiscent of everyday life experience, and the user is able to elaborate imaginations with emotional responses at multiple cognitive levels. First, the artifact allows the user to perform motor input and perceive instant sensory feedback or feedforward. During these reactive moments, the user's action and perception are coupled up in a continuous sensorimotor feedback loop (Figure 2(a)). When this loop evokes a slice of everyday life (e.g., holding and tilting a bottle of water), it elicits imaginative and affective responses from the user at the immediate, pre-reflective level (e.g., seeing water "inside" the phone). Secondly, the user is able to perceive additional changes (like the descending water level), which are apparently not an immediate response to the user input. The motor input to the loop is temporarily faded in the user's mind (Figure 2(b)). The changes seem to be contingent upon other variables such as time or location, bringing a sense of narrative (e.g., how much water is gone in just the morning). During these contingent moments, the user can elaborate imagined narratives from the experience at hand at the metaphorical, reflective level. When noticing the water level descending, the user may elaborate from this into a scenario of finding insufficient drinking water in a container (e.g., a carry-on bottle). Further emotional responses, like anxiety, may result.

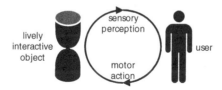

Fig. 2. (a) Continuous feedback loops between users and lively interactive objects during reactive moments

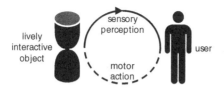

Fig. 3.   (b) Additional changes seemingly unrelated to user input implies contingency

2.2   Imaginative Blends

When the continuous feedback loop evokes a slice of life, a pervasive cognitive operation called "conceptual blending" takes place. Gilles Fauconnier and Mark Turner [3] argue that conceptual blending is a basic mental operation that generates new meanings by integrating two or more concepts. Blending is pervasive in common sense meaning making, and some blends can be so commonly exercised in everyday life that they become automatic and unnoticed. Fauconnier has cited the computer interface phenomenon as an example of this kind of immediate blend [4] (pp. 264-265). A computer user dragging a window on a computer desktop slides the mouse on a real horizontal desk. Meanwhile, the user's eyes track the vertically-oriented movement of the graphics on the screen. There are a set of mappings between the physical space and the screen space, including from the mouse to the window, from the mouse click to the act of "picking-up" the window, from forward to up, from backward to down, and so on. Most users, however, feel that they are directly manipulating the window, because of the unnoticed immediate blend between the computer interface and the experience of sliding a sheet of paper or a physical notebook on a desk.

For a lively interactive artifact during reactive moments, the continuous feedback loop is analogical to certain sensorimotor experience in everyday life. They have similarities but also subtle differences (e.g., tilting and seeing water waves inside the phone differs from doing so on a bottle of water in weight and force feedback). It is because of these nuances an immediate blend takes place. The similarities are compressed to relations in the blend (e.g., tilting and seeing waves), while the differences are selectively projected to the blend (e.g., the phone is selected but force feedback is left out). The output is an embodied imaginary concept (e.g., a water-filled phone). During contingent moments, lively artifacts continue to show changes apparently unrelated to user input. The perception of change brings to the user's mind narrative elements. A user may invoke a past experience comparable to the current experience and blend them to form imagined narratives (e.g., I am consuming the water "inside" the phone) at higher cognitive levels, which Author 1 and 2 call metaphorical blends.

2.3   Emotional Appraisals

In the sensorimotor feedback loop, motor action embodies a user's intention, desire, and also emotion. Maurice Merleau-Ponty believes that through repeated practice our bodies can "absorb" motor knowledge from the environment we inhabit and turn it into situated motor habits [5] (pp. 146-147). He called this the "intentional arc," which is the "power of laying out a past in order to move toward a future" [5] (pp. 135-136). The intentional arc forms the repertoire that directs our bodily actions beneath the level of reflective thought. Michelle Maiese believes that these pre-reflective actions driven by impulsive desires underpin our emotions [6] (pp. 62-63). When one feels a need or want, the body spontaneously performs the corresponding movement that embodies the desire (e.g., shake the phone to cancel a call).

In addition to desire, appraisal constitutes the core of our affect. James A. Russell [7] believes that "core affect is a continuous assessment of one's current state." This kind of appraisal is done via perception by users of lively artifacts during both reactive and contingent moments. As Roberta De Monticelli writes, "feeling is essentially the perception of values" of things [8] (pp. 65-66). Paul Ekman has described appraisal of a current event as one of the characteristics of emotion too [9, 10]. He points out that the appraisal mechanism can operate automatically at the primary level, or sometimes take place more reflectively at higher cognitive levels. The two mechanisms, namely automatic and extended as Ekman calls it, suggest appraisals of the enduring changes of lively artifacts during reactive and contingent moments respectively (e.g., seeing reactive water waves and seeing the water level descending), resulting in varied emotional responses.

2.4   Embodied Interaction, Reflective Design, and Behavior Change

Lively interactive artifacts enable interactions that are reminiscent of everyday life experience, which can be designed for making meaning, including reflection and then persuasion. Paul Dourish's notion of embodied interaction built upon phenomenology argues that designing interactive systems for people should consider their experiences in the mundane world and how they make meaning of it [11] (p. 126). Yet, Dourish seems to talk about meaning in a "work world," and his initial discussion focuses largely on the practical and functional meaning of everyday world objects or tools rather than reflective or critical meaning. Phoebe Senders and her colleagues consider the idea of non-utility in computing and explicitly introduce what they call "reflective design" [12]. Grounded in critical theory, the design notion emphasizes critical reflection as a means of exposing people's unconscious assumptions about everyday technologies and inviting them to look at possibilities, from perspectives of both designers and users, other than the norm. It integrates a range of related approaches, including critical design and ludic design. Reflective design attempts to balance between meaning production and utility via a set of design principles and guidelines, which designers can follow not only to stay in focus questioning entrenched practices but also to keep reminding users of the same.

Designing lively interactive artifacts can be a phenomenological approach to reflective design. Toward enabling interactions reminiscent of everyday experience, designers are required to attend to people's mundane practices (e.g., people might check availability of limited resources like battery power or drinking water quite often) and inevitably undergo critical reflection in their creative minds. The designed interactions also become evocative and affective to the user. Meanwhile, the subtle differences in the analogy (e.g., the water "inside" the mobile phone is not consumed by drinking) render possible the imaginative blends. Together with the desires and appraisals that come along, the user engages mentally and emotionally with the interactions, making meaning from the immediate, pre-reflective to the metaphorical, reflective levels during and after use. According to B. J. Fogg's behavior model [13], the imagined narratives can bring hope or fear as motivation to behavior change (e.g., one will suffer from lack of water), if the imaginative blends are vivid enough. The enduring changes presented by the artifacts can also function as compelling signals or uneasy reminders for taking action (e.g., need to consume less due to not enough drinking water). Hence, designing lively interactive artifacts emphasizes not only utilitarian values of physical interactions with objects (e.g., holding a bottle of liquid) but also the reflective and persuasive meaning generated from imagination (e.g., how much has been consumed).

3   Introducing Swing Compass

The first author have conducted cognitive and interpretive analyses on a wide range of lively interactive artifacts [1]. Meanwhile, we have been developing an interactive and generative computing system, Swing Compass. The system turns a tablet computer into a compass-like decision-making device with artificial intelligence based on an analogy and moderation engine. The engine is implemented with reference to the computational framework of the earlier Generative Visual Renku (GVR) project co-developed by Author 1 and 2 [14, 15] [16] (pp. 60-62). It takes a semi-structured database of images annotated with categorical information in different dimensions, for example, eating or doing, work or play, hedonic or eudemonic, and others, to compute and prioritize the matches between one image (currently selected) and every others (choices for the next selection) according to a set of moderation rules. The engine keeps record of the user's latest selections and moderates between the link (to the same category) and shift (to another category) patterns. The so-called "best matches" to the current selected image would be shown to the user at different directions (i.e., north, east, west, and south) on the compass rose (Figure 3) as suggested options. With configurable moderation rules and changeable images with varied annotations, variants of the compass can be instantiated, such as "daily activities advisors" or "app-launching guides", to make people aware of their unconscious practices or dispositions of making everyday choices, like addiction or decidophobia. During the development process, the research team has also pondered the hidden assumptions underlying a user's decision. This embodies the notion of reflective design.

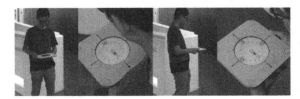

Fig. 4. Swing Compass tracks user selection and limits available options to "prompt" the user to "swing" and become aware of unconscious practices of making everyday choices

Swing Compass – The Status Messenger

We have been testing at least two variants of Swing Compass. The Status Compass can be a tool for users to update status in terms of daily activities. The activities in the given image database are annotated as either "eating" or "doing" on the superficial, perceptual dimension, and either "hedonic" (related to happiness, pleasure) or "eudemonic" (related to human potentials, virtue) [17] on the deep, conceptual dimension. The compass suggests options of next activities in one particular conceptual category (either hedonic or eudemonic) with alternating eating and doing. For another conceptual category, the user can re-orient with the compass to make a shift. If the user sticks with hedonic (or eudemonic) activities too often, the compass "prompts" a shift by limiting the number of options, and the user has to turn in order to uncover more choices in the other conceptual category (Figure 4).

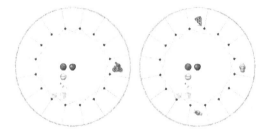

Fig. 5. A user selected eudemonic activities (apple, basketball, rice, etc.) too often, and only one option (cycling) was offered unless making a physical turn into hedonic activities (pizza, ice-cream, candy)

Swing Compass – The App Launcher

Another variant is the App Launching Compass, which functions like an app launcher on common gadgets. It suggests the type of apps the user "should" launch by displaying the app icons as options. The app icons in the database are marked as either "casual" (including social networking and entertainment apps) or "serious" (including news and productivity apps). Without a turn, the compass provides the same kind of app. When the user sticks with one kind too often, the compass reduces the number of available option as a subtle signal for a shift to another kind (Figure 5), which implies a switch between play and work.

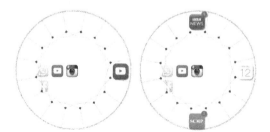

Fig. 6. A user selected casual apps (Instagram, Facebook, WhatsApp, etc.) too often, and only one option (YouTube) was offered unless making a physical turn into serious apps

In both variants, the compass "disrupts" the user's habitual engagement in activities (because using an app implies a kind of activities) through manipulating the set of available choices. Meanwhile, it drives the user actually "swing" the body (to reorient the compass) to shift to other kinds of activities. There is an embodied analogy between a turn in physical action and a shift in behavior. We hope that this analogy will emerge in the user via imaginative blends with affective responses. The expected process is delineated at the two moments.

Reactive Moments

Given a set of options, the user may tap what is wanted; otherwise one turns the compass left or right to look for other options. Rotating incrementally, one can see the old set fading out and the new fading in. The user may impulsively turn back for the old set or continue to turn further, which instantly depends on the appraisal of the new.

The impulsive desire to turn and automatic appraisal of status mobilize the sensorimotor feedback loop that is reminiscent of one's physical experience of looking around for a target. With the compass, the act of turning around is analogical to the act of moving and looking around, and the immediate blend results in an embodied imaginary concept of turning around to look for options. Figure 6(a) shows the blend with desire and appraisal. It is based on Fauconnier and Turner's integration diagrams [3]. An integration diagram consists of circles representing mental spaces, each of which contains conceptual elements of a scenario, such as actors, objects, actions, or relations. The two horizontal circles (mental spaces) are input for the blend, while the one below is the output. The horizontal solid lines between the two input spaces are links connecting the counterparts respectively. These outer-space links are compressed into inner-space relations inside the blended space. Other elements are selectively projected from either input to the blend. We add to the integration diagram the sensorimotor feedback loop, which envelops motor action and sensory perception in the mental space. The left input is the current experience enabled by a lively interactive object featuring a loop mobilized by impulsive desire and automatic appraisal, which is analogical to a past experience denoted by the right input. The result is an immediate blend. The texts in red represent imaginary thoughts and feelings of the user.

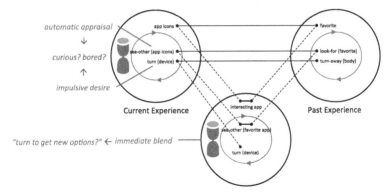

Fig. 7. (a) Impulsive desire, automatic appraisal, and immediate blend triggered by Swing Compass at reactive moments

Contingent Moments

After several rounds of selection, the user may wonder about the changing pattern of the compass's recommendation. One might not be aware that the system actually responds to one's track record. Some users might see the compass like an intelligent guide, while others might feel it set them limits, or just put them in sort of dilemma. This provokes probably different imagined narratives via different metaphorical blends. After extended appraisal, the user may feel thankful to the device for the suggestion, or conversely displeased with the limitation. Figure 6(b) illustrates a possible blend. The loop is partly faded in the user's mind, but perceivable change continues in the lively interactive object. An interpretation frame (in red) is invoked by the user, and a metaphorical blend results. This gives rise to an imagined narrative (in red) and elicits emotions (in red).

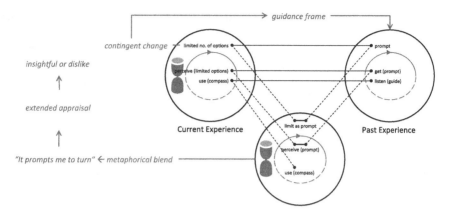

Fig. 8. (b) A metaphorical blend and extended appraisal enabled by Swing Compass during contingent moments

4   User Experience Study of Swing Compass

4.1   Methods and Participants

User experience tests on the compass were conducted in order to collect empirical data for the above framework. Each test was conducted with one participant at a time. It consisted of a questionnaire session, a series of activities, followed by an in-depth interview. The questionnaire was designed to probe the participant's adoption of digital and mobile technologies (e.g., how often one installs new apps, how many gadgets, whether play games or listen to music on the smartphone, etc.) and the prior experience of similar kinds of products (e.g., the objects one found most useful versus those most meaningful). It aims to identify their assumptions about technology between functionality and meaning.

There are three consecutive activities with different variants of Swing Compass. Each of them lasted five to ten minutes. The first activity served as a warm-up exercise. The participant was introduced to the compass (the variant is like a mini-game) and told that images were displayed at different directions as options for one to tap. The center part of the compass showed the selection record. The participant was not informed of the turning feature, and was asked to sit on a rotatable task chair. We hoped one could discover the turning feature during the process. The second activity was about the Status Compass. The participant was first shown with the images of all available everyday activities (22 out of 42 are eudemonic, while the others are hedonic), and was asked to identify those he or she likes or usually does. The participant was then invited to use the compass as if one updated status on social media intermittently or sometimes frequently during the day. This experiment required the participant to stand. Finally, the participant dealt with the App Launching Compass in the third activity. Before using it, one was given the icons of all available apps (totally 20, separated in 4 categories: social media, entertainment, news, and productivity), and was asked to fill out the one-day app usage map with those given apps according to one's own past experience. The participant then used the compass as if it was the only way of launching apps. The participant was asked to do think-aloud during all activities, which took place in our usability study room. The whole process was videotaped, and the researchers observed the participant behind the one-way mirror.

The in-depth interview was semi-structured. The outline reflected the timeline of the expected user experience from reactive moments to contingent moments. The questions for the reactive moments included those related to immediate blends, impulsive desires, and automatic appraisals. The questions for the contingent moments started with those about contingent changes, imagined narratives, metaphorical blends, and extended appraisals. Sometimes, more elaborate questions were raised for further discussion. Table 1 summarizes the questions according to the framework.

Table 1. Questions asked during interviews refer to the theoretical framework

Immediate blends (and embodied imaginary concepts)	• *Which activities have you selected? What apps have you launched? Why?* • *How did you know the turning feature?* • *To turn or not to turn, what are the reasons behind?* • *Do you recall anything similar in everyday life?*
Impulsive desires and automatic appraisals	• *How did you feel before and after a turn?* (Emoticons are used to cross-check verbal descriptions)
Contingent changes (and past experiences)	• *Did you notice any patterns from the options?* • *Could you relate to any scenarios in daily life?*
Metaphorical blends (and imagined narratives)	• *Do you prefer guidance or reminders?* • *How do you feel about intelligent agents?* • *Facing a dilemma, would you consult friends, mentors, fortunetellers, or even spiritual means?*
Extended appraisals	• *How did you feel about the compass's behavior? What would you say about the compass?*

Currently six participants (W, B, A, C, M, and I) have taken the tests. W, C, M, and I are graduate students, B is undergraduate (but relatively mature in his age), and A is university technical staff. B and M are at the age between 18 and 25. W, A, C, and I are at the age between 25 and 35. They come from various disciplines, including Computer Science (B), Architecture (W), Design (C, M, and I), and Medicine (A). Their cultural backgrounds are diverse with five participants influenced by Chinese cultures (Hong Kong, Mainland, Taiwan) and one participant from Nigeria. They all grew up in urban cities, with good exposure and accessibility to digital and mobile technologies.

4.2   Qualitative Findings

This study concentrates on qualitative data such as participants' bodily action and gestures during the tests, and their quotes, which reveal their thoughts and feelings, during the interviews. This section only summarizes a few major findings.

Turning the body

Most participants mostly turned their bodies together with the compass, though it was mentioned tiring. Actually, turning the body is an important act in the design of Swing Compass. It brings users an embodied meaning: one has to pay effort in order to discover other possibilities.

Discovering the turning feature

All participants discovered the turning feature very quickly.

Reasons behind a turn (impulsive desires and automatic appraisals)

Most of their reasons to turn include dissatisfaction and boredom of the available options. They turned in order for something new or different.

Immediate blends (and embodied imaginary concepts)

Participants spoke about what they recalled from the act of turning, revealing nuanced imaginary concepts of the action in their minds. Some quotes include:

… *"Turning around when I got stuck in a lecture, in order to find a solution. Turning the body, turning my mind."*… (B)

… *"Seeing it like a desk or table. I stop paying attention to those behind after a turn."*… (M)

… *"Exploring inside a bookstore. I might not look for something particular, or something similar instead. … Just to get a book as fast as possible. I became aware of something else."*… (W)

… *"It's like shopping! If you don't like the items in a shop, or you haven't seen those before, you turn away!"*… (C)

… *"It reminds me of attending seminar conference last week. Even though I found a presentation boring, I was hesitant whether to move to another concurrent panel. Just like I would not turn because the compass was heavy."*… (I)

… *"Waiting a bus for too long. Should I make an "extra" turn? Walking to the MTR (mass transit railway) station?"*… (A)

Contingent changes and extended appraisals

Participants tried to make sense of the varied options they were given, expressing their overall feelings. An example:

… *"It's like I hit the limit and need to relax."*…

… *"I don't like someone set limit on me."*… (W)

Metaphorical blends (and imagined narratives)

Participants tried to describe the compass, first literally and then metaphorically, showing their imagined scenarios of using it. Examples include:

… *"It helps people know about themselves. Sometimes it's difficult to choose. (Decidophobia?) Yes! Single option notifies you to turn, to think out of the box. Life is not only one way out."*…

… *"It's like at a crossroad. Sometimes you have to choose between options. Turn to explore, to get over obstacle."*…

... "Consult horoscope, even tarot cards. It might shed light, give a vision."...

... "(The Status Compass) is an inspiration for your life!"... (B)

... "(The App Launching Compass) reflects what I do, and then I reflect on it as I take its suggestion. ... like friends of similar taste. 'Hey you should check this out!', 'Last time you like Korean food, how about ...' It's mutual influence between friends."... (M)

... "It's like a companion, going with you everything. The suggestions might not necessary be the right one. It's no harm to listen. Just selective listening."...

... "It can be up-selling, like those in fitness center, about personal training."... (A)

5   Discussion

5.1   Reactive Moments

All six participants were able to "act out" the meaning of a turn. If they could not see their targets, or they found the options not interesting or boring, which is in fact an immediate appraisal on the offers, they had an impulsive desire to turn. The appraisals result in emotions (e.g., frustrated, confused, bored, hesitant, satisfied, grateful, appealed, etc.) and actions (e.g., turn vs. stay, change vs. accept). The sensorimotor feedback loop evoked varied slices of life in the participants, including contemplating a problem, working on stuff on a physical desktop, walking inside a bookstore or a shopping mall, choosing among concurrent presentations, and waiting for a bus. Since some participants (e.g., A and I) found turning with the compass rather tiring, the mental images provoked in their minds involved certain physical hurdles, which include getting out of a seminar room or walking away from a bus stop toward some uncertainties. One would not know if another presentation or transportation would be better or worse. This kind of dilemma was not obvious in the imaginations of other participants (e.g., walking inside a bookstore or a shopping mall). The immediate blends here tend to be divided into two kinds of decision-making, those you cannot revert versus those you can always come back.

5.2   Contingent Moments

Not all participants were fully aware of the compass's moderation logic. Participant B and M noticed the contingent changes that actually prompted a turn. Participant B imagined being at a crossroad with the interpretive frame of decidophobia invoked. On the other hand, Participant M invoked the interpretive frame of companion and thought of mutual influence between friends of similar taste. Both of them felt very positive (e.g., inspired, content, etc.) toward the compass after extended appraisals of the imagined narratives (being at a crossroad, influencing friends) resulted from metaphorical blends. Other participants (W, I, and A), though did not fully understand the patterns, they to a certain extent felt that the compass had an agenda. Participant W thought it set a limit like what a regulator does, which he/she disliked. Participant I saw a guide who made subtle advice just right. Participant A on one hand felt no harm listening to a companion's second opinion but uneasy facing a persuasive salesperson on the other. The interpretive frames they invoked seem to vary from full autonomy to advisory and persuasion, showing a continuum of power relations between users and agents.

6   Future Work

Based on a rigorous theoretical framework, we have been conducting user experience study of selected artifacts. The target number of participants for each artifact is 20. Now we have done six for Swing Compass, and promising initial results are summarized in this paper. As a reflective device, the compass generally disrupts a user's habitual engagement and might cause discomfort and confusion at the beginning. Yet, negative emotions can be an effective, though uneasy, trigger for behavior change through reflection and exposure of unconscious assumptions. We hope our continuing work will further enrich the evidence of imaginative and affective responses triggered by lively interactive artifacts.

Acknowledgments. We gratefully acknowledge the grant GRF from Hong Kong Research Grants Council (PolyU 5412/13H). Swing Compass was generated from another project funded by The Hong Kong Polytechnic University (A-PL94).

References

1. Chow, K.K.N.: Animation, embodiment, and digital media human experience of technological liveliness. Palgrave Macmillan, Basingstoke (2013)
2. Chow, K.K.N.: Sharing Imagination and Emotion Through the Use of Lively Interactive Products. In: Proceedings of 9th International Design and Emotion Conference (2014)
3. Fauconnier, G., Turner, M.: The way we think: conceptual blending and the mind's hidden complexities. Basic Books, New York (2002)
4. Fauconnier, G.: Conceptual Blending and Analogy. In: Gentner, D., Holyoak, K.J., Kokinov, B.N. (eds.) The Analogical Mind: Perspectives from Cognitive Science, pp. 255–285. MIT Press, Cambridge (2001)
5. Merleau-Ponty, M.: Phenomenology of perception. International library of philosophy and scientific method. Routledge & Kegan Paul, London (1962)
6. Maiese, M.: Embodiment, emotion, and cognition. New directions in philosophy and cognitive science. Palgrave Macmillan, Basingstoke (2011)
7. Russell, J.A.: Core Affect and the Psychological Construction of Emotion. Psychological Review 110(1), 145–172 (2003)
8. Monticelli, R.D.: The Feeling of Values: For a Phenomenological Theory of Affectivity. In: Bagnara, S., Smith, G.C. (eds.) Theories and Practice in Interaction Design, pp. 57–76. Lawrence Erlbaum, Interaction Design Institute Ivrea, Ivrea, Mahwah (2006)
9. Ekman, P.: An Argument for Basic Emotions. Cognition and Emotion 6(3), 169–200 (1992)
10. Ekman, P.: All Emotions Are Basic. In: Ekman, P., Davidson, R.J. (eds.) The Nature of Emotion: Fundamental Questions, pp. 15–19. Oxford University Press, Ltd., New York (1994)

11. Dourish, P.: Where the Action Is: The Foundations of Embedded Interaction. MIT Press, Cambridge (2001)
12. Sengers, P., et al.: Reflective Design. In: Proceedings of 4th Decennial Conference on Critical Computing (2005)
13. Fogg, B.J.: A Behavior Model for Persuasive Design. In: Proceedings of Persuasive 2009 (2009)
14. Harrell, D.F., Chow, K.K.N.: Generative Visual Renku: Poetic Multimedia Semantics with the GRIOT System. Hyperrhiz: New Media Cultures (Special Issue: Visionary Landscapes) (2009)
15. Chow, K.K.N., Harrell, D.F.: The Generative Visual Renku Project: Integrating Multimedia Semantics, Animation, and User-Interface Design. In: Proceedings of CHI 2010 (2010)
16. Harrell, D.F.: Phantasmal media: an approach to imagination, computation, and expression. MIT Press, Cambridge (2013)
17. Ryan, R.M., Deci, E.L.: On Happiness and Human Potentials: A Review of Research on Hedonic and Eudaimonic Well-Being. Annual Review of Psychology 52, 141–166 (2001)

Does Trigger Location Matter? The Influence of Localization and Motivation on the Persuasiveness of Mobile Purchase Recommendations

Frank Basten[1], Jaap Ham[1(✉)], Cees Midden[1], Luciano Gamberini[2], and Anna Spagnolli[2]

[1]Human-Technology Interaction Group, Eindhoven University of Technology, P.O. Box 513 – 5600 Eindhoven, The Netherlands
[2]Human Technology Lab, Department of General Psychology, University of Padova Via Venezia, 8 – 35131, Padova, Italy
ftwbasten@gmail.com, {j.r.c.Ham,c.j.h.midden}@tue.nl, {luciano.gamberini,anna.spagnolli}@unipd.it

Abstract. Thanks to the ubiquity of wireless network, location has become an easily available resource to exploit when sending purchase recommendations. We rely on Fogg's Behavior model (FBM; Fogg, 2009) and on previous research to study whether the appearance of such recommendations when the user spatially approaches a target item improves the recommendation persuasiveness. We created a virtual supermarket, where products images are displayed on posters and customers can scan products' QR codes with a tablet to buy them. The persuasiveness of triggers co-located or not with the target product was examined, in conditions of high vs. poor motivation to purchase that product. Confirming our hypotheses, triggers co-located with the target product lead to higher sales of that product. Furthermore, participants who received a co-located trigger that also contained a motivating message purchased more items than participants in other conditions. Therefore, setting triggers to appear at a specific location proximal to the target item can change behavior, especially for motivated subjects.

Keywords: Persuasive technology · Fogg behavior model · Triggers · Motivation · Location-based · Virtual supermarket

1   Introduction

Purchase recommendations represent a persuasive feature often exploited in e-commerce in order to orient the lay customers' decision process by both increasing the interest in a certain product and reducing the information overload due to examining a large offer of products [16]. Recommendations are generally based on preferences expressed by customers similar to the users, on the users' past choices or on the users' characteristics (respectively through collaborative filtering, content-based filtering and knowledge-based recommendation, [3]). Recommender systems have a large application in on-line shopping, but the advances in ubiquitous technology also

© Springer International Publishing Switzerland 2015
T. MacTavish and S. Basapur (Eds.): PERSUASIVE 2015, LNCS 9072, pp. 121–132, 2015.
DOI: 10.1007/978-3-319-20306-5_11

allow recommendations to be sent to the customers' mobile device when shopping in a physical store; once the user identifies a given item via barcode, QR code or RFID chip (e.g., [9]; [15]; [7]), recommendations can be generated and sent to his/her mobile device to affect subsequent actions.

Most research on recommendation systems focused on the algorithm that generates the recommendation [16], thus the research space for design issues related to the users' reception of the recommendation is still largely unexplored (althoug see: [17]; [18]. Persuasive technology has started investigating recommender systems to account for the factors that make recommendations effective (e.g., [2]; [8]; [11]). From a persuasive technology point of view, a recommendation provided by the system is supposed to work as an action trigger, that is, it must encourage the execution of a given action (Behavioral Model, [4]). In the case of shopping, a trigger can encourage the customers to purchase a given product or class of products. Triggers can simply remind customers of the availability of the product ("signals"), include some motivating cue ("spark") or provide some resource to simplify the purchase ("facilitator") 4].

Location is one resource that recommender systems can use to adapt the timing and content of the recommendation as well as to provide directions to the target ([1]. Location-aware recommender systems, in particular, can use the position of the user and of the target to send the trigger when the customer arrives at a certain location. Fogg [4] maintains that a trigger is successful under conditions of optimal localization: when it can be noticed, when it is associated with target behavior and when it presented at the right moment. Thus exploiting location information might improve the successfulness of the trigger.

Hühn and colleagues [6] provided a first empirical support for this claim; they tested in a virtual environment if a trigger located near the product (fit) compared with one located far from the product (misfit) influenced the purchase intention, finding that the localization fit of the trigger positively influenced buying intention. A study by Gröppel-Klein et al. [5] on the effect of in-store triggers on impulse buying behavior, however, found that a location fitted trigger increased sales, but this effect only held for some products. In their study, participants bought more milk when they received a location fitted trigger for a particular kind of milk in the store, but did not buy more chocolate when they received a location fitted trigger for a particular kind of chocolate. The reason for the different effectiveness of a trigger with different product types might be a different motivation for buying the product [4]. Therefore we decided to study the effect of triggers location on the purchase behavior and its interplay with motivation, which have never been studied in conjunction before to our knowledge.

To investigate the interaction of motivation and co-location, participants in our study were asked to do a simulated shopping task, during which they received action triggers to buy two different target products (a plain organic yoghurt and 'ziti', a type of pasta). In one condition the trigger was received near the target product (fit), and in another condition the trigger was received when the participants were far from the target product (misfit). The location fit/misfit per target item was counterbalanced within participants. In addition, one half of the participants received triggers with a motivating text (spark) while the other half received a trigger without a motivating component (signal).

The setting recreated in the laboratory was a virtual supermarket. Virtual supermarkets consist of posters showing items and prices (or coupons), allowing customers to buy products (or getting coupons) by scanning the QR code of the posted item via their smartphone or other mobile device. Such stores are found at metro stops in the US, South Korea, UK, Italy, the Netherlands and Spain (e.g., [13]) and represent an interesting and efficient case study for e-commerce and recommender systems.

In the following sections we will describe the hypotheses of the study, the study method and results, and will conclude with a discussion section.

1.1 Hypotheses

Previous research on location-based persuasive triggers suggests that the co-location of the trigger and the target item has a positive effect on sales. Hühn et al. [6] found an increase in buying intention when a trigger was presented close to the target product in a VR setting and Gröppel-Klein et al. [5] found this effect in a real shopping situation. Also, Fogg [4] claims that triggers will only succeed when given in the right context. Having the trigger co-located with the target item increases the opportunity [12] or the facilitating conditions [14] for performing the action of buying that product. Therefore, we expected participants who received a trigger co-located with the target item (fit) to buy more target items than the participants in the opposite condition (misfit).

H1: Participants who received the trigger when co-located with the target item (location fit) would purchase more target items than participants who received the trigger when distant from the target item (location misfit).

As mentioned before, according to Fogg [4] the effectiveness of persuasive technology (that employs triggers) is based on motivation, ability and the presence of a trigger. Therefore we expected that the number of people deciding to purchase a target product would increase when motivation was increased. In this experiment we used a spark (increased motivation) vs. signal (prompting message without motivational aspect) type of trigger to manipulate motivation. We also measured self-assessed motivation to purchase.

H2a: Participants who received a high motivation trigger (spark) would purchase more target items than participants who received the low motivation trigger (signal).

Finally, according to Fogg's behavior model [4], an 'activation threshold' needs to be surpassed before triggers can provoke actions but at the same time an action will not take place without a person being aware of an opportunity to act. Therefore we expected an interplay between motivation and trigger.

H3: Participants with high motivation and a co-located trigger are expected to purchase more and have higher buying intention compared to the three combined other conditions.

2 Method

2.1 Design and Participants

The study had a 2 (trigger localization: fit vs. misfit) X 2 (motivation: low vs. high) mixed design. Trigger localization was a within participants factor and motivation was a between participants factor. Each participant received two triggers with either high or low motivation texts. One of the triggers would appear close to a target product, the other far away from the target product. The trigger fit was counterbalanced between target products, so the design had a total of 4 conditions (Table 1).

We chose a sample of 61 participants to complete our experiment (G-power; effect size = 0.3, beta = 0.9 and alpha = 0.05). Ages ranged from 19 to 34 years ($M = 23.69$, $SD = 2.56$ years). The participants were randomly assigned to one of 4 conditions. Participants were recruited near the university campus in (city name anonymized for review) and received a 3€ compensation for their participation.

Table 1. Number of participants per conditions

		Participants		
		Women	Men	total
High motivation	Fit-Misfit	7	8	15
	Misfit-Fit	9	7	16
Low motivation	Fit-Misfit	8	7	15
	Misfit-Fit	8	7	15
		29	32	61

2.2 Setting

Virtual supermarket. The QR-shop consisted of four double-sided poster stands. The poster contained a title referring to a shop section (e.g., sauce) and three shelves with the images of two to four different products each, accompanied by their QR-code. Several types of food products were used: breakfast cereals, chocolates, pasta sauces, bread and pasta, pizza, dairy products and drinks. Stands were positioned so as to create a cross (Figure 1a) forcing the user to walk around all posters in order to access all items. This ensured that items in the misfit condition were not visible while triggered. The position of the target items is illustrated in Figure 1c.

Companion to the virtual supermarket was an on-line shop accessible from the participant's tablet. This on-line shop included information for each of the 56 different types of product displayed on the posters. Each product page offered a picture of the product (the same as on the poster), a description of the product and the option to buy the product (Figure 1b).

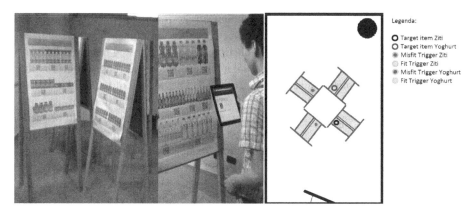

Fig. 1. a. The four two-sided poster stands of the virtual supermarket. **b.** One participant checking the product description on the on-line shop in front of a poster stand of the virtual supermarket. **c.** Map of the target items in the two-sided poster stands location in the virtual supermarket.

From the product page participants could either go back to the code acquisition page or the cart. No navigation from and to products was possible in the web shop; products could only be accessed by scanning the QR-codes on the poster. The number of products already in the cart could be adjusted at the participant's will.

Target products. The target products for which triggers were sent were two; a kind of pasta ('ziti') and an organic low fat yoghurt. The products were located in opposite sections of the QR-shop (Figure 1c).

Triggers. The trigger was a page appearing on the participants' tablet after scanning a specific product on his/her shopping list, which was positioned in a pre-defined location of the supermarket either close or far from the product refereed to in the trigger. The trigger page contained in vertical order: (a) The word 'Advertising' as a page title. (b) The name of the target product. (c) A text, which in the low motivation condition stated: 'Buy <name of target item>', while in the high motivation condition promised several health benefits of the item over comparable items plus a better taste. (d) A picture of the item, the same as in the poster. (e) A big button that read: "Click here to continue to the item you scanned" allowing to buy the product.

All text was in Italian. The whole setting was especially created for this study by using WordPress for the webstore with woocommerce plugin, a free online code generator to create QR codes, and Scan by Sca.Inc v. 1.5.3 for reading the codes. The tablet used in the study was an Apple iPad running Ios 7.1.2.

2.3   Procedure

After agreeing to participate, participants first received a short briefing and read the informed consent form. After signing the form, they were handed an instruction sheet and a shopping list containing 13 items (not the two target products) and entered the room with the virtual supermarket. As they finished reading the instructions, the researcher repeated explanations aloud and showed the functions of the web shop on the iPad (scanning, ordering the product and checking the content of the shopping cart) at least once per participant. These functions were executed by pointing the front camera of the iPad at a specific QR-code on a poster, which was then scanned by the QR-code scanning application running on the iPad. The display of the iPad then displayed the related on-line shop page. It was specified that multiple items of the same type could be put in the chart and that the number of items in the cart could be modified at will. Afterwards, the cart was emptied and the tablet handed to the participant, who was asked to scan one item, to order the products and to go back to scanning. This process continued until the participant could perform these tasks autonomously. Participants were told to knock on the lab door in case they had questions during the experiment, so the experiment leader could come in and answer (only a handful needed more info after the extensive instructions given). After the instruction phase, the experiment leader would leave the room.

The participants had to get all items on the list and seven more items to their own liking, which could be additional units of the items they already bought. While providing a specific shopping list allowed to administer the manipulation, the seven additional items freely chosen by the participant allowed to see if the triggers received affected his/her choices.

As the task was completed and the participant had the 13 + 7 items in the cart, s/he was asked to fill out the questionnaire. After the questionnaire, the participant was debriefed, given the compensation and thanked. No actual groceries were handed out to participants. Their shopping data was saved and sent to the server for later analysis.

The shopping task took an average of 8 minutes and 32 seconds and participants completed the survey in 5 to 10 minutes on average.

The procedure was described in details and approved by the Ethical Committee of the (anonymized institution name) hosting the study.

2.4   Data

The data collected consisted in the list of items bought by the participant, saved in the participant's cart and sent to the server, and in the answers to an *ad hoc* questionnaire. For this study, only manipulation check items of the questionnaire will be considered: one item ascertaining whether the participant did notice the trigger and having a yes/no answer format (i.e., 'Did you receive a pop-up message on [target product]?'); two statements checking whether the fit-misfit manipulation succeeded, to which participants could express their agreement on a Likert scale (i.e., 'The popup message related to [product] was shown at the proper time'; 'The popup message related to [product] was well positioned with respect to [product]'); and one item estimating the participant's motivation to buy the target product during the experiment (i.e., 'I felt motivated to buy [product]').

3   Results

3.1   Manipulation Check

Participants declared to have received a popup message on the product (95.1%). They also agreed that the message was shown at a proper time and was close to the target product more strongly in the fit condition (Table 2).

Table 2. Results of t-tests for independent samples comparing the responses to the questionnaire items in the fit and misfit conditions; 1 = means complete disagreement, 5 = complete agreement

		FIT	MISFIT			
		Mean (SD)	Mean (SD)	t	df	sig
The popup message related to [product] was shown at the proper time	yoghurt	3.32 (1.3)	2.72 (.84)	-2.071	58	.043
	ziti	3.25 (1.01)	2.61 (.96)	-2.490	55.68	.016
The popup message related to [product] was well positioned with respect to [product]	yoghurt	3.65 (1.0)	3 (1.1)	-2.351	56.78	.022
	ziti	3.36 (.68)	2.68 (1.01)	-2.995	57	.004

3.2   Effect of Motivation (Manipulated and Self-assessed) and Location-congruence

For our 2 x 2 mixed model design we preformed a MANOVA, with dependent variables (all distrubutions not deviating from normality) number of purchases for ziti, purchases for yogurt and combined sales (yogurt and ziti), independent variables location (fit vs. misfit) and motivation (high vs. low), and covariates self-assessed motivation.

In line with Hypothesis 1 about *location-congruence*, the MANOVA analysis indicated that participants who received the trigger close to the target product ($M = 0.541$, $sd = 0.765$) purchased the product more often than participants who received the trigger further away from the target product ($M = 0.1639$, $sd = 0.454$), $t(120) = 3.309$, $p = 0.001$. The hypothesis is also supported by the data of the separate target products. That is, more ziti was purchased in the location fit condition ($M = 0.53$, $sd = 0.819$) than in the misfit condition ($M = 0.10$, $sd = 0.301$), $t(59) = 2.780$ and $p = 0.007$ (Figure 3a). And, more yoghurt was purchased in the location fit condition ($M = 0.55$, $sd = 0.723$) than in the misfit condition ($M = 0.23$, $sd = 0.568$), as suggested by a marginally significant difference, $t(59) = 1.888$ and $p = 0.064$ (see Figure 3b).

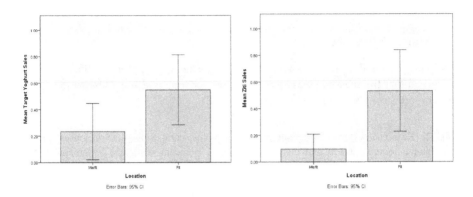

Fig. 3. a. Mean sales for Target yogurt split by trigger location fit. **b.** ,Mean sales for Target Pasta (ziti) split by trigger location fit.

As for the effect of *motivation*, we found no proof for Hypothesis 2a for the combined sales of both target products (yoghurt and ziti pasta): participants who received a motivating text did not purchase more target products than participants in the low motivation condition ($F < 1$).

We also assessed self-reported motivation to buy the product, although only after participants had bought the product. Therefore, this measure of motivation might certainly be influenced by response tendencies. Still, considering self-reported motivation to buy the product, results showed that participant's self-assessed motivation to buy a certain product (collected after the experimental session) had predictive value for the number of that target product a participant bought. In other words, participants self-assessed motivation to buy yoghurt showed a positive regression coefficient with the amount of target yoghurt bought, $B = 0.188$, $t = 2.964$, $p = 0.004$. Similarly, participants self-assessed motivation to buy ziti, showed a positive regression coefficient with the amount of ziti bought, $B = 0.233$, $t = 3.445$, $p = 0.001$.

Finally, using the MANOVA we found no proof for an *interaction* effect between the levels of motivation (spark vs. signal) in the trigger and trigger location (fit vs. misfit). However, in line with Fogg's behavior model (FBM; [4]), we expected to find a contrast effect when directly comparing the high motivation/ fit condition and all other positions. Confirming this expectation and in line with Hypothesis 3, a contrast analysis showed this contrast effect for the combined sales of target items (yogurt and ziti). That is, participants who received a location congruent and motivating trigger purchased more target items ($M = 0.63$, $sd = 0.85$) than in the other conditions ($M = 0.26$, $sd = 0.551$), $t(120) = 2.781$, $p = 0.006$ (see Figure 4).

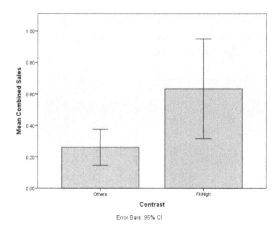

Fig. 4. Contrast effect fit/high vs. others on mean combined sales

This contrast effect was also found for the separate target items. That is, participants who received a location congruent, high motivation trigger for ziti purchased more ziti ($M = 0.60$, $sd = 0.91$) than others ($M = 0.22$, $sd = 0.52$), $t(59) = 2.042$, $p = 0.046$, and participants who received a location congruent, high motivation trigger for yoghurt purchased more target yoghurt ($M = 0.67$ with $sd = 0.82$) than others ($M = 0.30$ with $sd = 0.59$), as suggested by a marginally significant difference, $t(59) = 1.869$, $p = 0.067$.

Although of an exploratory nature, the contrast effect for high motivation plus well-located triggers vs. other conditions was also significant for self-assessed motivation. To analyze this contrast, we assigned participants who scored 4 and 5 on self-assessed motivation in a high self-assessed motivation group and those who scored 1-3 on self-assessed motivation to buy the target product in a low self-assessed motivation group. More ziti was purchased by participants who were highly motivated (self-assessed) and received a location congruent ($M = 1.00$, $sd = 0.926$) compared to participants in other conditions ($M = 0.09$, $sd = 0.288$), $t(58) = -5.884$, $p < 0.001$. Also, more yogurt was purchased by participants who were highly motivated (self-assessed) and received a location congruent trigger ($M = 1.00$, $sd = 0.866$) compared to participants in the combined other conditions ($M = 0.29$, $sd = 0.572$), $t(59) = 3.179$ $p = 0.002$.

3.3   Other Findings

For marketing purposes it is interesting to analyze whether effective triggers (that led to an increase of the sales of the target product) also led to a decrease of sales of other products in the same category. We observed that the increase in triggered product sales in the location-congruent condition was not at the expense of products in the *same* category but, rather, led to a decrease of sales of products of *different* categories. Figures 5a,b show the number of products of a same category as the one mentioned in the trigger that was bought in the fit vs. misfit condition. It can be observed that in the fit conditions, where the highest increase in sales of triggered products was found, there was no statistically significant decrease in selling similar products in the same category compared with the misfit condition.

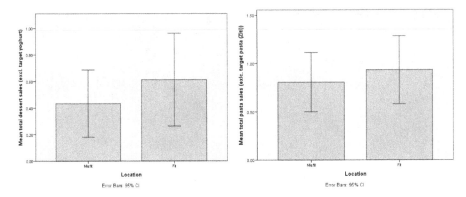

Fig. 5. a. Dessert sales exc. target item split by location fit of (natural) yoghurt trigger. **b.** Total sales for pasta per location.

4   Discussion and Conclusion

The current research investigated the effect of triggers location on the purchase behavior and its interplay with the motivation of the customer for buying a product. In a lab study, products were displayed in a virtual supermarket and persuasiveness of triggers co-located or not with the target item was examined, in conditions of high vs. poor motivation to purchase that item. In line with our first hypothesis, we found that participants who received the location congruent (fit) trigger purchased more target items than participants who received the location incongruent (misfit) trigger. This finding is in line the findings of Hühn et al.`s [6], who studied the effect of location congruency of a trigger on purchase intention. The present study, in addition, proved this effect on behavior, finding that participants who received the trigger near the item purchased the item more often than other participants.

The hypothesized combined effect of motivation and location-congruence (H3) was also found: participants who received a high motivation, location-congruent trigger bought more target items than participants in the other conditions. This finding is in line with the Fogg behavior model [4]. That model claims that increased motivation leads to a lowered action line, and a well located trigger should thereby lead to increased counts of target behavior when motivation is increased. Our results show an important interplay between trigger fit and consumer motivation: especially for highly motivated customers, trigger fit will lead to higher sales. This result might be crucial for application in real-store environments: triggers might be effective, but when people are interested. Curiously, this dependency of trigger effectiveness on motivation is even found when triggers are presented subliminally (studied in a completely different context, independent of localization by [9]), and might diminish worries about the usage of triggers that may arise from an ethical perspective: without inherent motivation, customers might not be influenced that easily.

Furthermore, independent of our manipulation of trigger location, the motivational text included in the trigger alone did not motivate participants enough to cause a difference in sales. Based on reactions of participants we argue that this is most likely because our participants might not have read it all the times, as is customary with pop-up messages and advertising in general. It is then even more interesting that the trigger worked, regardless of the ineffectiveness of the text, just because of its being contextually located with the target product, namely because it appeared while the user was close to the target product.

Although we asked questions to measure self-assessed motivation only after participants bought the products (allowing for response tendencies), results suggested that (self-assessed) motivation has a positive effect on purchase decisions. This finding is in line with [4], which claims that motivation is one of three key variables when it comes to decision-making.

For studies and applications of persuasive technology, our results suggest that emphasis on the context of a trigger is very important for effectiveness of persuasive designs. For e-commerce, they suggest hat investments in location-based persuasion/advertising can be very fruitful. Interestingly for a store manager, increase in one product sale will not necessarily be compensated by a decrease in the sale of other products of the same category, as one would intuitively expect.

4.1   Limits and Future Work

The main limit of this study is that it was carried out in a lab, and future research may investigate the generalizability to real shopping situations. Motivation is probably quite different under such conditions just as attention paid to the trigger, which might be covered by other cues and signals in a real grocery store. However, having selected the virtual grocery context as a setting for the study, the number of other in-store stimuli and the relevance of the digital trigger for a user already handling a smartphones to make the purchase might be higher than in traditional shops with real products and without QR-fed information.

Future research might also extend the current study to more diverse participants. Participants in the current study all had much experience with handheld digital devices such as the iPad used in the study. This might limit the generalization of the results to populations with a different age or a different level of familiarity with digital technologies. Message exposure and thereby influences on motivation might be different to an older or inexperienced population.

Future research might also take into account the shopping goals of a shopper. That is, for shoppers with the goal to buy a certain product, product-relevant triggers and trigger location may have different effects than for shoppers without that goal.

Finally, our findings show that context-relevant triggers can induce a target behavior, but are especially effective when participants were also motivated. Thereby finding a way of motivating a recipient of the trigger is the next important hurdle to successful persuasion with location based triggers. A strategy could be to personalize the trigger, which is quite easy if the purchase is made with a handheld QR device, which can keep track of the user's profile.

References

1. Bohnenberger, T., Jameson, A., Krüger, A., Butz, A.: Location-aware shopping assistance: Evaluation of a decision-theoretic approach. In: Paternó, F. (ed.) Mobile HCI 2002. LNCS, vol. 2411, pp. 155–169. Springer, Heidelberg (2002)
2. Felfernig, A., et al.: Persuasive recommendation: serial position effects in knowledge-based recommender systems. In: de Kort, Y.A.W., IJsselsteijn, W.A., Midden, C., Eggen, B., Fogg, B.J. (eds.) PERSUASIVE 2007. LNCS, vol. 4744, pp. 283–294. Springer, Heidelberg (2007)
3. Felfernig, A., Jeran, M., Ninaus, G., Reinfrank, F., Reiterer, S., Stettinger, M.: Basic approaches in recommendation systems. In: Recommendation Systems in Software Engineering, pp. 15–37. Springer, Berlin (2014)
4. Fogg, B.J.: A behavior model for persuasive design. In: Persuasive 2009; 4th International Conference on Persuasive Technology, Claremont, CA, USA, April 26-29 (2009)
5. Gröppel-Klein, A., Broeckelmann, P.: The influence of location-aware mobile marketing messages on consumers' buying behavior. In: Diamantopoulos, A., Fritz, W., Hildebrandt, L. (eds.) Quantitative Marketing and Marketing Management, pp. 353–377. Springer, Wiesbaden (2012)
6. Hühn, A.E., Khan, V.J., van Gisbergen, M., Ketelaar, P., Nuijten, K.: Mobile= location= effect. The effect of location on perceived intrusion of mobile. Esomar Publication Series C11, 315–322 (2011)
7. Kamei, K., Shinozawa, K., Ikeda, T., Utsumi, A., Miyashita, T., Hagita, N.: Recommendation from robots in a real-world retail shop. In: ICMI-MLMI 2010: International Conference on Multimodal Interfaces and the Workshop on Machine Learning for Multimodal Interaction. ACM, New York (2010)
8. Kaptein, M., Eckles, D.: Selecting effective means to any end: Futures and ethics of persuasion profiling. In: Ploug, T., Hasle, P., Oinas-Kukkonen, H. (eds.) PERSUASIVE 2010. LNCS, vol. 6137, pp. 82–93. Springer, Heidelberg (2010)
9. Karremans, J.C.T.M., Stroebe, W., Claus, J.: Beyond Vicary's fantasies: The impact of subliminal priming and brand choice. J of Exp. Soc. Psy. 42(6), 792–798 (2006)
10. Kowatsch, T., Maass, W.: In-store consumer behavior: How mobile recommendation agents influence usage intentions, product purchases, and store preferences. Computers in Human Behavior 26(4), 697–704 (2010)
11. Masthoff, J., Langrial, S., van Deemter, K.: Personalizing triggers for charity actions. In: Berkovsky, S., Freyne, J. (eds.) PERSUASIVE 2013. LNCS, vol. 7822, pp. 125–136. Springer, Heidelberg (2013)
12. Ölander, F., Thøgersen, J.: Understanding of consumer behavior as a prerequisite for environmental protection. Journal of Consumer Policy 18(4), 345–385 (1995)
13. Steadman, I.: Tesco brings 'virtual grocery stores' to the UK, Wired (August 7, 2012), http://www.wired.co.uk/news/archive/2012-08-07/tesco-virtual-store
14. Triandis, H.C.: Values, attitudes, and interpersonal behavior. In: Page, M.M. (ed.) Nebraska Symposium on Motivation, pp. 195–259. U. of Nebraska Press, Lincoln (1979)
15. van der Heijden, H.: Mobile decision support for in-store purchase decisions. Decision Support Systems 42(2), 656–663 (2006)
16. Xiao, B., Benbasat, I.: E-commerce product recommendation agents: use, characteristics, and impact. Mis Quarterly 31(1), 137–209 (2007)
17. Tintarev, N., Masthoff, J.: Evaluating the effectiveness of explanations for recommender systems. UMUAI 22, 399–439 (2012)
18. Pu, P., Chen, L., Hu, R.: Evaluating recommender systems from the user's perspective: survey of the state of the art. UMUAI 22, 317–355 (2012)

Understanding Communities

Adaptive Reminders for Safe Work

Matthias Hartwig[1](✉), Philipp Scholl[2], Vanessa Budde[1], and Armin Windel[1]

[1]Federal Institute for Occupational Safety and Health, Dortmund, Germany
[2]Technical University Darmstadt, Darmstadt, Germany

Abstract. In working context, new information and communication systems like head-mounted displays are often established to increase productivity. However, new technology can also potentially assist users to increase their health and well-being by encouraging safe behaviour, as they offer rich potential for persuasive elements and are highly adaptive to the respective situation. A setup is presented that evaluates the persuasive effect of a head mounted display-based assistance system on safe behaviour during a task in a laboratory simulation. In a randomised experimental design, the results show that the persuasive assistance system led to a significant and substantial reduction of safety violations compared to a traditionally designed warning sign. The findings suggest to design reminders not only according to ergonomic aspects, but also to consider persuasive effects on behavior. Furthermore, the results highlight the opportunities of mobile devices for assisting healthy behaviour in working environments.

Keywords: Head mounted display · Occupational safety · Laboratory safety · Assistance system · Persuasive technology · Anthropomorphic agent

1   Background

When it comes to new information and communication technology (ICT) used in working contexts, head mounted displays (HMD) have received a lot of attention during the last decades. Being able to display information not only independent of the position of the user, but also of the specific movement of the head, they can be used to present important information at the most relevant moment. As an additional advantage, they can be used hands-free, enabling the person to continue working with both hands while interacting with the display. A large body of literature deals with classical usability aspects of HMDs, such as visual devices and optical engineering (for a review, see [1]). More recent studies also evaluate ergonomic aspects under certain application fields [2].

In work context, new forms of technological assistance like head mounted displays are often introduced by companies to increase productivity. Little attention, however, is paid to the effects of modern assistance systems in working environments on employee safety. This is not adequate, since modern ICT offers an important potential in this area, which is especially true for systems oriented to the technological vision of ambient intelligence. This technology paradigm is based on the idea of "ubiquitous computing" [3]. The central features are context awareness, personalization, adaptive

© Springer International Publishing Switzerland 2015
T. MacTavish and S. Basapur (Eds.): PERSUASIVE 2015, LNCS 9072, pp. 135–140, 2015.
DOI: 10.1007/978-3-319-20306-5_12

behaviour and anticipation [4]. In working environment, ICT systems to support users with these adaptive capabilities are referred to as "adaptive work assisting systems" [5], a concept that explicitly considers not only the effect on efficiency, but also on work safety.

Computer interfaces, purposely designed to have an impact on the attitude and/or the behaviour of users can be subsumed under the term persuasive technology [6]. While there are numerous possible applications of persuasive technologies in private sector like e-commerce, environmental protection or private healthcare, there are only few approaches on how persuasive technology can be applied in the working environment for occupational safety [7], for exceptions see [8,9].

When it comes to computer-generated persuasive reminders, it is still a matter of discussion whether their outward appearance is critical for the impact on behaviour. [10] were able to show that users involuntarily attribute human characteristics to computer interfaces with human-like appearances. Therefore, computers can provide similar social cues as other humans do. If this implies similar effects and action mechanisms as in social persuasion, is subject of an on-going debate (for examples see [11]). In a predecessor study on static work assistance systems [12], an anthropomorphic agent presented on a static monitor was proved to be effective to facilitate safe behaviour within an electric working task, operationalised as the adequate use of isolating gloves.

One of the more dangerous working environment areas is work in chemical and biological laboratories. Work in these laboratories is often complex and involves materials which can be hazardous. Safe working with such materials therefore often requires a certain appropriate behaviour like usage of protective equipment or adequate stowage of the materials. However, during the often complex procedures and strict timeframes of laboratory tasks, there is a risk of neglecting these safe behaviours. Therefore, work in laboratories might benefit from computer-generated reminders on the right safety behaviour. A laboratory is also a working environment that often includes multiple working stations and movement between them. Therefore, an assistance system based on reminders to facilitate safe behaviour should not be static, since the user might not perceive the feedback in the crucial moment while currently working at a different physical space. Applying these elements, a mobile work assistance system based on persuasive reminders by an avatar was developed and tested in an experimental setup to evaluate its persuasive impact on safe behaviour. In addition, subjective attitudes towards the safety behaviour were measured to gain insight into the psychological mechanisms that lead to the respective behaviour change.

2   Method and Experimental Setup

The test setup was modelled on a typical chemical laboratory workplace containing the necessary equipment for the task, as shown in Fig. 1 (right). At the start of each simulation, all participants were given detailed standardised instructions on using the HMD (Google Glass), which provided a step by step protocol for the main task. After that, participants were instructed to manually extract DNA from two different vegetables (an onion and a tomato) and to make it optically visible. Doing this required a fixed sequence of classic basic laboratory working steps like blending and separating liquids in different laboratory vessels and heating or cooling the substances, none of which required any special training.

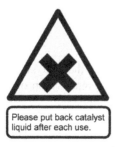 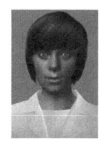 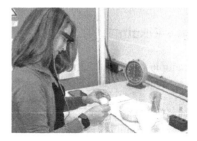

Fig. 1. Warning sign (left), anthropomorphic virtual agent (middle), experimental setup (right)

To include the safety aspect, the participants were informed that to facilitate the chemical reaction, a catalyst liquid has to be added to the chemical solution at eight certain working steps. The liquid was introduced as chemically irritant (which was in fact not the case), and leaving the bottle open over a period of time at room temperature might lead to evaporation which could irritate eyes, skin, and mucous membranes. Therefore, safe use of the catalyst liquid included closing the bottle and storing it in the correct marked box, which in turn had to be placed in a certain spot in a freezer after each use. The freezer was positioned approximately five meters away from the main working area. This additional distance, the burdensome design of the bottle box and the hard to reach shelf of the box in the freezer made the appropriate stowage of the liquid purposely inconvenient and time consuming, slowing down the participants and disrupting the workflow. This way, a conflict was created between smooth and fast working procedure and supposedly safe behaviour. The participants therefore had to choose between fulfilling the working task as fast and easy as possible, or following the safety instructions, as this is often an issue when it comes to the violation of safe behaviour in real working conditions.

The participants were randomly assigned into one of two experimental groups. In the control group, the participants were reminded of the safe storage by a classically styled warning sign (Fig. 1, left), positioned at the main working desk. As this is common practice in laboratory to facilitate safe behaviour, this group was designed to simulate the established standard of workplace safety measures. In the other experimental group, the participants were reminded of the safe liquid stowage by a persuasive designed reminder presented on Google Glass as a mobile work assistance system. To make sure they receive the reminder at the very moment the safe behaviour is relevant, it was scripted to appear 10 sec. after the user reached the respective working step instruction mentioning the catalyst liquid. Concerning its optical appearance, a female virtual agent (Fig. 1, middle) was used, which has been used as a persuasive interactive feature in a former study [11]. The picture of the female anthropomorphic avatar was shown for 5 sec. and accompanied by a short text message

(„please put back catalyst liquid after each use"). The reminders were accompanied by a very short bell sound, to make sure that they were recognized. In order to explore possible mechanisms of persuasion, the participants were asked after the simulation to rate their subjective necessity of the safe behaviour as well as the subjective hindrance by it on a 5 point Likert scale.

3   Results

A sample of 58 participants (43 male, 15 female) were included in the analysis and their mean age was 28.69 (SD = 8.79). All subjects received a compensation of 10 Euro (~12,45 USD) for participating. The average time for task completion was ~ 45 minutes. Table 1 shows the correlations of all experimental variables. There is a significant correlation between experimental group and safety violations and a significant negative correlation between perceived necessity and hindrance of the safety behaviour.

Table 1. Correlations of all experimental variables

	Gender	Experimental group	Time pressure	Necessity for safe behaviour	Hindrance of safe behaviour	Number of violations
Age	.152	.114	.064	.016	.073	.017
Gender		-.019	.040	-.038	-.038	-.162
Group			.080	-.186	-.023	-.273
Time pressure				.041	.229	.143
Necessity for safe behaviour					-.408**	-.015
Hindrance of safe behaviour						.023

**Correlation is significant at the 0.01 level (2-tailed)
*Correlation is significant at the 0.05 level (2-tailed)

Main research question of the study was to evaluate the persuasiveness of the mobile assistance system to encourage safe behaviour. A T-test was therefore conducted to compare the average number of safety violations in the two experimental groups. The differences are highlighted in Figure **2**. On average, the participants in the control group with the static standard safety sign committed 2.00 (SD = 2.67) of eight possible safety violations. The participants in the second group with the mobile emotional reminder committed an average of 0.71 (SD = 1.84) violations. A T-test for independent samples revealed a significant difference between the two groups ($t(52)$ = 2.15, $p < 0.05$). To explore possible psychological routes of persuasion, further T-tests compared the average ratings between the two experimental groups concerning subjective necessity and hindrance of safe behaviour. Participants in the control group rated the subjective necessity for safe storage on average 4.03 (1 = not necessary at all, 5 = very necessary, SD = 0.93). Participants in the persuasion group rated an average of 3.68 (SD = 0.98). No significant differences were found between the groups after comparing them via T-test ($t(56)$= 1.41, p > 0.05). Concerning the subjective hindrance of safe behaviour, no significant difference was found between the control group (M = 2.77, SD = 1.14) and the persuasion group (M = 2.71, SD = 1.21) via T-test $(t(56) = 0.17, p > 0.05)$.

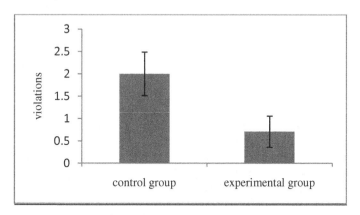

Fig. 2. Mean and standard error of the mean of safety violations in the two experimental groups

4   Discussion

The results of this study concerning the safety violations indicate a significant and substantial impact of the persuasive assistant system on behaviour of the participants. Compared to the traditionally designed warning sign, participants reminded by the persuasive agent committed only one third of the violations. This indicates a causal persuasive effect between the optical appearance of the safety reminder and safety behaviour. At the moment, the design of safety signs is often limited to classic ergonomic aspects like comprehensibility and perceptibility, completely neglecting the possible persuasive impact of design. For workplace design, the results strongly suggest to take the appearance of safety signs from a persuasive perspective into account. The same conclusion applies to the use of new technology devices in working environments. The results also highlight the possibilities of mobile work equipment like HMD for persuasive intentions because the user can be influenced at the most critical moment regardless of their current position. Therefore, when developing and introducing new technical systems for workplace applications, one should not only focus on using new technology to increase an efficient work processes, but also consider persuasive aspects, for example in increasing safety and health of working individuals. However, the results of the current study cannot differentiate between these two factors. The difference between the groups could be the result of the optical appearance, the adaptive timing or a combination of the two. An Interaction effect between shape and timing might also be a relevant factor.

This experiment did not show any evidence for the mechanism how the participants were influenced by the persuasive reminder, as no difference in the perception of the safety behaviour between the groups was shown. Therefore, it will be subject of a follow up study to determine which attitude alteration leads to the changed behaviour. A third limitation of the study concerns the temporal stability of the persuasion. Participants in the persuasion group worked about 45 minutes and were reminded 8 times during the task. A longer working time with the reminder might either lead to habituation and a decreasing persuasive effect, or to a permanent behavioural change that does not need continual reminders at all. Therefore, an upcoming study will also evaluate the temporal stability of the persuasion.

References

1. Rolland, J.P., Thompson, K.P., Urey, H., Thomas, M.: See-Through Head Worn Display (HWD) Architectures. In: Chen, J., Cranton, W., Fihn, M. (eds.) Handbook of Visual Display Technology. LNCS, pp. 2145–2170. Springer, Heidelberg (2006)
2. Theis, S., Alexander, T., Mayer, M.p., Wille, M.: Considering ergonomic aspects of head-mounted displays for applications in industrial manufacturing. In: Duffy, V.G. (ed.) HCII 2013 and DHM 2013, Part II. LNCS, vol. 8026, pp. 282–291. Springer, Heidelberg (2013)
3. Weiser, M.: The Computer for the 21st Century. Scientific American 265, 66–75 (1991)
4. Aarts, E.H.L., Harwig, H., Schuurmans, M.: Ambient Intelligence. In: Denning, J. (ed.) The Invisible Future, pp. 235–250. McGraw Hill, New York (2001)
5. Windel, A., Hartwig, M.: New Forms of Work Assistance by Ambient Intelligence. In: Paternò, F., de Ruyter, B., Markopoulos, P., Santoro, C., van Loenen, E., Luyten, K. (eds.) AmI 2012. LNCS, vol. 7683, pp. 348–355. Springer, Heidelberg (2012)
6. Fogg, B.J.: Persuasive Technology: Using Computers to Change What We Think and Do. Morgan Kaufmann, San Francisco (2003)
7. Hamari, J., Koivisto, J., Pakkanen, T.: Do Persuasive Technologies Persuade? - A Review of Empirical Studies. In: Spagnolli, A., Chittaro, L., Gamberini, L. (eds.) PERSUASIVE 2014. LNCS, vol. 8462, pp. 118–136. Springer, Heidelberg (2014)
8. De Boer, J., Teeuw, W.B., Heylen, D.K.J.: Applying the Behaviour Grid for Improving Safety in Industrial Environments. In: Berkovsky, S., Freyne, J. (eds.) CEUR Workshop Proceedings, p. 6. CEUR, Sydney (2013)
9. Zhang-Kennedy, L.: Persuading Secure User Behaviour at ork. In: 9th International Conference, PERSUASIVE 2014, Padua, Italy, pp. 127–129 (2014)
10. Reeves, B., Nass, C.: The Media Equation: how people treat computers, television, and new media like real people and places. University Press, Cambridge (1996)
11. Schulman, D., Bickmore, T.: Persuading users through counseling dialogue with a conversational agent. In: Persuasive 2009 Proceedings of the 4th International Conference on Persuasive Technology. ACM, New York (2009)
12. Hartwig, M., Windel, A.: Safety and Health at Work through Persuasive Assistance Systems. In: Duffy, V.G. (ed.) HCII 2013 and DHM 2013, Part II. LNCS, vol. 8026, pp. 40–49. Springer, Heidelberg (2013)

"For Your Safety"

Effects of Camera Surveillance on Safety Impressions, Situation Construal and Attributed Intent

Thomas J.L. Van Rompay[✉], Peter W. De Vries, and Manon T. Damink

Faculty of Behavioural, Management and Social sciences, University of Twente,
P.O. Box 217, 7500 AE Enschede, The Netherlands
t.j.l.vanrompay@utwente.nl, p.w.devries@utwente.nl,
m.t.damink@student.utwente.nl

Abstract. Based on the assumption that monitoring technology in environmental settings impacts people's state of mind and subsequent perceptions, the current study examines the influence of security camera's on safety perceptions and citizen wellbeing. Participants watched a video of city streets that featured (versus not featured) security cameras. In the camera condition, their safety ratings were significantly higher than in the camera-less (control) condition. In addition, the camera condition caused more positive ("safe") interpretations of an ambiguous situation than the control condition. Finally, results suggest that attributed intent underlying camera usage is a key construct to reckon with when considering camera placement. In discussing these findings, the conditions under which camera surveillance contributes to citizen wellbeing are elaborated on.

Keywords: Security cameras · Safety perceptions · Environmental design · Perceived intent

1 Introduction

In many western societies, closed-circuit television (CCTV) or video surveillance has become a fact of life. Many societies aim to safeguard their citizens against evildoers by installing watchful eyes, and probably none more so than the UK. According to BBC Newsnight television program, the City of London (London's financial district) has a total number of cameras of 619, on a population of about 9 000 – almost 69 cameras per 1000 inhabitants. Many other European countries appear to be following suit. Although accurate estimations are largely missing, the omnipresence of security cameras at airports, in bus and train stations, large shops, malls, offices, industrial areas, etc., are an indication that 'big brother' is closely watching over its citizens.

The dominant goal of video surveillance is the prevention of crimes and misdemeanors such as burglary, theft, pickpocketing, intimidation, violence, and vandalism, and, thus, maintaining an environment in which citizens feel safe and sound. There are various indications in literature, however, suggesting that the mere presence of

© Springer International Publishing Switzerland 2015
T. MacTavish and S. Basapur (Eds.): PERSUASIVE 2015, LNCS 9072, pp. 141–146, 2015.
DOI: 10.1007/978-3-319-20306-5_13

cameras has additional psychological effects on citizens, which usually receive limited attention by policy makers and law enforcers. For instance, in lab studies camera presence has been shown to promote prosocial behaviors [e.g., Van Rompay, Vonk, & Fransen] as the resultant of people's need for approval in front of an 'audience' [e.g., Latané, 1981; Leary & Kowalski, 1990]. Additionally, cameras may elicit suspicion (*Why am I being watched?*) and trigger 'acting out' behaviors (e.g., hooligans acting out in front of cameras, suggestive of defiance and rebellion). In other words, how people react to camera placement seems to vary depending on contextual influences such as the type of setting and people's attributions of intent.

By consequence, the conditions under which cameras actually induce feelings of safety are likewise debated. Whereas some have found that CCTV increases feelings of safety [Gill & Spriggs, 2005], others have argued that this applies only to those among the public who already feel safe [Ditton, 2000]. In line with such an argument, cameras could also make people more aware of safety threats, especially those already ill at ease or suspicious, and may therefore negatively influence safety perceptions [Gill & Spriggs, 2005]. Inspired by this controversy, the current research aims to shed light on the influence of CCTV camera presence (in a Dutch city center) on feelings of safety and environmental perceptions. In addition, it seeks to explore the role of attributed intent as a potential mediator of effects of camera surveillance on safety impressions.

1.1   Environmental Design and Perception

In addition to research highlighting social feelings and interpersonal consequences of camera surveillance (e.g., helping behavior; Van Rompay et al., 2009), another line of research that is highly relevant to current undertaking concerns priming research in social psychology [Aarts & Dijksterhuis, 2003; Aarts, Dijksterhuis, & De Vries, 2001; Kay, Wheeler, Bargh, & Rossa, 2004]. For instance, Kay et al. [2004] showed that people who had been exposed to objects common to the domain of business (e.g., fountain pens, conference tables and brief cases) tended to interpret ambiguous social situations as more competitive in nature than those who had not been exposed to such stimuli. Similarly, primed individuals also behaved more competitive by keeping more money to themselves in a so-called 'ultimatum game'. Apparently, exposing people to objects associated with specific norms or values (e.g., self-interest, competition) may cause people to behave in line with such context-specific norms.

Along a similar line of reasoning, Aarts and Dijksterhuis [2003] showed that exposure to pictures of library environments (in which silence or keeping one's voice down so as not to disturb other is considered appropriate) made participants talk less loud, again showing that people tend to behave in line with associations tied to objects. These results show that objects in an environment may steer an individual's perceptions and behaviors in line with meanings associated with these stimuli. However, as hinted at, it is an open question whether cameras foremost evoke safety perceptions or whether they rather induce perceptions and feelings related to vandalism and related transgressions. In the latter case, cameras would rather elicit negative affect and feelings of unease.

Arguably, which of these two routes prevails also depends on people's attributions; perceiving camera surveillance as a sign of care and genuine concern for civilian safety arguably triggers a qualitatively different experience than framing camera presence as a sign of distrust towards citizens and 'big brother'-like control. The study presented in the next section was designed to address these research questions.

2   Method

2.1   Participants and Design

Seventy-six students of two Dutch universities took part in this study; 52 participants were female, and 24 were male (Mean age: 22 years). The study employed a one-factor, between-participants design. The independent variable "Camera presence" consisted of two levels, present versus absent (control).

2.2   Procedure

Participants entered the lab and were told that they would evaluate a city environment based on video footage presented on a LCD screen. They were randomly assigned to one of the two conditions. In the Camera present condition they were shown video footage recorded while walking through the streets of a small local city. The footage comprised streets in the city center, the shopping area, and several alleys (all outdoor settings). All of these streets had CCTV cameras installed. In the Camera absent (control) condition, participants were shown the same footage, but this time all frames in which CCTV cameras were visible were removed. This was done to create two identical videos, the only difference between them being the visibility of cameras. Afterwards, participants filled out a questionnaire comprising the dependent measures.

2.3   Dependent Measures

Affective evaluation of environment. In order to measure participants' overall affective evaluation of the environment, they indicated on 5-point rating scales the extent to which they considered the environment depicted in the video safe, agreeable, cozy, warm and orderly (alpha = .68).
Interpretation of ambiguous situation. In order to test the presumed effect of camera surveillance on participants' interpretation of an ambiguous situation, participants provided a story-script to a scene involving an encounter between a man and woman in a foggy setting (see Figure 1). Subsequently, participants' responses were categorized into four categories ranging from 'very negative' to 'positive' by three independent coders (Cohen's kappa's > .72).
Attributed intent. In order to measure participants' 'attributed intent' underlying camera placement, they indicated to what extent they agreed with the statements 'policy makers have a keen eye for things going on here' and 'policy makers have taken adequate measures to make these streets safe' (r = .55).

Familiarity with city streets. In order to control for feelings of familiarity (covariate), participants indicated (yes/no response) whether they were familiar with the city streets depicted.

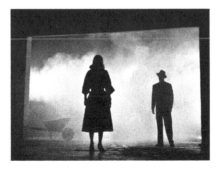

Fig. 1. Ambiguous situation portrayal

3   Results

A univariate analysis of variance with camera presence as independent variable, affective evaluation of the environment as dependent variable, and familiarity with city streets as covariate, revealed a significant effect of camera presence; $F (1,73) = 4.43$, $p < .05$, showing that participants in the video surveillance condition entertained a more positive affective evaluation of the city center (M = 2.50, SD = .68) compared to participants in the no-camera, control condition (M = 2.22, SD = .43).

In line with these findings, the same analysis, but this time with 'interpretation of ambiguous situation' as dependent variable, showed that participants in the camera condition framed the ambiguous scene in more positive terms compared to the control condition (F $(1,73) = 5.03$, p < .05). To illustrate, participants in the camera surveillance condition were more likely to provide positive, or affectively neutral, evaluations of the depicted scene (e.g., "A man and a woman have taken a walk at night and have come across an industrial workplace", "A man and a woman have a rendezvous in a stable on a foggy evening") compared to the no-camera condition (e.g., "A young woman is being chased by a perpetrator", "There has been an explosion and a man and woman are watching events unfold from a distance").

Finally, a significant effect emerged on 'attributed intent' (F $(1,73) = 33.66$, $p <$ .001), showing that participants in the video surveillance condition were much more likely to infer that law enforcers in the city act on behalf of citizen safety (M = 3.68, SD = .52) compared to participants in the no-camera condition (M = 2.65, SD = .95).

In order to test whether camera presence positively impacts participants' affective evaluation of the environment *because* it is interpreted as a sign of good intent, mediation analyses (Baron & Kenny, 1986) were conducted. In addition to the already established effect of camera surveillance on participants' affective evaluation of the environment, regression analyses also revealed a significant effect of the mediator (attributed intent) on the dependent variable (affective evaluation of the environment; $\beta = .55$, t $(73) = 5.63$, $p <$ .001. For mediation to apply, the effect of the independent variable (camera surveillance) should become non-significant, whereas the mediator should remain significant, when both are entered simultaneously in the regression analysis as predictors of the dependent variable 'affective evaluation of the environment'. The respective regression analysis showed this to be the case; the effect of camera presence was no longer significant; $\beta = .10$, t (73) = .84, $p = .40$, whereas the effect of the mediator (attributed intent) remained significant; $\beta = .60$, t (73) = 5.13, $p < .001$.

Hence, camera surveillance positively affects the affective evaluation of the environment because it is perceived as a sign of positive, well-meant intent.

4   Conclusions and Discussion

These combined findings underscore the potential of camera surveillance to positively impact citizens' affective experience comprising safety feelings and feelings of being 'at ease'. In line with these impressions (generated by camera presence), participants framed an ambiguous interaction in more positive terms compared to those in the no-camera condition. This finding indicates that effects of camera presence extend beyond mere perceptions and may also impact social evaluations and related behaviors. Hence, in follow-up research, it would be interesting to study whether effects of camera presence also transpire in actual behaviors. For instance, if camera presence enacts more positive social evaluations, does this also transpire in a more open, forthcoming attitude towards strangers, and thus perhaps in heightened willingness to initiate, for instance, small talk?

Importantly, the results presented also underscore the importance of people's inferences with respect to camera presence. That is, in the current study, camera presence elicited positive inferences reflecting law enforcers and policy makers (e.g., *"They know what is going on, they know what they are doing, and they do it with citizen safety in mind"*). Arguably, such inferences came natural in the context central to current undertaking (i.e., city streets). An interesting question to be addressed by follow-up research is what would happen in situations wherein the rationale for camera presence is less obvious (e.g., in indoor environments such as retail centers or town halls, or in public parks). That is, when and where is camera presence framed as a sign of distrust or control rather than an outcome of genuine concern for citizen safety?

To address these and related questions, different types of environments (varying in the extent to which camera presence therein is perceived as natural) could be pitted against each other. Alternatively, framing of camera presence could be varied within one and the same environment. For instance, accompanying camera presence we may sometimes find video surveillance signs stating *"For your safety"*, *"Warning, video surveillance in progress"*, or *"Smile, you are being videotaped"*. How do such different messages varying in verbal aggressiveness ("Warning!"), indication of genuine concern ("For your safety"), or humor ("Smile...") guide inference making and behavior? Insights in effects of contextual variables (e.g., type of environment) and framing of camera presence may very well make the difference between a suspicious, irritation-prone, anti-social civilian and a citizen feeling at ease, cared for, and open towards others. Ideally, such effects should be tested in a real-world setting in cooperation with policy makers.

Finally, in terms of intra-psychological processes, research indicates that watchful eyes make one more self-aware: *The mechanism underlying the effect of the presence of others is a process in which the person becomes aware of the reception of his image as an object by another. This awareness causes the person's attention to be focused upon the self* (Wicklund & Duval, 1971, p. 322). In some cases, this may inspire prosocial behavior (e.g., Van Rompay et al., 2009). However, in other cases this may also inspire 'acting out' and less positive impression management behaviors (e.g., hooligans showing off their toughness in front of cameras). Clearly the conditions under which such effects occur should be further pinpointed in follow-up research in field studies in which actual behaviors can be observed.

References

1. Aarts, H., Dijksterhuis, A.: The silence of the library: Environment, situational norm, and social behavior. Journal of Personality and Social Psychology 84(1), 18–28 (2003)
2. Aarts, H., Dijksterhuis, A., De Vries, P.: On the psychology of drinking: Being thirsty and perceptually ready. British Journal of Psychology 92(4), 631–642 (2001)
3. Baron, R.M., Kenny, D.A.: The moderator-mediator variable distinction in social psychological research: Conceptual, strategic, and statistical considerations. Journal of Personality and Social Psychology 51(6), 1173–1182 (1986)
4. BBC (2009), http://news.bbc.co.uk/2/hi/uk/8159141.stm
5. Ditton, J.: Crime and the city: Public attitudes to CCTV in Glasgow. British Journal of Criminology 40, 692–709 (2002)
6. Gill, M., Spriggs, A.: Assessing the impact of CCTV. Home Office Research Study 292. Her Majesty's Stationary Office, London (2005)
7. Kay, A.C., Wheeler, S.C., Bargh, J.A., Rossa, L.: Material priming: The influence of mundane physical objects on situational construal and competitive behavioral choice. Organizational Behavior and Human Decision Processes 95(1), 83–96 (2004)
8. Latané, B.: The psychology of social Impact. American Psychologist 36(4), 343–356 (1981)
9. Leary, M.R., Kowalski, R.M.: Impression management: A literature review and two-component model. Psychological Bulletin 107(1), 34–47 (1990)
10. Van Rompay, T.J.L., Vonk, D.J., Fransen, M.L.: The eye of the camera: Effects of security cameras on prosocial behavior. Environment and Behavior 41(1), 60–74 (2009)
11. Wicklund, R.A., Duval, S.: Opinion change and performance facilitation as a result of objective self-awareness. Journal of Experimental Social Psychology 7(3), 319–342 (1971)

Gender, Age, and Responsiveness to Cialdini's Persuasion Strategies

Rita Orji[✉], Regan L. Mandryk, and Julita Vassileva

Computer Science Department,
University of Saskatchewan,
Saskatoon, SK. S7N 5C9, Canada
rita.orji@usask.ca, {regan,jiv}@cs.usask.ca

Abstract. Research has shown that there are differences in how males and females respond to persuasive attempts. This paper examines the persuasiveness of the six persuasive strategies - *Reciprocity, Scarcity, Authority, Commitment* and *Consistency, Consensus* and *Liking* developed by Cialdini with respect to age and gender. The results of the large-scale study (N = 1108) show that males and females differ significantly in their responsiveness to the strategies. Overall, females are more responsive to most of the strategies than males and some strategies are more suitable for persuading one gender than the other. The results of our study also reveal some differences between younger adults and adults with respect to the persuasiveness of the strategies. Finally, the results show that irrespective of gender and age, there are significant differences between the strategies regarding their perceived persuasiveness overall, shedding light on the comparative effectiveness of the strategies.

Keywords: Persuasive technology · Behavior change · Gender · Age · Persuasive strategies · Persuasiveness · Individual differences · Susceptibility

1 Introduction

Persuasive Technology (PT) is a term used to define a class of technologies that are intentionally designed to change people's attitude or behavior [1] using various strategies. In the last few decades, the attention of PT researchers has focused on developing technologies and strategies to influence people's behaviors. As a result, several persuasive strategies have been developed that could be employed to motivate desired behavior change [1–3]. However, people differ in how they are motivated; a strategy that motivates one type of person to change her behavior may actually deter behavior change for another type of person [4, 5]. It is only recently that researchers have started to investigate how various users' characteristics and individual differences mediate the persuasiveness of the strategies and hence the need to tailor the strategies to increase their effectiveness [4–7].

In choosing approaches for group-based tailoring, research has shown that gender is a reliable characteristic [8]. Research has also established gender and age differences in many areas including the perception of different behavioral determinants [9],

© Springer International Publishing Switzerland 2015
T. MacTavish and S. Basapur (Eds.): PERSUASIVE 2015, LNCS 9072, pp. 147–159, 2015.
DOI: 10.1007/978-3-319-20306-5_14

gameplay, and health behavior [5, 10]. However, the effect of gender and age on the persuasiveness of the six strategies highlighted by Cialdini [3] have not been explored quantitatively.

In this paper, we investigate how the responsiveness to Cialdini's six persuasive strategies varies by gender and by age group (younger adults and adults). To achieve this, we conduct a large-scale study involving 1108 participants where we investigated the perceived persuasiveness of the six strategies - *Reciprocity, Scarcity, Authority, Commitment and Consistency, Consensus and Liking* – developed by Cialdini [3]. We adopted the Susceptibility to Persuasion Scale (STPS) developed by Kaptein et al. [4]. The results of our study show that males and females differ significantly in persuadability – with females being more responsive to most of the strategies. The results also reveal some significant differences between the age groups. Finally, the study provides a quantitative validation of the persuasiveness of the strategies overall. Irrespective of gender and age groups, there was significant variability in the perceived persuasiveness of the six strategies.

Our three main contributions are: first, we conducted a large-scale quantitative study to validate the six persuasive strategies developed by Cialdini. Second, we established that there are gender differences in the perceived persuasiveness of the strategies. Third, we show that age influences the persuasiveness the strategies.

2   Background

Persuasive strategies are techniques that can be employed in PTs to motivate behavior and/or attitude change. Over the years, a number of strategies for persuading people to perform the desired behavior have been developed. For example, Fogg [1] developed seven persuasive tools, and Oinas-Kukkonen [2] built on Fogg's strategies to develop 28 persuasive system design principles.

The six persuasive strategies developed by Cialdini – *Reciprocity, Scarcity, Authority, Commitment and Consistency, Consensus and Liking* – are among the oldest and most widely employed strategies [3]. The six strategies are:

1. **Reciprocity:** People by their nature feel obliged to return a favor and to pay back others. Thus when a persuasive request is made by a person the receiver feels indebted to, the receiver is more inclined to adhere to the request [11].
2. **Scarcity:** People tend to place more value on things that are in short supply. This is due to the popular belief that less available options are of higher quality.
3. **Authority:** People defer to experts [3]. Therefore, individuals are more likely to comply with a request when it is made by a person or people they perceived as possessing high levels of knowledge, wisdom, or power [12].
4. **Commitment and Consistency**: People by their nature strive to be consistent with previous or reported behavior to avoid cognitive dissonance.
5. **Liking:** People can be easily influenced or persuaded by someone they like. Factors such as: similarity, praise, and attractiveness can reliably increase the effectiveness of the liking strategy [3].
6. **Consensus:** We often observe the behaviors of others to help us make decisions. This is because "a large majority of individuals are imitators rather than initiators,

and therefore make decisions only after observing the behaviors and consequences on those around them [12]."

In summary, empirical evidence shows that people differ in their general responsiveness to persuasive appeals as well as in their response to certain persuasive strategies [4–6, 8, 13, 14]. Studies have shown that applying inappropriate strategies may be counterproductive – resulting not only to refusal to comply to persuasive attempts, but even leading to adverse changes in behavior [4, 5]. Responsiveness to persuasive strategies can be predicted on the basis of demographic characteristics and personality traits [8, 14]. On that same note, Cialdini et al. [15] showed that the commitment and consistency strategy is only effective for individuals that have a high Preference for Consistency (PFC). Hence, there is need to investigate for other factors that may influence the effectiveness of the strategies.

3   Study Design and Methods

The data reported in this paper is part of a project aimed at investigating the effectiveness of persuasive strategies for various user groups and hence, develop guidelines for tailoring PTs to increase their effectiveness.

To achieve this, in this paper we adopt the well-established strategies (*reciprocity, scarcity, authority, commitment and consistency, and liking*) developed by Cialdini [3]. We focus on these strategies because they are simple and widely applicable both in technology-mediated persuasion and in human-mediated persuasion.

3.1   Measurement Instrument

To collect data for our study, we adapted the Susceptibility to Persuasive Strategies Scale (STPS) developed by Kaptein et al. [4, 13]. The items were used to assess participants' responsivess to Cialdini's six persuasive strategies. The questions were measured using participant agreement with a 7-point Likert scale ranging from "1 = Strongly disagree" to "7 = Strongly agree". The STPS scale has been shown to adequately predict participant susceptibility to individual strategies and the efficacy of the strategies for motivating behavior change in real life in various domains [4, 13]. We also included questions for assessing participants' demographic information (such as age, gender, geographical territory). Furthermore, we employed attention questions to ensure that participants were actively considering their answers.

3.2   Participants

We recruited participants for this study using Amazon's Mechanical Turk (AMT). AMT has become an accepted method of gathering users' responses [16]. It allows access to a global audience, ensures efficient survey distribution, and high quality results [16, 17]. We followed the recommendations for performing effective studies on the AMT by Mason and Suri [16] and before the main study, we conducted pilot studies to test the validity of our study instruments.

We collected a total of 1,384 responses and retained a total of 1,108 valid responses, which were included in our analysis. Incomplete responses and responses from participants who got the attention questions incorrect were discarded Demographic information is shown in Table 1.

Table 1. Participants' demographic information

N = 1108	
Gender	Females (533, 48%), Males (575, 52%).
Age	18-25 (418, 38%), 26-35 (406, 37%), Over 35 (284, 25%).
Education	Less than High School (12, 1%), High School Graduate (387, 35%), College Diploma (147, 13%), Bachelor's Degree (393, 35%), Master's Degree (141, 13%).
Country	Canada (40, 4%), India (148, 13%), Italy (23, 2%), United States (714,64%), United Kingdom (38, 3%), others (145, 13%)

4   Data Analyses

The goals of this paper are to determine whether significant differences exist between males and females and between younger adults (18-25) and adults (Over 35) with respect to the perceived persuasiveness of the strategies and to compare the persuasiveness of the strategies overall. Below, we present the various steps taken to analyze our data.

4.1   Instrument Validity

We begin our analysis by validating our study instrument. To determine the validity of our survey instrument we performed Principal Component Analysis (PCA) using SPSS. Before conducting PCA, the Kaiser-Meyer-Olkin (KMO) sampling adequacy was determined and found to be 0.72, well above the recommended 0.6. The Bartlett Test of Sphericity was significant at ($\chi^2(55) = 3792.0$, $p < 0.0001$). These two measures indicate that the data was suitable to conduct factor analysis [18].

Indicator reliability can be assumed because Cronbach's α of the strategies are all higher than a threshold value of 0.7 [19] except for liking and consensus strategies which showed a Cronbach's α of 0.56 and 0.45 respectively. This is acceptable because according to Peter [25], Cronbach's α should be ≥ 0.7, but for variables with 2-3 indicator, a Cronbach's $\alpha \geq 0.4$ is acceptable. The liking and consensus strategies contains 2 indicators each, therefore, Cronbach's α is within the acceptable range of ≥ 0.4.

After establishing the suitability of our data, we computed the average score for each strategy and then performed Repeated-Measure ANOVA (RM-ANOVA) with the strategies (reciprocity, scarcity, authority, commitment and consistency, and liking) as within-subject factors and gender and age as between-subject factors to explore for significant differences between the groups as well as to compare the overall persuasiveness of the strategies. The analysis was performed after validating our data for ANOVA assumptions, with no violations. When the sphericity assumption was violated, we used the Greenhouse-Geisser method of correcting the degrees of freedom. Following findings of significant effects, we performed post-hoc pairwise comparisons, using the Bonferonni method for adjusting the degrees of freedom for multiple comparisons, to determine the groups that significantly differ from each other.

5   Result

We present the results for the overall persuasiveness of the strategies followed by the effects of gender and age on the persuasiveness of the strategies.

5.1   Overall Persuasiveness of the Strategies

Our results show significant main effects of strategy type ($F_{4.14, 4576.54}=324.9$, p≈.000, $\eta^2=.227$) on persuasiveness. This means that there are significant differences between the strategies with respect to their perceived persuasiveness overall. Regardless of gender and age group, commitment and reciprocity emerged as the most persuasive (significantly different from all other strategies as shown by the Bonferonni-corrected pairwise comparisons), whereas consensus and scarcity were the least persuasive (also significantly different from all others). The rest of the strategies (authority and liking) were in the middle, with liking leading the group, see Table 1.

In general, participants perceived all of the strategies as persuasive, well above the neutral rating of 3.5, see Figure 1.

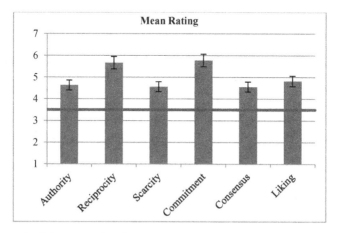

Fig. 1. A bar graph of the mean of individual strategies, showing their overall persuasiveness. Error bars represent a 95% confidence interval.

5.2   Gender Effects

The results of the RM-ANOVA showed a significant main effect of gender on persuasiveness ($F_{1,1106}=7.3$, $p\approx.007$, $\eta^2=.007$). Overall, females rated the strategies as more persuasive than men. See Figure 2 and Table 2.

5.3   Interaction Between Gender and Strategies

The results of the RM-ANOVA showed a significant interaction between gender and strategy ($F_{4.138,4576.55}=3.2$, $p\approx.011$, $\eta^2=.003$). Pairwise comparisons showed that females found three out of the six strategies significantly more persuasive than males: reciprocity ($F_{1,1106}=9.2$, $p\approx.003$, $\eta^2=.008$); commitment ($F_{1,\ 1106}=9.1$, $p\ \approx.003$, $\eta^2=.008$); and consensus ($F_{1,1106}=10.6$, $p\approx.001$, $\eta^2=.010$), see Figure 2 and Table 2.

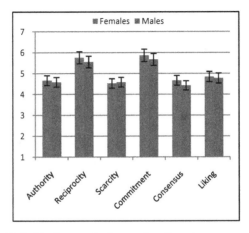

Fig. 2. Paired mean of individual strategies by gender. Error bars represent a 95% confidence interval.

Table 2. Mean and Standard Deviations (SD) for the strategies by gender. Bolded means are significantly different across males and females.; p<.005.

N = 1108					
Strategies	Authority	Reciprocity	Scarcity	Commitment	Consensus	Liking
	mean(SD)	mean(SD)	mean(SD)	mean(SD)	mean(SD)	mean(SD)
Females	4.67(1.29)	**5.76(1.10)**	4.53(1.46)	**5.87(1.04)**	**4.67(1.22)**	4.85(1.13)
Males	4.59(1.24)	**5.56(1.18)**	4.59(1.36)	**5.68(1.10)**	**4.43(1.19)**	4.78(1.14)

5.4   Age Effects

For the purpose of this study, we defined three age categories: 18-25, 26-35, and above 35. However, because we aimed at groups with a considerable age difference, we selected only participants within the 18-25 (younger adults) and above 35 (adults) age categories for this analysis. Also to avoid comparing groups with unequal sample sizes we undersampled the younger adults group using SPSS random sampling. After, the random sampling, the dataset contains 298 younger adults and 284 adults.

The results of the RM-ANOVA showed no significant effect of age on the overall persuasiveness of the strategies ($F_{1, 580}=2.4$, $p\approx.125$, $\eta^2=.004$). This means that the age groups did not perceive the strategies differently overall, establishing that there were no group-level differences in the ratings by the two age groups.

5.5 Interaction Between Age and Strategies

The results of the RM-ANOVA showed a significant interaction between age and strategy ($F_{4.118,2388.338}=10.7$, $p\approx.000$, $\eta^2=.018$). Pairwise comparisons showed that adults found commitment ($F_{1,580}=9.0$, $p\approx.003$, $\eta^2=.015$) significantly more persuasive than the younger adults, while younger adults found scarcity to be significantly more persuasive than adults ($F_{1,580}=20.7$, $p\approx.000$, $\eta^2=.034$), see Figure 3 and Table 3.

The results show no significant three-way interaction between age, gender, and strategy ($F_{4.172,2912.37}=0.672$, $p\approx.618$, $\eta^2=.001$).

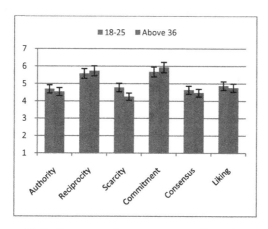

Fig. 3. Paired mean of individual strategies by age group. Error bars represent a 95% confidence interval.

Table 3. Mean and Standard Deviations (SD) for the strategies by age group. Bolded means are significantly different across the age group; p<.05.

N = 1108					
Strategies **Authority**	**Reciprocity**	**Scarcity**	**Commitment**	**Consensus**	**Liking**
mean(SD)	mean(SD)	mean(SD)	mean(SD)	mean(SD)	mean(SD)
18-25 4.70(1.20)	5.58(1.11)	**4.78(1.36)**	**5.68(1.11)**	4.64(1.16)	4.88(1.11)
Above 35 4.54(1.32)	5.74(1.10)	**4.26(1.44)**	**5.94(0.94)**	4.47(1.19)	4.76(1.06)

6   Discussion

This study presents the results of a large-scale study investigating gender and age differences in the persuasiveness of Cialdini's six persuasive strategies. It also provides a quantitative validation of the persuasive strategies overall.

The results of the analysis show that there are significant differences between the strategies with respect to their perceived persuasiveness overall. This means that the strategies are not equally persuasive – some of the strategies are perceived as more persuasive than others. In line with previous research, there are differences in the persuasiveness of the strategies across the gender and age groups. Below, we discuss the persuasiveness of the strategies individually.

6.1   Authority

According to Cialdini [3], establishing and revealing expertise can help to convince the persuadee. In this context, showing some expert endorsement of a PT could help increase its appeal [2]. Although authority is a widely-employed strategy, the results of our study show that it is not one of the best strategies with respect to the persuasiveness. It is significantly less persuasive than commitment and reciprocity. One explanation for this can be found in the statement by Rhoads and Cialdini [20]: "when feeling overwhelmed by a complicated and consequential choice, most individuals still want a fully considered, point by point analysis of it—an analysis they may not be able to achieve except, ironically enough, through a shortcut: reliance on an expert." This means that the persuasiveness of authority is contingent on many other factors including the persuadee's mode (in the case "feeling overwhelmed"). In addition, there has been an erosion of the culture of expertise in the past decade, and this change in how people perceive expertise could contribute to the lower persuasiveness of the strategy of authority [21].

Regarding gender differences, there was no significant difference between males and females with respect to their responsiveness to the authority strategy. Similarly, age has no significant impact in the participants responsiveness to the authority strategy. Younger adults and adults show a similar response to the authority strategy. This means that PTs employing the authority strategy in their design will persuade both gender (males and females) equally and both age groups (younger adults and adults) equally. However, it is important to note, that authority is not among the best strategy for any of the groups considered.

6.2   Reciprocity

Reciprocity is based on the idea that people by their nature feel obliged to return favor, to pay back. Thus when a persuasive request is made by a person the receiver feels indebted to, the receiver is more inclined to respond positively to the request Cialdini [11]. Although, reciprocity is not among the widely-employed strategies in PT design because of possible difficulty in operationalizing it in system design [4], the result from our study shows that reciprocity is among the best strategies that is capable of motivating users to take a desired action. It is second to commitment in persuasiveness overall. Therefore, it could be employed to create compelling PTs. For example, it can be employed in PTs used for asking for academic favours such as a paper review request, requesting for answers from experts in a domain in forums like ResearchGate.

With respect to gender differences, reciprocity is one of the strategies that is perceived differently across the gender groups. Females are significantly more responsive to reciprocity strategy than males. This is probably because females tend to be more relational and community-oriented. For example, Billy and Udry [22] showed that compared to males, females maintain stronger relationships. These results are in line with [23–25], who found that women are more inclined to reciprocate. The finding indicates that females feel more indebted and obliged to pay back favor than men. However,there was no significant difference between younger adults and adults with respect to their responsiveness to the resprocity strategy.

6.3   Scarcity

The scarcity strategy is based on the principle that people tend to place more value on things that are in short supply. For example, announcing that a product or service is scarce will favor its evaluation and consequently increase the chance of purchase [26]. This is due to the popular belief that less-available options are of higher quality than those options that are more available. As a result, scarcity is one of the frequently-employed strategies in PT design, especially in the marketing domain. Surprisingly, the results of our study show that scarcity is among the least persuasive strategies overall – only slightly better than consensus.

Regarding gender and age, there was no significant difference between males and females with respect to their responsiveness to the scarcity strategy; however, there was a significant difference between the age groups, with younger adults being more responsive to the scarcity strategy than adults. This suggests that younger people have a greater tendency to evaluate the persuasive appeal via the pheripheral route (without thoughtfully considering the arguments) compared to the adults. This implies that an emotional persuasive approach may work well for younger adults [8].

6.4   Commitment and Consistency

People naturally strive to be consistent in their statements and behaviors [3]. According to Cialdini [3], people are more inclined to comply to a persuasive request that aligns with their previous behavior. Commitment emerged as the most persuasive of all the strategies for all the groups considered.

Our results suggest that females are more responsive to the commitment strategy than males and that adults are more responsive to the commitment strategy than younger adults. One possible explanation is that females and adults care more about their public image and strive to manage and maintain the impression that they have created to avoid feeling of inconsistency [27]. Another possible reason is that females and adults tend to experience higher cognitive dissonance, i.e., the discomfort that is experienced when new information conflicts with existing beliefs, ideas, or values, and are therefore more responsive to the commitment strategy [28, 29]. The results suggest that persuasive approaches that require users to make any kind of commitment such as those that requires users to set a daily or weekly goal and compare achievement with set goal (as in Fish'n'Steps [30]) should be emphasized.

6.5   Consensus

According to the consensus principle, we often observe the behaviors of others to help us make decisions. Therefore, when a persuasive request is made, people are more inclined to comply if they are aware that others have complied [11]. This is one of the widely-employed strategies, however, the results of our study shows that consensus has the lowest persuasiveness of the six strategies

A possible reason for this shortfall in persuasiveness of the consensus strategy relative to the other strategies can be found in Cialdini's [3] statement that consensus is particularly impactful in situations of high uncertainty or ambiguity, when others are viewed as similar to oneself, and when there is substantial risk involved. This means that there are antecedent conditions (e.g., are others similar to me? How risky is the action?) that contribute to the persuasiveness of the consensus strategy. These conditions are not always present in all persuasive attempts. These results are similar to the research findings that show that social influence is not a significant determinant of healthy behavior [8].

With regards to gender and age, consensus is one of the strategies that is significantly different across genders. Females are more responsive to the consensus strategy than males; however, there is no effect of age on the response to the consensus strategy. The results are also similar to the research finding that females are more receptive to social influence than males [8], suggesting that females are more responsive to socially-driven strategies (such as consensus) than males.

6.6   Liking

The principle of liking states that individuals can be easily influenced or persuaded by someone they like. In relating this strategy to PT design, Oinas-Kukkonen [2] said "a system that is visually attractive for its users is likely to be more persuasive." The results from our study show that liking is not one of the best strategies with respect to the persuasiveness. In fact, it is significantly below commitment and reciprocity in overall persuasiveness.

With regards to gender and age effect, there is no significant difference between males and females and there is also no significant difference between younger adults and adults with respect to their responsiveness to the liking strategy. This means that PTs employing the liking strategy in their design will be equally persuasive for both males and females and for both younger adults and adults. However, it is important to note that liking is not among the best strategy for any of the groups.

6.7   Summary

Our study compares the persuasiveness of six persuasive strategies proposed by Cialdini and compares the effects by gender and age group. We present a summary of our findings in Table 3. It can guide designers in choosing the right strategy to motivate behavior change in both a one-size-fits-all approach or in a tailored approach that targets individual groups.

Table 4. Summary of persuasiveness to persuasive strategies. The strategies presented in descending order of persuasive strength (underlined is the highest).

Group	Strategy
Females	Commitment, Reciprocity, Liking, Consensus, Authority, Scarcity
Males	Commitment, Reciprocity, Liking, Scarcity, Authority, Consensus
Younger Adults	Commitment, Reciprocity, Liking, Scarcity, Authority, Consensus
Adults	Commitment, Reciprocity, Liking, Authority, 'Consensus', Scarcity
Overall	Commitment, Reciprocity, Liking, Authority, Scarcity, Consensus

7   Limitations

This study examined the perceived persuasiveness using self-reported measures; however, actual persuasiveness may be different when implemented and used in an implementation of a persuasive technology system. In addition, just like other population-based personalization, our results will apply to the majority of the group; however, there may be outliers who do not respond in the predicted manner.

8   Conclusions and Future Work

This paper presented the results of a large-scale study with three major goals: (1) to investigate the comparative persuasiveness of the six persuasive strategies (*reciprocity, scarcity, authority, commitment* and *consistency, and liking*) proposed by Cialdini; (2) examining for possible gender effects in the persuasiveness of the strategies; and finally (3) examining for possible age group differences in the persuasiveness of the strategies.

Our results show that in general, regardless of gender and age group, commitment followed by reciprocity emerged as the most persuasive strategies (significantly different from all the other strategies), whereas consensus followed by scarcity were the least persuasive strategy (also significantly different from all others). The rest of the strategies (authority and liking) were in the middle, with liking leading the group, see Table 3.

We found that males and females differ significantly with regard to the responsiveness to three out of the six strategies. Specifically, females found reciprocity, commitment, and consensus more persuasive than males. This implies that females can be more easily persuaded using these strategies. It also implies that females may respond more favorably to persuasive attempts that offer some kind of reward to them even before they perform the desired behavior (reciprocity) or those that require them to commit to a long-term or short-term goal (in line with goal setting theory) than males. It also suggests that peer pressure may work better for females than males. Overall, females are more responsive to all the strategies except the scarcity than males. This implies that females are more persuadable than males with respect to the persuasiveness of the strategies overall.

Similarly, younger adults and adults differ significantly with regard to their responsiveness to two out of the six strategies. Specifically, adults found commitment more persuasive than younger adults, whereas younger adults perceive scarcity as more persuasive than adults. However, younger adults have a slightly higher persuasiveness score overall than adults.

Although future work should design and compare the effectiveness of the strategies in actual persuasive implementation, our study contributes important findings about population differences that are relevant to designers of persuasive technology interventions.

References

1. Fogg, B.J.: Persuasive Technology: Using Computers to Change What We Think and Do. Morgan Kaufmann (2003)
2. Oinas-Kukkonen, H., Harjumaa, M.: Persuasive systems design: Key issues, process model, and system features. Commun. Assoc. Inf. Syst. 24, 28 (2009)
3. Cialdini, R.: Harnessing the science of persuasion. Harv. Bus. Rev. 79, 72–79 (2001)
4. Kaptein, et al.: Adaptive Persuasive Systems. Trans. Interact. Intell. Syst. 2, 1–25 (2012)
5. Orji, R.: Design for Behaviour Change: A Model-driven Approach for Tailoring Persuasive Technologies (2014)
6. Orji, et al.: Modeling the Efficacy of Persuasive Strategies for Different Gamer Types in Serious Games for Health. User Model. User Adapt. Interact. Spec. Issue Pers. Behav. Chang. 42, 453–498 (2014)
7. Kaptein, M., Lacroix, J., Saini, P.: Individual differences in persuadability in the health promotion domain. In: Ploug, T., Hasle, P., Oinas-Kukkonen, H. (eds.) PERSUASIVE 2010. LNCS, vol. 6137, pp. 94–105. Springer, Heidelberg (2010)
8. Orji, R.O., Vassileva, J., Mandryk, R.L.: Modeling Gender Differences in Healthy Eating Determinants for Persuasive Intervention Design. In: Berkovsky, S., Freyne, J. (eds.) PERSUASIVE 2013. LNCS, vol. 7822, pp. 161–173. Springer, Heidelberg (2013)
9. Orji, R., Mandryk, R.L.: Developing culturally relevant design guidelines for encouraging healthy eating behavior. Int. J. Hum. Comput. Stud. 72, 207–223 (2014)

10. Dawson, et al.: Examining gender differences in the health behaviors of Canadian university students. J. R. Soc. Promot. Health 127, 38–44 (2007)
11. Cialdini, R.B.: The Science of Persuasion. Sci. Am. Mind. 284, 76–84 (2004)
12. Clark, W.R., Tennessee, M.: Using the Six Principles of Influence to Increase Student Involvement in Professional Organizations: A Relationship Marketing Approach. J. Adv. Mark. Educ. 12, 43–52 (2008)
13. Kaptein, M., Markopoulos, P., de Ruyter, B., Aarts, E.: Can you be persuaded? individual differences in susceptibility to persuasion. In: Gross, T., Gulliksen, J., Kotzé, P., Oestreicher, L., Palanque, P., Prates, R.O., Winckler, M. (eds.) INTERACT 2009. LNCS, vol. 5726, pp. 115–118. Springer, Heidelberg (2009)
14. Halko, S., Kientz, J.A.: Personality and Persuasive Technology: An Exploratory Study on Health-Promoting Mobile Applications. In: Ploug, T., Hasle, P., Oinas-Kukkonen, H. (eds.) PERSUASIVE 2010. LNCS, vol. 6137, pp. 150–161. Springer, Heidelberg (2010)
15. Cialdini, et al.: Preference for consistency: The development of a valid measure and the discovery of surprising behavioral implications 69, 318–328 (1995)
16. Mason, W., Suri, S.: Conducting behavioral research on Amazon's Mechanical Turk. Behav. Res. Methods. 44, 1–23 (2012)
17. Buhrmester, M.D., Kwang, T., Gosling, S.D.: Amazon's Mechanical Turk A New Source of Inexpensive, Yet High-Quality, Data? Perspect. Psychol. Sci. 6, 3–5 (2011)
18. Hinton, et al.: SPSS Explained. Routledge (2004)
19. Chin, W.W.: The Partial Least Squares Approach to Structural Equation Modeling, http://www.bibsonomy.org/bibtex/276aba15e34b8d636650ed79f158 1f50b/naegle
20. Rhoads, K.V., Cialdini, R.B.: The business of influence: Principles that lead to success in commercial settings. In: The Persuasion Handbook: Dev. in Theory and Pract., pp. 513–542 (2002)
21. Pure, et al: Understanding and Evaluating Source Expertise in an Evolving Media Environment. In: Takševa, T. (ed.) Social Software and the Evolution of User Expertise: Future Trends in Knowledge Creation and Dissemination, pp. 37–51. IGI Global (2013)
22. Billy, J.O., Udry, J.R.: Patterns of adolescent friendship and effects on sexual behavior. Soc. Psychol. Q., 27-41 (1985)
23. Dohmen, et al.: Representative Trust and Reciprocity: Prevalence and Determinants. Econ. Inq. 46, 84–90 (2006)
24. Rau, H.A.: Trust and Trustworthiness: A Survey of Gender Differences. Psychol. Gend. Differ., 205–224 (2011)
25. Chaudhuri, A., Gangadharan, L.: Gender Differences in Trust and Reciprocity (2003)
26. West, S.G.: Increasing the attractiveness of college cafeteria food: A reactance theory perspective. J. Appl. Psychol. 6, 656 (1975)
27. Orji, et al.: Providing for Impression Management in Persuasive Designs. Persuas. Technol., 1–4 (2012)
28. Lackenbauer, S.D.: Do I Feel Dissonance Over You? Sex Differences in the Experience of Dissonance for Romantic Partners (2011)
29. Dare, B., Guadagno, R., Nicole Muscanell, M.A.: Commitment: The Key to Women Staying in Abusive Relationships. J. Interpers. Relations, Intergr. Relations Identity 6, 58–64 (2013)
30. Lin, J.J., Mamykina, L., Lindtner, S., Delajoux, G., Strub, H.B.: Fish'n'Steps: Encouraging physical activity with an interactive computer game. In: Dourish, P., Friday, A. (eds.) UbiComp 2006. LNCS, vol. 4206, pp. 261–278. Springer, Heidelberg (2006)

Using Individual and Collaborative Challenges in Behavior Change Support Systems: Findings from a Two-Month Field Trial of a Trip Planner Application

Johann Schrammel[1(✉)], Sebastian Prost[1], Elke Mattheiss[1], Efthimios Bothos[2], and Manfred Tscheligi[1,3]

[1] AIT – Austrian Institute of Technology, Vienna, Austria
{Johann.Schrammel,Sebastian.Prost,Elke.Mattheiss,
Manfred.Tscheligi}@ait.ac.at
[2] NTUA- National Technical University of Athens, Greece
mpthim@mail.ntua.gr
[3] University of Salzburg, Austria
manfred.tscheligi@sbg.ac.at

Abstract. Besides other popular strategies, such as feedback and (social) comparisons, challenges have been proposed and used to influence people's behavior towards a targeted goal. However, only very limited data on the effectiveness of such approaches and how to best design them is available yet. In this work we report the findings of a two months field study analyzing the effectiveness and perception of challenges in the context of influencing personal mobility. Individual and collaborative approaches towards challenges were studied, and specific focus was laid on what aspect makes users willing to participate in these challenges. Our findings suggest that both individual and collaborative challenges have the potential to sustain the interest of users in using behavior change support systems, that collaborative and individual challenges seem to not attract different types of users, that individual challenges in general are preferred, and that challenges are only a useful means for a subset of users. Also, ICT-competence seems to be an important aspect of being willing to participate in electronically organized challenges.

1 Introduction

Sustainable mobility choices are an important aspect of achieving a greener lifestyle. Within the last couple of years different behavior change support systems (BCSS) have been proposed and introduced addressing this issue, e.g. [1, 2]. A concept utilized in this context has been the introduction of challenges i.e. to provide users with a set of behavior-goals, were they can voluntarily decide whether to accept or decline the challenge. This approach is based on the background of goal-setting theory [3, 4]. Typically such implementations are combined with social comparisons, which allow users to participate and engage in pre-defined challenges posed by some mediating instance (typically the provider of the BCSS) and to compare their success (and compete) with others. Whereas such approaches are common, surprisingly few empirical data on their actual performance and empirically funded guidelines for the design of

T. MacTavish and S. Basapur (Eds.): PERSUASIVE 2015, LNCS 9072, pp. 160–171, 2015.
DOI: 10.1007/978-3-319-20306-5_15

such challenges exist. Questions like how to best frame these challenges, whether to better organize them in an individual or collaborative manner, how to tailor them towards specific user groups still remain largely unanswered from an empirical perspective.

We addressed some of these aspects in our work, and this paper reports the findings of an empirical study which researches the influence of different types of challenges and the user's characteristics on the effectiveness, perception and acceptance of challenges in the context of behavior change support systems in personal mobility.

In the following sections we first provide a review of relevant related work from different perspectives, especially persuasive strategies, goal-setting theory and behavior change in personal mobility. We then picture the PEACOX-System, which was used in the field trial and formed the basis for the conduction of this study. Next we describe the study methodology and report the main findings. The paper closes with the discussion of results and provides conclusions for future applications of and research on challenges in persuasive systems.

2   Related Work

Persuasion using technological support tools has been studied in depth for numerous years now, and a substantial body of knowledge has been generated. Different strategies to persuade people have been proposed and identified (e.g. [5, 6]), and have been applied in different application domains, e.g. health, energy consumption, personal mobility, etc. Torning and Oinas-Kukkonen [6] provide an overview and ranking of the most used design principles, and almost all strategies relevant for the design of challenges (e.g. feedback/self-monitoring, (social) comparisons, suggestions and personalization) are included within the top-ten of this list.

Sharing. Sharing ones progress with regard to set goals and making the commitment to achieving the goal public has been suggested as means for increasing the effectiveness of goal-setting approaches and has been used in numerous persuasive systems. Sharing has been found to have positive effects in several systems (e.g. [7, 8]), but research also showed that sharing with strangers is not always motivating and might sometimes be perceived as awkward [8].

Comparisons. Sharing ones results e.g. of participation in challenges also implies the possibility for social comparison. Persuasive systems frequently explicitly design for this aspect, e.g. by displaying the individual achievements contrasted with other users [11]. Comparisons have been especially popular in the field of energy consumption, and research studying the consequences of this approach comes to conflicting results [12]. There is indication that comparative approaches might increase the effectiveness in some cases, but also evidence has been presented that indicates direct comparison to other users actually might have detrimental consequences in unfavorable conditions. One possibility to avoid such negative effects is to tailor the interventions towards the user.

Personalization/Tailoring. Personalization and tailoring refers to the adaptation of the persuasive measures and approaches towards the individual person, situation and usage context. This strategy has been frequently suggested as means to increase both the impact and acceptance of persuasive systems [13]. Also research on identifying persuadability factors has been introduced in order to provide a solid framework for designing and applying tailoring and personalization in practice [14].

Challenges and goal-setting. Challenges are closely related to the concept of goal-setting, and can be understood as a special case thereof. Goal-setting theory was originally developed within an organizational context and showed that specific and hard goals lead to better performance results than easy and unspecific goals [3, 4]. Especially the question of how to define the goal is of major importance. Building on goal-setting theory Consolvo et al. [15] explored the preference of users on different goal sources (self-set, assigned, participatory, guided or group-set) and goal timeframes (fixed weekly scheme versus rolling time-window). Unfortunately no actual behavior data is available in this study, but an analysis of self-reported preferences indicates that self-set goals are preferred, but also that interesting design opportunities for guided and group-set approaches exist. Besides source and timeframe also the role of different defaults in the goal setting process has been researched recently [16]. In the context of energy saving in the household the study found that default goals can lead to significant savings, and that it is important to choose the right defaults as both too low and too high goals have detrimental effects on the behavior.

If the goal-setting is not done directly by the user, but the system presents the user with goals to achieve this is typically labeled challenges. Similar to classical goal-setting for challenges it seems to be important to achieve the correct level of difficulty as well as a close match to the user's intrinsic goals [22].

Using teams rather than individuals has also been suggested to improve persuasiveness [19]. Consequently, team-based challenges are used in several systems, however only very limited data on their performance or guidelines for their design exist.

Personal mobility and behavior change. In our work we research challenges in the context of influencing mobility behavior. Early systems in this domain typically tried to motivate behavioral changes by means of tracking the effects of existing mobility behavior and providing feedback on the ecological footprint of a given route, expressed in different ways, e.g. as gasoline consumption, CO_2 values, or associated emissions of other environmental pollutants, see e.g., [1] and [21]. Such approaches are now very common, and many commercial routing services and web sites already provide this information for everyday use. A common approach is to use these numbers to compute an overall score, which then can be expressed in a more appealing and persuasive way (e.g. a plant growing or the size of an ice floe [1], or a virtual fish [9], etc.). Reitberger et al. [20] use implicit and peripheral cues in the user's environment that provide indicators about the environmental pollution to influence mobility decisions. Also, elements of gamification have been used in the context of personal mobility. For example, Jylhä et al. [22] designed a system that implements personalized challenges which are constructed through automated sensing of travel behaviors whereas Broll et al. [23] describe a system that provides visualizations which illustrate users' performance with regard to saved money, CO2, health, and collected points derived from mobility data.

3   The PEACOX System

PEACOX [26] is a mobile travel planning application, which builds upon the de-scribed approaches. Its main design goal is to support the user in engaging in more sustainable travel mode decisions. The PEACOX app allows the user to perform a multi-modal search for a route, which is tailored to the user's individual preferences and behavior patterns. In general, it works like a common journey planner. An origin and a destination are specified and then possible routes are suggested. When routes are requested in PEACOX the available alternatives are enriched with emission in-formation. The enriched results are then ranked and personalized by a recommender engine [10]. Recommendations are partially based on the users' individual trip history that is detected from recorded GPS and accelerometer data. Selected eco-friendly route options are promoted by adding an encouraging message. When clicking on a route all details are displayed, that is walking-, driving- and waiting times, public transport line and schedule. After that the routes can also be viewed on the map. Indi-vidual statistics regarding the used trip modes and produced CO_2 can be accessed, and the user's relative performance compared to their own previous behavior is measured and represented by a growing or shrinking tree.

The journey planner is implemented as a smartphone application for the Android platform version 4.0 and higher. Challenges were implemented as part of this overall system and were integrated with the rest of the functions. A specified screen within the application provided all necessary information (cf. Figure 1 below). Messages informing the users about new challenges or the outcome of prior ones could be pushed to the users. Messages were also shown in the Android notification bar and supported links, which could be easily followed by a tap.

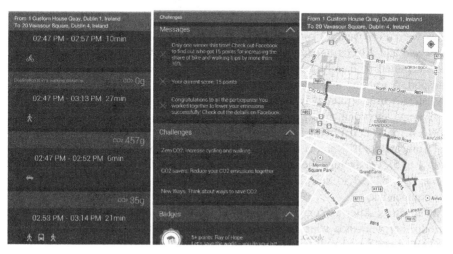

Fig. 1. Screenshots showing key elements of the PEACOX system. Route search results screen (left), overview-screen related to challenges (middle), and route in map view (right).

4   Research Questions and Method

As described above the PEACOX-System provided the basis for the study in order to address our research goals. In detail we wanted to answer the following main research questions with our work:

a) Are challenges a successful means to sustain interest and motivation of users for engaging with behavior change support systems?

b) Is there a main difference in whether challenges are framed on an individual or a collaborative level?

c) How do different types of individuals react to different types of challenges, and what are the design implications of such differences?

In order to answer these questions und to test the overall acceptance and impact of the system we conducted a two month field trial (August & September 2014) with 37 participants in two European cities (Vienna and Dublin). Collaborative and individual challenges were organized, and data regarding usage, success and subjective experience was collected. In the following paragraphs we provide the details on this study.

Participants. Participants were recruited from a database of people interested in taking part in usability and user experience studies and by open calls for participation promoted in university lectures and university mailing lists. Prospective participants had to fill in a screening questionnaire, and only were recruited in case they fulfilled the following predefined criteria: age 18 or older, living and working/studying in the test area (Vienna respectively Dublin metropolitan area), users of an Android smart phone (running Android OS 4.0 or newer) for at least three months, must have an associated data plan with a minimum of 500 MB per month, and during the eight weeks of trial plan to be absent (e.g. holiday outside of the study regions) for no more than one week.

Altogether 37 participants (14 female, 23 male; 20 from Vienna, 17 from Dublin) between 19 and 69 years (mean=32.92, SD=12.48) took part in the study. 16 participants were employed, 12 were students, 4 were unemployed or retired, 3 were self-employed and 2 were on parental leave. Regarding their main transportation means 6 users reported to mainly use car or motorbike, 6 to use bicycles, 11 stated public transport, 5 walking and 9 didn't provide data on this question. A majority of users (29) already used a journey planning app prior to the study.

Average environmental concern [18] of the participants was moderately high (Mean 4.15, STD 0.68 on a scale from 1 low to 5 high). Scores on importance of social comparison [17] are in the medium range (Mean 3.19, STD 0.84, again scale from 1 to 5). On average the user group also had a rather high ICT-competence [25]: Mean 1.99, STD 0.50, scale poled inverse to prior ones with 1 indicating high and 5 low competence.

Procedure. After agreeing to take part in the trial, participants were invited to an introductory workshop which focused on instructing the users on the trial procedure, explaining the functionality and handling of the app and how participants were expected to use it. Participants were instructed to enable GPS-positioning and logging on their smartphones and to regularly charge the device.

During the field trial, after about three and six weeks of usage qualitative in-depth interviews concerning the usage of the app and the experiences made were conducted with most users (some were not reachable for the first interview). At the end of the trial participants were invited to focus groups to reflect on the experiences made.

Additionally online questionnaires were sent three times during the trial: at the beginning, in the middle and at the end. The questionnaires focused on demographic data, mobility behavior, application usage and and attitudes towards different transportation means and environmental issues.

Challenges. There were two different types of challenges used in the study. In the individual challenges participants had to achieve a defined goal on their own. In collaborative challenges participants could join a group, which had to achieve the defined goal together, with each participant contributing to the overall goal. Altogether there were three pairs of challenges; these pairs differed from each other only in the individual or collaborative aspect. All six challenges were presented to the participants.

Challenges were designed so they can be achieved by all mobility types. The following three challenges either framed in an individual or collaborative way have been used in the trial:

Challenge #1: Identify 2 (for individual) respectively 10 (for collaborative) specific possibilities to save CO_2 in personal transport. Please post your findings to the Facebook group.

Challenge #2: Try to lower your (individual or collaborative) CO_2 emissions by 10 percent compared to last week or try to reach a value below 20g/km.

Challenge #3: Try to increase your (individual or collaborative) kilometers for cycling and walking by 10% or try to walk or cycle 50% or more of your kilometers.

Participants were instructed that taking part in the challenges is voluntary. To announce the challenges to the participants, we set up Facebook groups and events and asked the participants to join them. To counterbalance the sequence of individual and collaborative challenges we created four Facebook groups (two for each study site), one starting with an individual challenge and one starting with a collaborative challenge. The challenges were posted as Facebook events in the groups. Additionally participants got a notification through the app with a link to the Facebook event.

During the field trial, every week (except in week one and five) a challenge was proposed to the participants. Each challenge lasted for five to seven days. The travel behavior of the participating users was analyzed in the middle and end of the challenge period. In the middle of the challenge period, we presented an intermediate result to the participants by posting in the respective Facebook event site. For each challenge we measured how many participants took part in them and how many succeeded.

All participants who wanted to take part in a challenge had to accept the event invitation. As a reward for succeeding in a challenge participants could earn points, which defined the reputation level of each participant. By winning challenges the participants could rise from "wannabe" to "eco guru". In order to support motivation of participating in the challenges information regarding their status was made visible on the Facebook group page.

5   Results

5.1   General Usage and Perception of the Application

Before we analyze the data regarding our main research questions we want to report some general information on the overall usage and perception of the application in order to provide a sound background for the detailed understanding of the specific findings.

Usability and Satisfaction. The overall usability of the application was rated average to well in the middle of the trial (3.57 ± 1.09 on a scale from 1 – totally disagree to 5 – totally agree on the statement "The system is easy to use"), and improved until the end of the field trial (3.97 ± 0.84). Similarly the experienced usefulness ("The system is useful") improved from 3.73 ± 0.96 to 4.06 ± 0.68. This increase in perceived usability and usefulness is probably related to the increased familiarity of the users with the application.

Application Usage. After the trials participants were asked how often they accessed two important system parts: the summary feedback provided by the tree, and the general statistics page. Answer categories were the following: 1 - never, 2 - once, so far, 3 - once a month, 4 - once every other week, 5 - once a week, 6 - several times a week, 7 - every day. Reported usage frequency for both system parts was in the order of once per week (tree 5.35 ± 1.64, statistics 4.58 ± 1.50).

Additionally, access to different parts of the system was automatically logged. Figure 2 below shows the evolution of usage for the whole trial period. The data show only a slight decline of usage over time. This decline is much less pronounced than with prior versions of the system (which did not including challenges and statistics) tested in the field in similar conditions a year earlier. Also, logged access data is not 100% conform to the reports of the users. This is probably related to the fact that what might be perceived as one action actually results in several screen accesses.

The graph also shows comparatively small amount of screen accesses to the challenges overview screen. This should not be misinterpreted as lack of interest as all information presented there was also accessible either on the Facebook group page or as Android system messages. Access to these elements unfortunately could not be logged due to technical restrictions.

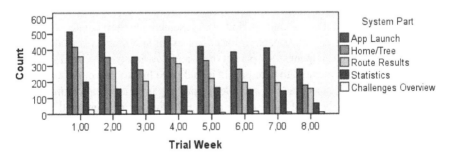

Fig. 2. Logged access numbers to different system parts during the trial period

5.2   Challenges

Overall Perception and Participation. Overall the challenges were perceived well by the participants, and a substantial amount of users participated in the challenges, although participation was voluntary. However, there seems to be a subgroup of users which did not like the challenges. Of our 37 participants 14 did not take part in a single challenge. Possible reasons for this behavior are analyzed in the section discussing factors influencing willingness to participate on the next page. Table 1 below provides an overview on the number of users that participated in the challenges over the duration of the field trial split according to individual versus collaborative challenge, and also provides information on how many of the accepted challenge were actually won.

Table 1. Participation and achievements in challenges

	Individual				Collaborative			
	Participated	%	Won	%	Participated	%	Won	%
Challenge #1	13	35.1	11	84.6	10	27.0	7	70.0
Challenge #2	15	40.5	8	53.4	12	32.4	9	75.0
Challenge #3	10	27.0	5	50.0	16	43.2	4	25.0
Total	38	34.3	24	63.2	38	34.3	20	52.6

Interest in participation in the challenges fluctuates somewhat (as has to be expected considering the limited number of users), but generally seems to continue over time and does not decline as might be expected. This is especially remarkable, as the app usage however slightly drops. This seems to indicate that challenges have the potential to better stimulate the long-term interest of users.

This interpretation is also supported by qualitative feedback collected in the interviews. Several users stated that the announcement of challenges worked as a reminder for them to keep using the app. As one user puts it: „It is motivating when you get 5 or 15 points as a reward. This is a motivational boost to keep using the app".

Moreover, the challenges helped some users to spur goals for greener mobility: "I'm trying to fit it in, to exercise, to see how much more exercise I can do compared to using the car. The challenges were enabling me to use the bike. It's good to do exercise and take part in a challenge".

Overall most participants liked the idea of the challenges, as they were seen as a way to raise awareness and rethink existing behavior patterns. The challenges were seen as an aid to make new experiences by pushing you to try out alternative modes of transport or routes: "[I participated] because it was fun […], because one is motivated to do things different, stop doing things by the book. […] You are encouraged to try something new. [Normally,] you just do these things out of habit".

Also, several users liked that the challenges posed also personal goals: "It was something to aim for. It's always nice to have targets, […] because you can't achieve anything without goals. So I tried to set myself little objectives, […] to be proud of achievements".

Individual versus Collaborative Challenges. Another question of our study was whether individual versus collaborative framing of challenges influences the willingness to participate in them. Table 1 above shows the average number of challenges the participants took part in. As is already obvious from the identical means paired samples t-test does not show any difference at all (t_{36}=0, p=1.00). Participation in collaborative challenges was highly correlated with participation in the individual challenges (r=0.833).

We also explicitly asked which type of challenges the users preferred. 14 stated that they did not look at the challenges closely and therefore cannot answer the question. About half of the remaining users did not have a preference (8) or didn't notice the difference (4). 8 participants clearly preferred individual challenges, and only 3 users favored collective ones.

A very similar trend is present in the qualitative data. While during the interviews users were not explicitly asked about the two different types of challenges, none made an explicit statement differentiating between the two. All statements mentioned above refer to the challenges in general, not a particular type. When referring to challenges, many participants did, however, implicitly express a preference to individual challenges. Users were complaining that in group challenges other participants did not show enough engagement to complete the challenge: "[Regarding] the challenges with ideas [...]: Most of the suggestions in the group work are mine. I would have wished more collaboration from the others." Also, the overall participation in the challenges was perceived as low by some: "I'm surprised so few participate. For me, if I say yes to something I say yes to the whole of it." This behavior can be explained by the fact that the participants mostly did not know each other before the trial and therefore social pressure to work together as a group was low. As has been suggested before [24], collaborative and competitive mechanisms work better if participants know each other: "There is another guy that I know who is participating in the study. So, I'm only just checking to make sure I'm ahead of him. [...] There's lot of people [...] I wouldn't know, so I'm not that interested in them".

We also analyzed the success rates of the two types of challenges. On average the individual challenges were successful in 60% of cases, whereas the collective ones only were successful in 49.21%. This difference however is not statistically significant (paired-samples t-test with 18 users that participated in individual and collective Challenges, t_{17}=0.772, p=0.451).

Due to the fact that most users did not distinguish between the two types of challenges, and no clear differentiation is visible in the data, in the following analysis steps we do not distinguish between the two types of challenges anymore.

Factors Influencing Willingness to Participate. In order to further explore which factors actually underlie the users willingness to participate in challenges we analyzed the data using a multiple linear regression approach with the number of challenges participated as independent variable. As dependent variables we used basic demographics (sex, age), ICT-competence, Environmental concern (measured using the scale provided in [18]) and a score of importance of the dimension of social comparison (based on [17]). This resulted in an overall marginally significant model ($F_{5,31}$=2.326, p=0.066, adjusted r^2=0.156). As shown in Table 2 below only ICT-competence had a significant influence on the willingness to participate in challenges. The more competent users were the more likely they are to participate in challenges.

Motivations for Participation. Some users remarked that the reward scheme through points and achievement levels was motivation for them: "There were no real rewards waiting, but you could get virtual points, a form of reward. [...] I thought

Table 1. Summary of multiple linear regression model

	B	Std. Error	t	p
Constant	1.539	3.296	0.467	0.644
Age	0.015	0.027	0.563	0.578
Sex	-0.686	0.740	-0.927	0.361
ICT Competence	-1.790	0.630	-2.839	**0.008****
Environmental Concern	0.565	0.527	1.071	0.292
Social Comparison	0.548	0.402	1.364	0.182

that was fun". Also, not gaining points can be motivational factor: „I didn't take part in the first [challenge]. I didn't get any points in the second group challenge. Then I thought, that can't be it, can it? And so I tried in the third and fourth if it is possible to achieve a little something using [different] modes of transport".

Others did not share this excitement about virtual rewards. Just collecting points was not motivation enough. They would have wanted "real" value in order to change their transport behavior: "Which grown-up person changes his behavior because of four points?". A number of users also explicitly expressed their disinterest in the game-like aspects: "I'm not the player type. This has never interested me". Also, the competitive character of challenges was sometimes rejected: "I'm not the competitive type. When I do something then I do it. Not because I want to trump someone".

Reasons for not Participating. Participation in challenges does require users to commit additional effort. A number of users stated that they did not find the time to participate in challenges. Some of them stated they rarely use Facebook and therefore missed the challenge, despite the app notification that was sent out. For most users, the reason why they wouldn't find the time for the challenges, was that they were simply too busy in their lives. Others, however, blamed their own laziness: "To be honest, I was too lazy. It was not immediately obvious how this works. There was too much to look at for joining. [...] I thought I can't change my modes of transport anyway, because I will not cycle to work".

6   Discussion and Conclusion

In our research we were interested in exploring the role and possibilities of challenges in persuasive technology. Our findings suggest that challenges have the possibility to sustain the interest in using persuasive systems for a longer time compared to approaches that rely merely on feedback strategies. In order to maximize this effect known design principles especially the correct match of challenge difficulty and users' needs should be applied. Also, timing is important, and measurements of a users' activity level should be considered to decide when to prompt challenges to users. Alternatively, the possibility to postpone challenges in a simply manner could be a good design solution to allow the users to better fit challenges into their busy lives.

Our data suggest that individual challenges are the more appropriate means for organizing challenges, if there is no intrinsic collaborative aspect present. This is mainly linked to the users' possibility to feel in charge of the outcome (Self-efficacy). However, this finding does not mean that one should approach challenges in an isolated manner. Sharing of results of individual challenges was perceived as supportive, and has been shown to can have positive effects when designed well [8].

Participation in challenges was correlated with ICT competence. This is surprising, as a selection criterion for participating in the study was regular use of an up-to-date Android phone, which excluded technology-avoiding users. Even though the system was easy to use according to the feedback from our participants, users confident in dealing with new technologies seem to be more willing to engage in digital challenges. Consequently, it is even more important to design the challenges as user friendly as possible. Also providing different access means for users might be a good design solution, as this allows users' to rely on known technologies.

Another unexpected find was that environmental concern was not related to the number of challenges the user participated in. Concerned users might focus their energy on changing their lifestyle, and playful means such as challenges are not needed to support this as they already are willing to do so. However, more data and research is needed to confirm (or disprove) this conjecture.

Some users explicitly rejected challenges as they dislike games and competitions. Therefore designers need to carefully consider their use. Gamification elements should be voluntary, so that users can simply ignore them. Regarding the persuasiveness of a system, elements like social comparison, competition and virtual rewards should not be the only strategy to be included, as some users will not respond to them.

Conclusions. In conclusion we can say that challenges seem to present an important possibility to sustain interest in interacting with persuasive technology, even though this is only true for a subset of users. Further research is needed regarding the question of how challenges can be made more attractive to these users, or to identify other approaches that better address the needs of them.

Our results also suggest that individual challenges seem to be preferable over collaborative ones, especially in application contexts were the users are not personally known to each other, and where there is no intrinsic collaborative aspect of the task.

References

1. Froehlich, J., Dillahunt, T., Klasnja, P., Mankoff, J., Consolvo, S., Harrison, B., James, A., Landay, J.A.: UbiGreen: investigating a mobile tool for tracking and supporting green transportation habits. In: Proc. CHI 2009. ACM (2009)
2. Carreras, I., Gabrielli, S., Miorandi, D., Tamilin, A., Cartolano, F., Jakob, M., Marzorati, S.: SUPERHUB: a user-centric perspective on sustainable urban mobility. In: Workshop Proc. Sense Transport 2012. ACM (2012)
3. Locke, E.A., Latham, G.P.: A theory of goal setting and task performance. Prentice-Hall, Englewood Cliffs (1990)
4. Locke, E.A., Latham, G.P.: Building a practically useful theory of goal setting and task motivation: A 35-year odyssey. American Psychologist 57 (2002)
5. Fogg, B.J.: Persuasive Technology: Using Computers to Change What We Think and Do (Interactive Technologies). Morgan Kaufmann Publishers Inc. (2003)
6. Torning, K.: Oinas-Kukkonen. H.: Persuasive system design: state of the art and future directions. In: Proc. Persuasive 2009. ACM (2009)

7. Consolvo, S., Everitt, K., Smith, I., Landay, J.A.: Design requirements for technologies that encourage physical activity. In: Proc. CHI 2006. ACM (2006)
8. Richardson, C.R., Buis, L.R., Janney, A.W., Goodrich, D.E., Sen, A., Hess, M.L., Piette, J.D.: An online community improves adherence in an internet-mediated walking program. Journal of Medical Internet Research 12(4) (2010)
9. Lin, J.J., Mamykina, L., Lindtner, S., Delajoux, G., Strub, H.B.: Fish'n'Steps: encouraging physical activity with an interactive computer game. In: Dourish, P., Friday, A. (eds.) UbiComp 2006. LNCS, vol. 4206, pp. 261–278. Springer, Heidelberg (2006)
10. Bothos, E., Prost, S., Schrammel, J., Röderer, K., Mentzas, G.: Watch your Emissions: Persuasive Strategies and Choice Architecture for Sustainable Decisions in Urban Mobility. PsychNology Journal 12(3) (2014)
11. Toscos, T., Faber, A., An, S., Praful Gandhi, M.: Chick clique: persuasive technology to motivate teenage girls to exercise. In: CHI 2006 Extended Abstracts. ACM (2006)
12. Petkov, P., Foth, M., Road, V.P.: Motivating domestic energy conservation through comparative, community-based feedback in mobile and social media. In: C&T 2011 (2011)
13. Berkovsky, S., Freyne, J., Oinas-Kukkonen, H.: Influencing individually: Fusing personalization and persuasion. ACM Transactions on Interactive Intelligent Systems 2(2) (2012)
14. Kaptein, M., Lacroix, J., Saini, P.: Individual differences in persuadability in the health promotion domain. In: Ploug, T., Hasle, P., Oinas-Kukkonen, H. (eds.) PERSUASIVE 2010. LNCS, vol. 6137, pp. 94–105. Springer, Heidelberg (2010)
15. Consolvo, S., Klasnja, P., McDonald, D.W., Landay, J.A.: Goal-setting considerations for persuasive technologies that encourage physical activity. In: Persuasive 2009. ACM (2009)
16. Loock, C., Staake, T., Thiesse, F.: Motivating energy-efficient behavior with green IS: an investigation of goal setting and the role of defaults. Mis Quarterly 37(4) (2013)
17. Busch, M., Schrammel, J., Tscheligi, M.: Personalized Persuasive Technology – Development and Validation of Scales for Measuring Persuadability. In: Berkovsky, S., Freyne, J. (eds.) PERSUASIVE 2013. LNCS, vol. 7822, pp. 33–38. Springer, Heidelberg (2013)
18. Worsley, A., Skrzypiec, G.: Environmental attitudes of senior secondary school students in South Australia. Global Environmental Change 8(3) (1998)
19. Staats, H., Harland, P., Wilke, H.A.: Effecting durable change a team approach to improve environmental behavior in the household. Environment and Behavior 36(3) (2004)
20. Reitberger, W., Ploderer, B., Obermair, C., Tscheligi, M.: The percues framework and its application for sustainable mobility. In: de Kort, Y.A.W., IJsselsteijn, W.A., Midden, C., Eggen, B., Fogg, B.J. (eds.) PERSUASIVE 2007. LNCS, vol. 4744, pp. 92–95. Springer, Heidelberg (2007)
21. MIT SENSEable City Lab, http://senseable.mit.edu/co2go (last retrieved January 12, 2014)
22. Jylhä, A., Nurmi, P., Sirén, M., Hemminki, S., Jacucci, G.: Matkahupi: a persuasive mobile application for sustainable mobility. In: UbiComp 2013 (2013)
23. Broll, G., Cao, H., Ebben, P., Holleis, P., Jacobs, K., Koolwaaij, S.B.: Tripzoom: an app to improve your mobility behavior. In: Proc. Conference MUM. ACM (2012)
24. Gabrielli, S., Forbes, P., Jylhä, A., Wells, S., Sirén, M., Hemminki, S., Jacucci, G.: Design challenges in motivating change for sustainable urban mobility. Computers in Human Behavior 41 (2014)
25. Weiss, B., Wechsung, I., Marquardt, S.: Assessing ICT user groups. In: NordCHI 2012. ACM (2012)
26. Schrammel, J., Busch, M., Tscheligi, M.: Peacox – Persuasive Advisor for CO2-Reducing Cross-modal Trip Planning. In: 1st International Workshop on Behavior Change Support Systems, BCSS (2013)

Towards a Framework for Socially Influencing Systems: Meta-analysis of Four PLS-SEM Based Studies

Agnis Stibe[✉]

MIT Media Lab, Cambridge, MA, USA
agnis@mit.edu

Abstract. People continuously experience various types of engagement through social media, mobile interaction, location-based applications, and other technologically advanced environments. Often, integral parts of such socio-technical contexts often are information systems designed to change behaviors and attitudes of their users by leveraging powers of social influence, further defined as socially influencing systems (SIS). Drawing upon socio-psychological theories, this paper initially reviews and presents a typology of relevant social influence aspects. Following that, it analyzes four partial least squares structural equation modeling (PLS-SEM) based empirical studies to examine the interconnectedness of their social influence aspects. As a result, the analysis provides grounds for seminal steps towards the development and advancement of a framework for designing and evaluating socially influencing systems. The main findings can also deepen understanding of how to effectively harness social influence for enhanced user engagement in socio-technical environments and guide persuasive engineering of future socially influencing systems.

Keywords: Socially influencing systems · Framework · Persuasive technology

1 Introduction

The dynamic evolution of social media, mobile connectivity, and a digital economy is continuously reshaping how businesses approach and engage customers [1]. Rapidly growing connectedness not only provides new methods for organizations to retain existing relationships with consumers, but also opens new ways to enrich customer engagement experiences and foster innovation [21]. Along the way, businesses and customers tend to naturally follow new market trends and steadily develop an understanding of the spectrum of opportunities provided by emerging technologies. People seamlessly acquire new habits of interaction and consumption behavior, which then set their expectations about how products and services should be designed [34].

Customers increasingly demand products and services that better match their needs and individual preferences [29]. Therefore, businesses face a need to continuously understand the individual and evolving expectations of their customers [26]. Thus, organizations stand to benefit from systems that are designed to reach customers more proactively and provide convenient ways for interaction [32].

© Springer International Publishing Switzerland 2015
T. MacTavish and S. Basapur (Eds.): PERSUASIVE 2015, LNCS 9072, pp. 172–183, 2015.
DOI: 10.1007/978-3-319-20306-5_16

The Internet has become increasingly mobile and social over the last decade [1]. Social media has rapidly expanded and businesses tend to use social media more often for the development of customer relationships. Simultaneously, these advancements exert various effects on everyday life by changing human behavior in both virtual and physical spaces. For example, it has become common for people to use social media through mobile devices [10]. The combination of socially dynamic and technologically advanced contexts has gradually introduced unique modes for businesses to engage customers almost instantly. Such socio-technical spaces often comprise information systems designed to change behavior and attitudes of their users by leveraging powers of social influence, further described as socially influencing systems [38].

To enrich an understanding of how to effectively harness social influence for enhanced user engagement through socio-technical environments, this paper continues with the following sections. In the next, a social cognitive perspective on human behavior is described. Then, the paper introduces a concept of socially influencing systems and reviews a typology of relevant social influence aspects. Thereafter, it provides a meta-analysis of four empirical studies based on partial least squares structural equation modeling (PLS-SEM) methodology and reports seminal steps towards a framework structure for designing and evaluating socially influencing systems. Finally, implications of the main outcomes are discussed and conclusions drawn.

2   Social Cognitive Foundation

According to Ryan and Deci [36], whether people become proactive and engaged depends largely on the social environments in which they develop and function. Bandura [5] has extended this perspective by suggesting that human self-development, adaptation, and change are embedded in social systems. In such systems, according to social cognitive theory [4], personal, behavioral, and environmental factors all interact continuously, perpetually influencing each other and determining the effect of each. There is an endless dynamic interplay between people, their behavior, and the environments where their behavior occurs.

The described triadic reciprocal determinism unfolds multiple angles for studying behavioral change, including environmental and personal change. Human behavior alters environmental conditions and, in turn, is changed by the same conditions that it creates [4]. Along the same vein, social cognitive theory suggests exploring how ambient environments maintain aspects of social persuasion.

Theories of persuasion often aim at describing either influences on or changes in behavior and attitudes on individual, group, and societal levels [33]. According to Fogg [19], persuasive technologies can be designed as social actors and are therefore capable of social influence even in the absence of other people in an immediate physical space. When properly designed, such persuasive technologies can become very effective for inducing behavioral and attitudinal changes in novel socio-technical contexts. Exploring the ability of persuasive technologies and systems to engage users is an essential direction for future research [9].

3   Socially Influencing Systems (SIS)

Social influence, as a substantive phenomenon, has a longstanding history in psychology [12], providing insights on various forms of potential influences on human behavior by the actual, imagined, or implied presence of other people [35]. Along its history, social influence has often been associated with compliance, identification, internalization, obedience, and persuasion, although at the same time kept distinct from conformity, power, and authority. Recent research on social influence mainly has been addressing either minority influence in group settings, dynamic social impact theory, social influence in expectation states theory, or persuasion [8], the latter being broadly defined as change in behavior or attitudes due to information received from others [13-14].

Human beings can experience social influence not only from others in physical proximity around them, but likewise through information systems that are engineered to serve such purpose. Information systems can exert social influence through their design and user interfaces when augmented with relevant social influence aspects, such as *social learning, social comparison, normative influence, social facilitation, cooperation, competition,* and *recognition* [38]. An information system becomes socially influencing when it has been enriched with social influence aspects to facilitate changes in behavior and attitudes of its users (Fig. 1).

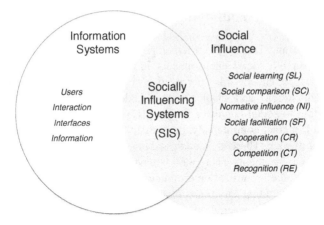

Fig. 1. Socially Influencing Systems

Besides a general comprehension of information system development and software engineering, designers of *socially influencing systems* are required to acquire or maintain a decent level of understanding about human behavior and social psychology. The foundation of the theory and research on socially influencing systems is underpinned by a list of fundamental theories originating from affined areas of social and cognitive psychology. The following are primary theories that are used in this research: social cognitive theory [4], social comparison theory [17], focus theory of normative conduct [13], social facilitation theory [20], cooperation theory [2], competition theory [15], and taxonomy of intrinsic motivators [25].

The listed theories suggest multiple sources of reference for the seven aforementioned social influence aspects that have the capacity to alter behavior and attitudes of users of socially influencing systems. Table 1 summarizes the descriptions, implementation examples, and relevant references of each aspect, while Fig. 2 provides more graphical representation of their sub-dimensions that are discussed and *highlighted* in the following sub-sections.

Table 1. Social influence aspects

Aspect	Description	Implementation example
Social learning (SL) [3-5]	Learning new behavior by observing how other people perform them.	Enabling users to see how others are using a system.
Social comparison (SC) [17], [40-42]	Comparing a behavior of an individual with behavior of others.	Names of active users grow larger as compared to passive users.
Normative influence (NI) [13], [16], [23]	People tend to follow norms and experience peer pressure.	Presenting normative statements or how a majority of others behave.
Social facilitation (SF) [20], [44]	Influence on an individual when surrounded or watched by others.	Displaying how many others are using a system at the same time.
Cooperation (CR) [2], [25], [27]	Activity aimed at achieving a common goal or working together.	Exposing results of cooperative efforts through a system.
Competition (CT) [15], [25], [28]	Endeavoring to gain what others are striving to gain at the same time.	Demonstrating a list of users who are ordered based on their performance.
Recognition (RE) [6], [25], [37]	Value that a person derives from gaining acceptance and approval from others.	Receiving a special title that is displayed to everybody through a system.

3.1 Social Learning

People learn from others by observing their behavior in social contexts [3]. This implies that the information from one individual to another can be transferred through imitation, teaching, and spoken or written language. According to Bandura [4], social learning is ubiquitous and potent, because it allows people to avoid the costs of individual learning. Accordingly, new behavioral patterns can be obtained through observational learning, for example, to share knowledge [11].

3.2 Social Comparison

When individuals use information about other people to evaluate themselves, they engage in social comparison [17]. Specifically, social comparison is described as the process of thinking about others in relation to the self [42]. This process affects motivation, because people tend to look for self-enhancement when comparing themselves *downward* with others who are worse off [40], or individuals look *upward* for self-improvement when seeking a positive example for comparison [41]. In any case, social comparison affects human attitude and behavior [31].

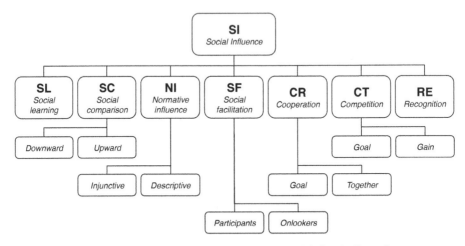

Fig. 2. Structure of the social influence aspects and their sub-dimensions

3.3   Normative Influence

Influence of other people also leads individuals conforming in order to be liked and accepted [16]. Such human action is guided by perceptions of the popularity of certain behavior, that is, by social norms. Research emphasizes that both injunctive and descriptive norms are effective in altering behavior and attitudes of people [23]. *Injunctive* norms inform individuals about what ought to be done, whereas *descriptive* norms refer to what most people actually do [13]. Thus, normative influence affects a wide range of behaviors, e.g. blog usage [22].

3.4   Social Facilitation

The mere or imagined presence of other people in social situations creates an atmosphere of evaluation, which enhances the speed and accuracy of well-practiced tasks, but reduces the performance of less familiar tasks [43]. These social facilitation effects occur in the presence of either passive *onlookers*, or people who are active *participants*, or both [20]. As a result, these effects influence human behavior [44].

3.5   Cooperation, Competition, and Recognition

Interpersonal factors of cooperation, competition, and recognition provide intrinsic motivation that would not be present in the absence of other people [25]. Competition and cooperation are directed toward the same social end by at least two persons [27]. On a social level, people cooperate when they are striving to achieve the same *goal* or are they are working *together*, but compete when they are trying to achieve the same *goal* that is scarce or are seeking to *gain* what others are endeavoring to gain at the same time [28].

Combining the scores of independent tasks performed by different people can encourage cooperation, but providing some salient metric for individuals to compare their performances can promote competition [25]. Meanwhile, recognition can be experienced after competing or cooperating with others [37] or can simply be enjoyed when gaining acceptance and approval from others [6]. The three motivating factors influence various behaviors, including learning [25] and the use of podcasts for generating a sense of community [18].

4   Meta-analysis

To enrich an understanding of how to effectively harness the previously reviewed social influence aspects for enhanced user engagement through socio-technical environments, this section presents a meta-analysis of four empirical studies conducted using partial least squares structural equation modeling (PLS-SEM) methodology.

The four studies (Table 2) were selected based on the shared methodological approach, context, and equal granularity in the exploration of three to seven of the social influence aspects [38]. To the best of accessible knowledge, there were no other comparable studies for inclusion into the present meta-analysis of four socially influencing systems.

Table 2. The list of analyzed studies [38]

Study	Description	Examined aspects
I	Empirical study involving 37 users of a socially influencing system designed for feedback collection through situated displays integrated with Twitter	SL, SF, CR, CT, RE
II	Empirical study involving 69 users of a socially influencing system designed for feedback collection through situated displays integrated with Twitter	SL, SC, NI
III	Empirical study involving 101 participants and a socially influencing system designed for collaborative engagement through situated displays integrated with Twitter	SL, SF, CR
IV	Empirical study involving 77 users of a socially influencing system designed for feedback collection through situated displays integrated with Twitter	SL, SC, NI, SF, CR, CT, RE

The analysis was performed in several consecutive steps. First, the structural models from all studies were reviewed in terms of the present social influence aspects and directed paths (arrows) interconnecting them (Table 3). Second, all seven aspects were mapped out into a single model and all arrows from original models were drawn into the new model. Third, if there were several arrows connecting a pair of aspects, i.e. same directed path originated from several studies (Table 3), only one arrow was kept to represent all of them.

Table 3. Summary of the directed paths from all studies

Directed path between aspects		From study
Social facilitation → Social learning	SF → SL	III
Social facilitation → Social comparison	SF → SC	IV
Social facilitation → Cooperation	SF → CR	I
Social facilitation → Competition	SF → CT	I
Social learning → Social comparison	SL → SC	II
Social learning → Normative influence	SL → NI	II
Social learning → Cooperation	SL → CR	I, III, IV
Social comparison → Normative influence	SC → NI	II
Social comparison → Competition	SC → CT	IV
Competition → Recognition	CT → RE	IV
Recognition → Cooperation	RE → CR	I, IV
Cooperation → Normative influence	CR → NI	IV

Fourth, to obtain deeper understanding of particular interaction effects between the social influence aspects, each arrow was reviewed separately before its inclusion in the final framework structure of the meta-analysis (Fig. 3).

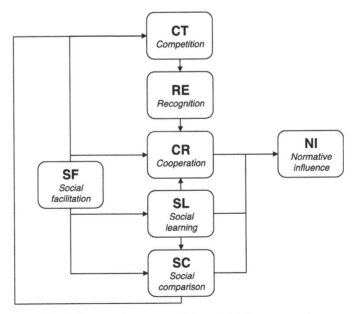

Fig. 3. Framework structure of the social influence aspects

In further analysis, the social facilitation [20] aspect was found to be the only aspect that has no inbound arrows from other social influence aspects in the original structural models. At the same time, the social facilitation aspect directly affected the social learning (study III), social comparison (study IV), competition, and cooperation (both in study I) aspects. The social learning [3-4] aspect was found as one of the most central aspects in all of the studies - having strong direct effects on the cooperation (studies I, III, and IV), normative influence (study II), and social comparison (study II) aspects. The social comparison [17] aspect was found to have strong direct effects on the normative influence (study II) and competition (study IV) aspects.

The competition [15] aspect was found to have strong direct effects on the recognition aspect (study IV). The recognition [6] aspect, in turn, was found to have a strong direct effect on the cooperation aspect (studies I and IV). But, the cooperation [2] aspect was found to have a strong direct effect on the normative influence aspect (study IV). Finally, the normative influence [13] aspect was found to be the only aspect that has no outbound arrows to other social influence aspects.

5 Towards a Framework for Socially Influencing Systems

The reviewed social influence aspects and the output of the meta-analysis provide grounds for making seminal steps towards the development of a solid framework for designing and evaluating socially influencing systems. The achieved results can help deepen understanding of how social influence aspects are affecting each other, and therefore advancing further theory development with regards to the role of each aspect in explaining and predicting how influential an envisioned socially influencing system will be.

5.1 How to Read the Framework

Designers of future socially influencing systems will find the structural framework (Fig. 3) beneficial with some additional guidance. Therefore, this section provides basic instruction for interpreting the presented interconnectedness of the social influence aspects. For example, the social facilitation aspect does not have any inbound arrows but has four outbound arrows directed to other aspects. This implies that social influence effects may commence as soon as other people are present [20]. In the presence of others [44], people can begin to learn from others [3-5], to compare themselves with others [17], and to cooperate [2] or to compete [15] with them.

Following the same logic, the arrow from the social comparison to the competition aspect implies that when people are able to compare themselves with others [17] they are likely to be prompted to compete [15] with those who are better than them, which also might create a sense of social norms [16]. The arrow from the competition to the recognition aspect explains that people who are ranked higher naturally receive some kind of public recognition [25] as others can see how well they have performed. Meanwhile, those who receive public recognition [6] can become more motivated to keep up their excellent performance, which means that they would continue contributing to a collective goal in a cooperative context [28].

Social learning has always played an important role in the evolution of mankind [3-5], because it helps kids to learn quickly just by observing what adults do, to put it simply. The performed meta-analysis reveals that the vast majority of arrows going out from the social learning aspect bear very strong, large, and highly significant effects on succeeding aspects. The framework presents that in a social context people can learn how to compare themselves to others [17], cooperate [27], and read or create an understanding about social norms [16]. Besides, the more people cooperate the more likely they will experience cooperation as a norm for the particular occasion.

In the framework, the arrows are not meant to be completely isolated, i.e. if there is an aspect which has both inbound and outbound arrows, then there is a high likelihood that the aspect also plays a mediating role. For example, besides the direct effect of the social learning aspect on the normative influence aspect, the reviewed studies [38] also reveal significant mediating effects of both the social comparison and cooperation aspects on the relationship.

5.2   Implications for Further Research

The results of the meta-analysis reveal the strength and prominence of social influence aspects in designing socially influencing systems for user engagement. While the world gets increasingly interconnected, such systems could help build novel socio-technical environments for active participation and contribution rather than for passive consumption [30].

The paper reviewed four socially influencing systems (Table 2) that are potentially applicable and useful for engaging people in a wide range of contexts, including business and education. According to earlier studies, socially influencing systems could enable organizations to facilitate innovative collaborations with customers [32], designing novel models for better anticipation of market changes [34], effective responses to customer needs, and catalyzing innovations [21]. In education, these systems could positively impact student learning and engagement [7].

Further research should focus on testing the current framework and expanding research into other potential social influence aspects. Such studies would contribute to a richer and more elaborate understanding of various social influence aspects and their effects when software features them in user interfaces. The next steps should also include a deeper analysis of how social influence aspects can explain the perceived persuasiveness of socially influencing systems and predict user involvement, participation, and engagement with such systems [38].

Another direction for further research would be to study the design of particular implementations of social influence aspects. The number of different designs for a single social influence aspect is limitless. Thus, this research direction would reveal new design patterns that might have increased potential to shape user behavior and attitude. These designs then should be applied and tested in various contexts to find their best fit.

6   Conclusions

The presented meta-analysis is a highly relevant and timely research effort, because it advances the methodology for engineering future socially influential systems [24]. Along these lines, the present paper provides both researchers and practitioners with richer insights on how social influence aspects can help them to build socio-technical environments aimed at facilitating behavioral and attitudinal changes.

Drawing upon a list of fundamental socio-psychological theories, such as social cognitive theory [4], social comparison theory [17], focus theory of normative conduct [13], social facilitation theory [20], cooperation theory [2], competition theory [15], and taxonomy of intrinsic motivators [25], this paper explored a list of seven social influence aspects and their interconnectedness. In achieving that, four empirical studies based on partial least squares structural equation modeling (PLS-SEM) approach were methodologically analyzed.

Main contributions of the meta-analysis include the reviewed background of social influence aspects and the originated framework structure for designing and evaluating socially influencing systems. These contributions supplement the existing body of knowledge and can be instrumental for scholars focusing on research related to persuasive engineering of socially influencing systems for behavior change.

For the future, socially influencing systems can open up new seamless and natural channels for businesses to engage with customers. These channels can potentially play a significant role in advancing customer relationships, as they enable immediate interaction at the place and time where customers acquire new experiences about certain product or services.

Presented research includes a limited number of empirical studies that were available for the current review. Thus, scholars are encouraged to conduct similar studies in order to extend the meta-analysis [38] and overall understanding of the role of social aspects in the typology of computer-supported influence [39].

References

1. Appleford, S., Bottum, J.R., Thatcher, J.B.: Understanding the Social Web: Towards Defining an Interdisciplinary Research Agenda for Information Systems. ACM SIGMIS Database 45(1), 29–37 (2014)
2. Axelrod, R.: On Six Advances in Cooperation Theory. Analyse & Kritik 22(1), 130–151 (2000)
3. Bandura, A.: Social Learning Theory. Prentice Hall, Englewood Cliffs (1977)
4. Bandura, A.: Social Foundations of Thought and Action: A Social Cognitive Theory. Prentice Hall, Englewood Cliffs (1986)
5. Bandura, A.: Social cognitive theory of mass communication. Media Psychology 3(3), 265–299 (2001)
6. Baumeister, R.F.: The self. In: Gilbert, D.T., Fiske, S.T., Lindzey, G. (eds.) The Handbook of Social Psychology, pp. 680–740. McGraw–Hill, New York (1998)

7. Blasco-Arcas, L., Buil, I., Hernández-Ortega, B., Javier Sese, F.: Using Clickers in Class. The Role of Interactivity, Active Collaborative Learning and Engagement in Learning Performance. Computers Science Education 13(2), 137–172 (2012)
8. Cacioppo, J.T., Petty, R.E., Stoltenberg, C.D.: Processes of Social Influence: The Elaboration Likelihood Model of Persuasion. In: Kendall, P.C. (ed.) Advances in Cognitive-Behavioral Research and Therapy, pp. 215–274. Academic Press, San Diego (1985)
9. Chatterjee, S., Price, A.: Healthy Living with Persuasive Technologies: Framework, Issues, and Challenges. Journal of the American Medical Informatics Association 16(2), 171–178 (2009)
10. Cheng, Y., Liang, J., Leung, L.: Social Network Service Use on Mobile Devices: An Examination of Gratifications, Civic Attitudes and Civic Engagement in China. New Media & Society (2014)
11. Chiu, C.M., Hsu, M.H., Wang, E.T.: Understanding Knowledge Sharing in Virtual Communities: An Integration of Social Capital and Social Cognitive Theories. Decision Support Systems 42(3), 1872–1888 (2006)
12. Cialdini, R.B.: Influence: The Psychology of Persuasion. HarperCollins e-books (2009)
13. Cialdini, R.B., Kallgren, C.A., Reno, R.R.: A Focus Theory of Normative Conduct: A Theoretical Refinement and Reevaluation of the Role of Norms in Human Behavior. Advances in Experimental Social Psychology 24(20), 1–243 (1991)
14. Crano, W.D., Prislin, R.: Attitudes and Persuasion. Annual Review of Psychology 57, 345–374 (2006)
15. Deutsch, M.: A Theory of Cooperation-Competition and Beyond. In: Handbook of Theories of Social Psychology, vol. 2, p. 275 (2011)
16. Deutsch, M., Gerard, H.B.: A Study of Normative and Informational Social Influences upon Individual Judgment. The Journal of Abnormal and Social Psychology 51(3), 629 (1955)
17. Festinger, L.: A Theory of Social Comparison Processes. Human Relations 7(2), 117–140 (1954)
18. Firpo, D., Kasemvilas, S., Ractham, P., Zhang, X.: Generating a Sense of Community in a Graduate Educational Setting through Persuasive Technology. In: 4th International Conference on Persuasive Technology, p. 41 (2009)
19. Fogg, B.J.: Persuasive Technology: Using Computers to Change What We Think and Do. Morgan Kaufmann, San Francisco (2003)
20. Guerin, B., Innes, J.: Social Facilitation. Cambridge University Press, Cambridge (2009)
21. von Hippel, E.: Democratizing Innovation: The Evolving Phenomenon of User Innovation. International Journal of Innovation Science 1(1), 29–40 (2009)
22. Hsu, C.L., Lin, J.C.C.: Acceptance of Blog Usage: The Roles of Technology Acceptance, Social Influence and Knowledge Sharing Motivation. Information & Management 45(1), 65–74 (2008)
23. Lapinski, M.K., Rimal, R.N.: An Explication of Social Norms. Communication Theory 15(2), 127–147 (2005)
24. Loock, C.M., Staake, T., Landwehr, J.: Green IS Design and Energy Conservation: An Empirical Investigation of Social Normative Feedback. In: International Conference on Information Systems, p. 10 (2011)
25. Malone, T.W., Lepper, M.: Making Learning Fun: A Taxonomy of Intrinsic Motivations for Learning. In: Snow, R.E., Farr, M.J. (eds.) Aptitude, Learning and Instruction: III. Conative and Affective Process Analyses, pp. 223–253. Erlbaum, Hillsdale (1987)
26. Mangold, W.G., Faulds, D.J.: Social Media: The New Hybrid Element of the Promotion Mix. Business Horizons 52(4), 357–365 (2009)

27. May, M.A., Doob, L.W.: Cooperation and Competition. Social Science Research Council Bulletin, 125 (1937)
28. Mead, M.: Cooperation and Competition among Primitive Peoples. McGraw-Hill, New York (1937)
29. Moeller, S., Ciuchita, R., Mahr, D., Odekerken-Schröder, G., Fassnacht, M.: Uncovering Collaborative Value Creation Patterns and Establishing Corresponding Customer Roles. Journal of Service Research 16(4), 471–487 (2013)
30. Mumford, E.: A Socio-Technical Approach to Systems Design. Requirements Engineering 5(2), 125–133 (2000)
31. Mumm, J., Mutlu, B.: Designing Motivational Agents: The Role of Praise, Social Comparison, and Embodiment in Computer Feedback. Computers in Human Behavior 27(5), 1643–1650 (2011)
32. Nambisan, S., Baron, R.A.: Virtual Customer Environments: Testing a Model of Voluntary Participation in Value Co-creation Activities. Journal of Product Innovation Management 26(4), 388–406 (2009)
33. O'Keefe, D.J.: Theories of Persuasion. In: Nabi, R., Oliver, M.B. (eds.) Handbook of Media Processes and Effects. Sage Publications, Thousand Oaks (2009)
34. Prahalad, C.K., Ramaswamy, V.: The New Frontier of Experience Innovation. MIT Sloan Management Review 44(4), 12–18 (2003)
35. Rashotte, L.: Social Influence. The Blackwell Encyclopedia of Social Psychology 9, 562–563 (2007)
36. Ryan, R.M., Deci, E.L.: Self-Determination Theory and the Facilitation of Intrinsic Motivation, Social Development, and Well-Being. American Psychologist 55(1), 68 (2000)
37. Schoenau-Fog, H.: Teaching Serious Issues through Player Engagement in an Interactive Experiential Learning Scenario. Eludamos, Journal for Computer Game Culture 6(1), 53–70 (2012)
38. Stibe, A.: Socially Influencing Systems: Persuading People to Engage with Publicly Displayed Twitter-based Systems. Acta Universitatis Ouluensis (2014)
39. Stibe, A.: Advancing Typology of Computer-Supported Influence: Moderation Effects in Socially Influencing Systems. In: MacTavish, T., Basapur, S. (eds.) Persuasive Technology. LNCS, vol. 9072, pp. 251–262. Springer, Heidelberg (2015)
40. Wills, T.A.: Downward Comparison Principles in Social Psychology. Psychological Bulletin 90(2), 245 (1981)
41. Wilson, S.R., Benner, L.A.: The Effects of Self-Esteem and Situation upon Comparison Choices During Ability Evaluation. Sociometry, 381–397 (1971)
42. Wood, J.V.: What is Social Comparison and How Should We Study It? Personality and Social Psychology Bulletin 22(5), 520–537 (1996)
43. Yerkes, R.M., Dodson, J.D.: The Relation of Strength of Stimulus to Rapidity of Habit-Formation. Journal of Comparative Neurology and Psychology 18(5), 459–482 (1908)
44. Zajonc, R.B.: Social Facilitation. Science 149, 269–274 (1965)

Acttention – Influencing Communities of Practice with Persuasive Learning Designs

Sandra Burri Gram-Hansen[✉] and Thomas Ryberg

Department of Communication and Psychology, Aalborg University, Aalborg, Denmark
{burri,ryberg}@hum.aau.dk

Abstract. Based on the preliminary results of implementing and testing a persuasive learning initiative in the Danish Military, this paper discusses and develops the notion of persuasive learning designs. It is suggested that the acquirement of new knowledge is fundamental to persuasion, and that persuasive learning designs distinguish themselves by leading to sustainable change to the learner's attitude and/or behaviour. A practical example of persuasive learning designs is provided in terms of the interactive location-based learning game Acttention, which has been developed and tested on behalf of the Danish Military and aims to motivate a sustainable environmental attitude and behaviour amongst army employees. The learning design was first implemented, tested and evaluated at the army base on Bornholm in November 2014. The study was conducted in accordance with the Design Based Research approach and the evaluation include both qualitative and quantitative results, based on observations, questionnaires, photo and video documentation and in situ interviews. The results presented in this paper indicate that it may be beneficial to consider different levels of learning when arguing towards a claim of persuasive design within this more established field of research and development. Rather than focus on improving learning technologies or motivating the interest in a subject, persuasive designs may be more efficient when used to influence the communities of practice in educational institutions.

Keywords: Learning · Kairos · Persuasive design · Learning games · Situation-based learning · Communities of practice · e-Learning · Persuasive learning Designs · Design based research · Energy and environmental behaviour · Sustainability

1 Introduction

In this paper, the notion of applying persuasive design in the development of learning designs in complex organisations is analysed and discussed based on the design process and preliminary results from on-going tests and evaluation of persuasive learning designs in the Danish Military. More specifically the environmental education provided to recruits in the Danish army. In November 2014, the Installation Management Command (IMC), a government agency for Military establishments conducted the first of a series of tests where a location and situation based game was used as a supplement or alternative to traditional learning methods.

© Springer International Publishing Switzerland 2015
T. MacTavish and S. Basapur (Eds.): PERSUASIVE 2015, LNCS 9072, pp. 184–195, 2015.
DOI: 10.1007/978-3-319-20306-5_17

The main contribution of this paper constitutes a combination of theoretical and methodological reflections, which lead towards an understanding of the potential of persuasive design in relation to learning. The literature on both learning designs and persuasion is vast, yet research in the cross field between these two fields show that the claim of persuasive design in relation to learning is not easily established. Many learning experts will argue that attitude and behaviour change is a core element in any learning design [1]. As a result, the approach taken to persuasive learning designs in this paper is founded in the rhetorical notion of Kairos [2], and the understanding of persuasive design as being a particular type of context adaptation. By considering persuasive design a meta-perspective, which can be applied to more established design fields such as learning, the persuasive contribution to the design constitutes a strong focus on the intended use context and on the ethical implications of the design [3]. The approach has lead us to the understanding that persuasive design may hold particular potential in relation to learning, when aiming to influence a community of practice in the intended use context, rather than focusing solely on the individual learner or optimizing existing learning technologies.

The energy and environment related challenges that the world is facing are well known to most. The Danish Military is one of the largest organisations in Denmark and as a result the Danish Ministry of Defence has presented an ambitious climate and energy strategy, which addresses ways in which the Danish Military actively wishes to lower the energy consumption level and minimize their influence on the climate [4]. Overall, the Danish Military aims to:

- Lower their energy consumption by 20% compared to 2006
- Increase the use of energy from sustainable sources by 60%
- Reduce Co2 waste by 40% compared to 1990

The Danish Military is a highly complex organisation with a combination of armed forces, technical staff and civilian employees. One of the primary roles of the Danish Military is to function as a particular type of educational institution, where soldiers are educated and trained. The educational engagement of the Danish Military does not only apply to those who chose to become professional soldiers in the Danish armed forces. In Denmark, all eligible young men above the age of 18 are drafted and based on a draw; some are called upon to serve as drafted recruits for 4 months basic Military training. Only 25% of the drafted recruits continue with a military education once their drafting session is complete, but the basic Military training is argued to produce valuable members of society. In light of the drafting policy, the recruits constitute a highly diverse target group, where some may be on their way to a university education, whilst others may struggle to read and write.

The goal to become a more energy and environment efficient organization has not been received solely positive by the employees in the Danish Military. Energy and environment related issues are not a core area for most employees in the Danish Military, and whilst many segments are positive towards the idea of an environment friendly workplace, some find that the strategic goals conflict with the primary tasks of the Military [5]. As such, ICM strives to not only promote an appropriate environment friendly behaviour, but also to motivate a positive attitude towards transforming the Military into a more "green" organisation.

The persuasive learning design discussed in this paper aims to educate the drafted recruits in appropriate waste management and action in case of accidents. The central element in this persuasive learning design is the location- and situation-based game *Acttention*, which has been designed and developed specifically to meet the requirements of the Danish Military. As such, the content is targeted directly towards the drafted recruits, whilst the game is designed to be flexible and easily adjusted to fit the needs of other employee groups.

1.1   On the Relation between Persuasion and Learning

Miller argues that persuasion is most often equated with behaviour change [6]. One reason for this may be that whilst behaviour change is easily identified and evaluated, as opposed to attitude change, which is harder to detect as it is most often expressed through statements regarding a topic and influenced by the given situation. The distinction between attitude change and behaviour change and in particular the recognition that behaviour change is traditionally considered the primary effect of a persuasive initiative is however fundamental to the discussion regarding the potential of persuasive design in relation to learning. In order to distinguish between behaviour changes shaped by persuasive initiatives, and behaviour changes in general, Miller argues that persuasion is to some extent based on learning [6].

Whilst behaviour in general may be influenced by a number of different things such as obstacles on the road, sensory perception or group dynamics, "being persuaded" calls for a deeper understanding of the given situation and an active decision to change behaviour - based on an attitude change. Thereby persuasion distinguishes itself from e.g. commercially based behaviour change and nudging, by constituting a more sustainable and voluntary change. More than simply adjusting behaviour in one given context, persuasion constitutes a behavioural and emotional change, which may potentially be transferred to other situations as it is based on a deeper understanding of appropriateness. For example, one could design a sensor system that would nudge people to take shorter showers, but would not encourage them to turn off the lights when leaving the bathroom. We argue that a persuasive learning design must exceed and transcend a purely behavioural response and should also include a change of attitude or perspective i.e. leading to a generally more environmental sensitivity and behaviour as well as further a shift from individual towards communal focus

In order for a person to change attitude towards a given subject, he or she must acquire new knowledge, either from personal experience or from provided information or a combination of the two. As such, learning becomes a founding element in a persuasive design as learning itself may be seen as the process of acquiring knowledge and adjusting attitude towards a subject accordingly.

As such our understanding of learning transcends training or mere acquisition of knowledge and aligns more with e.g. Wenger's understanding of learning as associated with identity and change of practice or similar notions of learning as transformation [7]. Wenger's social theory of learning and the concept of Communities of Practices departs from the notion that humans are inherently social beings. Learning is not only a matter of memorisation or knowledge but also a matter of becoming someone. A community of practice can be understood as a: "group of people who share a concern or a passion for something they do, and learn how to do it better as they interact

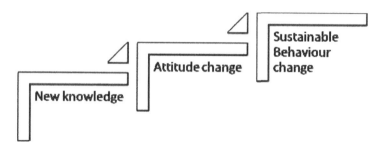

Fig. 1. New knowledge leads to attitude change, which leads to sustainable behaviour change

regularly."[8] This could be a group of physicist learning from each other, but it could equally be a group or platoon of recruits gradually developing a mutual engagement, joint enterprise and a shared repertoire and a sense of meaning with their practice of being new recruits and gradually becoming more experienced together. Further, the army can be understood more broadly as a community of practice in the sense of having certain recognisable practices (certain ways of doing and understanding the world) that sustain over time and which newcomers to the 'community' need to understand and become part of.

2   Design Based Research and the Development of Acttention

Design, implementation and evaluation of the Acttention learning design, is structured in accordance with the Design Based Research methodology (DBR). DBR is a recognised approach to development of learning designs, and distinguishes itself by an iterative approach to design and a distinct focus on participatory design (PD). Furthermore, several researchers have argued that Value Sensitive Design (VSD) and PD may hold particular potential in the development of persuasive technologies, as these approaches enable designers to address and incorporate user values in the design and implementation process [9, 10].

When considering Kairos a key concept in relation to persuasion, PD is argued to be essential to the design process, both due to the ethical implications of the design, and due to the need for a deeper understanding of *appropriate manner* within the intended use context [3].

As visualised above, DBR constitutes an iterative process where designs are developed, tested, evaluated and refined, based on an analysis of problems identified in practice. As participatory design has been argued to be of particularly relevance to persuasive design, both from a theoretical and a practical perspective [3, 9, 12], DBR has facilitated a learning design process where both learning perspectives and persuasive reflections have been equally considered. In the development of the Acttention learning design, participatory design was vital, as designers contributed with new perspectives on learning, whilst the army instructors, who work with the drafted recruits on a daily basis, are the ones with knowledge about the context and the learners. Furthermore, during the tests of the learning design, the involvement of the army instructors throughout the process, ensured credibility for both the learning material

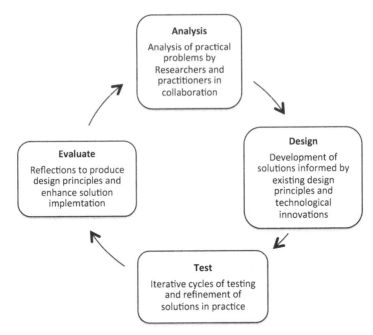

Fig. 2. Visualization of the iterative DBR process, inspired by Reeves (2006)[11]

and the learning design, which might otherwise have been hard to establish. Although the Military considers itself a particular type of educational institution, it is also an organisation with strong traditions, values and hierarchies, and the presence of respected instructors ensured the engagement of the involved platoons.

In the acknowledgement that the employees do not see energy and environment issues as core focus areas, the persuasive learning design has been developed with an intent to influence the community of practice in the Danish Military, rather than strive towards acknowledgement alongside core areas such as weapon management. Communities of practice are referred to as the mutual understanding of appropriate behaviour, which the employees in the Danish Military gain through interaction, reflection and collaborative learning [8]. Communities of practice already exist both on larger and smaller scales within the Military, and as new recruits join or new employees arrive, they are invited into these communities and taught through experience what is considered appropriate.

By moving from instructional learning design to a focus on adjusting practice, the learning design was expected to not only be efficient, but also particularly motivating, as the learning material was tailored specifically towards distinct learner communities [13]. Most importantly however, this approach clearly acknowledges that energy and environment concerns are not a core focus point for most employees in the Danish Military, and should as such not be presented alongside other primary learning topics.

Initially, the Acttention learning design consisted solely of the Acttention game. It was designed as a location based game where the recruits would interact with touch screens, be presented with waste management related questions and then sent to a relevant location on the Military base in order to link the content of the question to a specific location. However, very early in the design process, this solution was found inadequate both from a learning perspective and from a persuasive perspective. Learning wise the game lacked information regarding the appropriate action in different situations. Information which was a necessity if the game was to facilitate learning, rather than merely be a quiz game with 33% chance of answering correct. From a persuasive design perspective, the game lacked clearly defined persuasive intentions both with regards to the in-game situation and regarding the long-term effect.

The notion that persuasive design may be considered a particular type of context adaptation is closely linked to the rhetorical concept Kairos. Kairos is often referred to as an essential in relation to persuasion, and is most often described as the opportune moment to act or trigger a persuadee into changing attitudes or behaviour [2, 14]. The concept sums up the principle that any rhetorical approach is based upon the specific situation, and that comprehension of the context as such is one of the most vital resources when deciding upon which rhetorical means to apply to a given argument. Hansen specifies that the definitions of Kairos vary from narrow translations such as "particular point in time" and "specific circumstance", to wider concepts such as "situation", "occasion", and "opportunity". The narrow and wider definitions of Kairos are inseparable and must be considered in relation to each other [15].

The understanding of Kairos formed the foundation of a persuasive design meta-perspective, which was applied in the design process in order to strengthen both the learning potential and the persuasiveness of the Acttention game. An instructional film was created to ensure that all recruits were presented with knowledge regarding appropriate waste management. Consequently, the Acttention game transferred from being a learning game to being a tool for evaluating the recruits' knowledge about waste management, whilst placing them in a situation, which to some degree simulated the situation they might find themselves in when the acquired knowledge becomes relevant.

In the process of bridging from location- to situation-based learning, the notion of Kairos furthermore promoted reflection regarding not just the learning situation, but also the situation the recruits would likely find themselves in when needing to recall their knowledge about appropriate waste management. Accidents in relations to e.g. fuel spillage rarely happen when people are calm and focused, they more likely occur when attention is directed towards something else – such as a physical and mentally demanding army activity. In order to simulate a situation where the recruits are forced to focus on several challenges at the same time, the recruits are required to not only answer the Acttention questions correctly, they must also run to a designated destination, retrieve a three digit colour code and memorise the code until they return to their team's touch screen. Once the code is entered, the recruit is awarded points based on a combination of correct answer to the question, hastiness and entering the correct colour code. Answering the question correctly is weighed most heavily and points for hastiness and colour code are only awarded as bonus for a correct answer.

During the test iterations, the learning design was evaluated through a combination of qualitative and quantitative methods, ensuring that both the learning potential and the persuasiveness of the design were assessed. Preliminary findings indicate that combination of instructional film and location-based learning facilitate a transition from individual learning to collaborate learning. This blended learning approach and in particular the collaborative activities in the team-based learning game, ensured that all members of the platoon were able to engage in the learning experience and reflect upon the learning material.

Results from the first test show that more than 71% of the recruits completed with results that meet or exceed the expectations of the Defence Academy. From a persuasive perspective, the learning design was well received by the recruits, who found it particularly positive to be physically active while learning, and who found the competitive element to be highly motivating. After completing the game, 78% of the recruits indicated that they found the learning material relevant and useful, and 81% indicated that learning about appropriate waste management had been fun. In light of the previously mentioned negativity towards the subject, the feedback regarding the learning experience was received as highly positive and promising.

3   Reflections

The decision to focus on influencing the community of practice rather than insist on a more traditional approach to learning design, is further based on the previously described understanding of the relationship between learning and persuasion. In this situation, the intended attitude and behaviour change is not directly related to the overall educational aim (training soldiers), but instead related to motivating an attitude and behaviour amongst the recruits, which may optimize their ability to work in the Danish Military and in continuation become better learners within this particular context. The distinction between levels of learning is important for several reasons. First of all, by acknowledging that education takes place on several levels and cannot be related solely to defined courses or training sessions, the persuasive intention may be more clearly defined and thus better implemented in the design. Secondly, by acknowledging the different levels of learning and focusing on educating better learners, the more established field of learning and learning design is more appropriately acknowledged and not approached as an area requiring improvement. The aim of persuasive learning designs is not to ensure better learning in a traditionally defined course, but to facilitate the learning experience by motivating learners to engage in the learning experience and to motivate a sustainable behaviour change.

By bridging from location- to situation-based learning, the Acttention learning designs become more flexible and mobile and hold the potential to be applied to any army facility in Denmark or in contexts outside the Military. Whilst locations are still applied in form of the destinations where the recruits go to retrieve colour codes they are used simply as reference points and can be changed according to new contexts. The locations currently applied in the Acttention game are chosen because they are present on all Danish army bases (barracks, garage, recycling area etc.), but the distance between them and the way they are used in daily practice may differ from base to base. Questions in the game are related to the location on a contextual level i.e. questions regarding fuel spillage will result in the recruit being sent to one of the locations where this situation might occur.

The recruits' knowledge about waste management stems from their existing knowledge and experiences as well as their understanding of practice in the community they are already a part of. The knowledge is actualised and related to their current situation by the instructional film. As such, the learning design to some extent draws upon Piaget's understanding of learning as an assimilative process [16] Most recruits already had some knowledge about appropriate waste management, and the introduction film ensured that their knowledge was put in relation to army activities and adjusted when necessary.

One of the objectives in the design and development of the Acttention learning designs, was to motivate a more positive attitude towards energy and climate education in the Danish Military, by creating a learning design which is time efficient but also fun and engaging. In order to reach an appropriate balance between serious learning and fun, the Acttention learning design facilitates a transition from an instructional, individual learning focus to collaborative learning. This blend of pedagogical approaches does not only help ensure that more members of a highly diverse target group understand the learning material they are presented with, it also motivates an important change in the behaviour of recruits during the learning process. Work and education in the Military is generally dominated by strict discipline and a strong sense of hierarchy. The recruits are trained to focus and pay attention when instructions are given, and they are also educated to trust and respect the orders they are given – and to comply without further considerations. The latter is important in situations where soldiers take part in armed action, however with a learning design aimed to motivate a sustainable attitude change both within and beyond Military duty, reflections and deeper understanding of the material is believed to be a necessity - particularly as the acquired knowledge must be transferrable to different situations both in the Military context and in civilian life.

As the recruits watched the instruction film, they displayed the level of focus and commitment usually required by them. Once the instruction film was finished, the recruits were instructed to go to a designated location on the Military base, where the touchscreens had been set up. Here they were given further information about how to play the Acttention game, and divided in to smaller teams of 5-6 members. As the terms of the game and the team competition was explained, the recruits' seriousness was replaced with a more playful and relaxed attitude – still without losing focus on what was being required from them. The team spirit and the more relaxed and collaborative attitude was facilitated further by elements such as selecting a team name.

The element of competition was well received by the recruits, and during the evaluation it was emphasized as being a particular highlight of the learning design. Although the recruits were visibly exhausted after completing the game, several of them indicated that they would have liked more questions in the game – and some even asked if they could do another round right away.

More importantly however, the team element of the Acttention game also motivated the members to collaborate on answering the questions correctly. When two or more members of a team were present at the touchscreen at the same time, they would discuss the questions and the different solutions, knowing that they would all be faced with the same question at some point. Facilitating a dialogue was considered particularly important in consideration of the design intent to influence the community of practice. Besides from ensuring that all recruits were aware of appropriate environmental behaviour

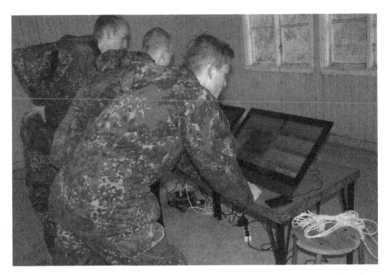

Image 1 - Recruits discuss the different solutions as they collaborate to complete the scenarios of the Acttention learning design

on the army base, the intent was also to motivate conversations about the different solutions. Part

The transition to a more relaxed and collaborative learning environment was important for two particular reasons:

1. The discussions amongst the recruits, and the articulation of why a certain answer was correct, required that the recruits actually reflect upon the questions. By demonstrating their ability to explain the correct answers while playing the game, the recruits also demonstrate that they not only know they answers they also understand why the answer is correct [17].
2. The collaboration between recruits also constitutes the situation where the community of practice was potentially influenced. Communities of practice are according to Wenger defined as a mutual understanding of appropriate behaviour, gained through reflection, negotiation and collaboration [8].

While we could focus on the individual recruit's acquisition of particular knowledge, the social and collaborative aspects of the game aim to leverage their shared negotiation of meaning. This to transform 'appropriate behaviour' from an abstracted checklist of correct answers towards a focus on lived experience of participation in a particular community of practice i.e. being a competent practitioner/recruit.

In general, the results of the first test iteration of the Acttention learning design were good and the design was well received by both recruits and the instructors who participated. In accordance with the DBR approach to this project, the instructors were involved throughout the entire iteration, including the evaluation of the iteration. From the perspective of the instructor, particular attention was directed towards other educational topics, which might also benefit from an Acttention inspired approach. Particular approval was given to the flexibility of the system, its ability to be implemented into scheduled activities such as physical training, and its versatility. Also, it was noted that the game requires very little guidance and as such demands very few instructors to be involved. The evaluation comments provided by the instructors were considered particular important with regards to the persuasive effect of the learning design, as this first iteration not only functioned as a test of the game but also aimed to motivate the instructors to take on a more positive attitude towards the requirements for environment education.

Although it may be intriguing to consider more areas to apply a well-received learning game, this was not found recommendable. Many games tend to become less interesting if they are played too often or for too long, and more importantly, not all learning material is suitable to be turned into game content. As mentioned, the Danish Military considers itself a particular type of educational institution, where soldiers are educated and trained. A core educational focus of this institution is to ensure that the soldiers are able to handle armed action in international missions, and as such the previously mentioned seriousness and focus of the recruits should not be compromised.

4   Future Research

Whilst the first iteration of testing the Acttention learning design has indicated the efficiency of the design both in relation to learning and in motivating an attitude change towards environmental education in the Military, future research will focus on transferability of knowledge and on a deeper understanding of the potential of persuasive design in relation to learning.

During spring 2015, two more test iterations are planned to take place. Iteration 2 will take place at one of the largest army bases in Denmark. The iteration will focus particularly on optimization of the learning design and on evaluating the mobility and flexibility of the design. It is considered a requisite that the learning design is applicable across different Military bases if Acttention is to be fully implemented as part of the educational program.

The third iteration aims to test the transferability and sustainability of knowledge. Recruits who have completed the Acttention learning design during their basic Military training and decided to continue with further Military education, will be asked to play the Acttention game again 3-4 months later without watching the instructional film. The goal is to evaluate the results in order to see if the recruits are still able to recall the correct answers even though they have not been confronted with the learning material for a while. If possible, the third iteration will take place outside the Military base at a location less familiar to the recruits. Thereby, the pressure to handle more situations at the same time will increase, as the recruits will not only have to answer the questions correctly, but also focus more on navigating in an unfamiliar location.

Previous research has indicated that the claim of persuasive design in relation to learning is not easily established due to the overlap between these two fields. Results from the first iteration of testing the Acttention learning design gives reason to consider that persuasive design may have a stronger claim, if aimed towards motivating an appropriate behaviour within a learning context, rather than a particular attitude towards a given subject.

The Acttention learning design and in particular the location- and situation-based learning game facilitates the learning, which relates to the communities of practice both on and beyond the Military bases. I.e. it does not aim to turn the primary elements in a basic Military education into a game, but to ensure that the recruits understand appropriate behaviour on and beyond the Military base. This is a focus on education, which may quite easily be transferred to other more classical educational institutions such as high schools or universities. Students who attend university do so to focus on getting a particular education or studying a particular subject (i.e. Medicine). However in order to become good students they also need to learn how to study and how to become a member of the community of practice that exists at their university. For some students the adjustment to learning at university level comes easy, but for others it is a large transition from what they have been used to previously.

Future research will include a further exploration of considering persuasive design a perspective which may facilitate better learning – not by producing better learning designs, but by motivating a more learning-oriented behaviour amongst students in educational institutions.

Acknowledgements. The practical example presented in this paper was arranged in collaboration with Boie Skov Frederiksen, Thomas Troels Klingemann and Thilde Møller Larsen from The Danish Ministry of Defence - Estates and Infrastructure Organisation, and with the support and collaboration of Senior Sargent Jan Meiner, Almegaard Kaserne, Bornholm. The Acttention game is developed in collaboration with experience design experts from Bunker43.

References

1. Gram-Hansen, S.B., Schärfe, H., Dinesen, J.V.: Plotting to Persuade - Exploring the theoretical cross field between Persuasion and Learning. In: Bang, M., Ragnemalm, E.L. (eds.) PERSUASIVE 2012. LNCS, vol. 7284, pp. 262–267. Springer, Heidelberg (2012)
2. Glud, L.N., Jespersen, J.: Leth Conceptual analysis of Kairos for Location-based mobile devices, pp. 17–21. University of Oulu. Department of Information Processing Science. Series A, Research Papers (2008)
3. Gram-Hansen, S.B., Ryberg, T.: Persuasion, Learning and Context Adaptation. Special Issue of the International Journal on Conceptual Structures and Smart Applications (2013)
4. Defence, D.M.O.: Forsvarets Klima og Energi. strategi (2012) [cited 2012]
5. Operate, Målgruppeanalyse og Segmentering (2012)
6. Miller, G.R.: On Being Persuaded, Some Basic Distinctions. In: Dillard, J.P., Pfau, M. (eds.) The Persuasion Handbook, Developments in Theory and Practice. Saga Publications, London (2002)
7. Engeström, Y.: Learning by Expanding: An Activity-theoretical Approach to Developmental Research. Orienta-Konsultit Oy (1987)
8. Wenger, E.: Communities of Practice - Learning, Meaning and Identity. Cambridge University Press (1998)
9. Davis, J.: Design methods for ethical persuasive computing. In: Proceedings of the 4th International Conference on Persuasive Technology. ACM, Claremont (2009)
10. Davis, J.: Generating Directions for Persuasive Technology Design with the Inspiration Card Workshop. In: Ploug, T., Hasle, P., Oinas-Kukkonen, H. (eds.) PERSUASIVE 2010. LNCS, vol. 6137, pp. 262–273. Springer, Heidelberg (2010)

11. Reeves, T.C.: Design research from a technology perspective. Educational Design research, pp. 52–66. Routledge, London (2006)
12. Davis, J.: Towards Participatory Design of Ambient Persuasive Technology. In: Pervasive 2008 Workshop Preceedings, Sydney, Australia (2008)
13. Fogg, B.: Persuasive Technology, Using Computers to change what we Think and Do. Morgan Kaufmann Publishers (2003)
14. Aagaard, M., Øhrstrøm, P., Moltsen, L.: It might be Kairos. In: Persuasive 2008. Springer, Oulu Finland (2008)
15. Hansen, J.B.: Den rette tale på det rette tidspunkt. RetorikMagasinet, 74 (2009)
16. Vejleskov, L.: Tænkningens udvikling - en introduktion til Piaget. Dansk Psykologisk Forlag, København (1999)
17. Bloom, B.S., et al.: Taxonomy of educational objectives: The classification of educational goals. In: Handbook I: Cognitive Domain. David McKay Company, New York (1956)

Ethical Challenges in Emerging Applications of Persuasive Technology

Jelte Timmer[✉], Linda Kool, and Rinie van Est

Rathenau Instituut, Anna van Saksenlaan 51, 2593HW, The Hague, The Netherlands
{j.timmer,l.kool,q.vanest}@rathenau.nl
http://www.rathenau.nl

Abstract. Persuasive technologies are gaining ground. As they enter into society they are being applied in more situations, and integrated with other technologies in increasingly smart environments. We argue that this development creates new challenges in designing ethically responsible persuasive technologies. Applications in social contexts like work environments raise the questions whether persuasion serves the interests of the user or the employer, and whether users can still voluntarily choose to use the technology. Informing the user and obtaining consent become complicated when persuasive systems are integrated in smart environments. To ensure that the autonomy of the user is respected, we argue that the user and provider should agree on the goal of persuasion, and users should be informed about persuasion in smart environments.

Keywords: Persuasive technology · Ethics · Autonomy · Smart environments

1 Introduction

Over the past years there has been growing interest in design strategies to change people's behavior. Governments are setting up 'nudging units' – such as the UK behavioral insights team – to design tax forms to increase payment rates [1]. And companies like Nike are employing badges and other game design features to stimulate Nike+ members to exercise more.

Such efforts can be described as persuasive technologies, defined by B.J. Fogg [2] as a brand of technologies designed explicitly to influence and change people's behavior or attitudes. Persuasive technology integrates insights derived from psychology and cognitive science into the design of information systems. We encounter persuasive technologies in cars, where ecodrive systems assist users in adapting environmentally friendly driving styles. Or in personal health, where apps like *RunKeeper* encourage users to exercise more. And even in personal finance where software like *You Need a Budget* promote a responsible approach to personal finances.

The use of persuasive technologies has inspired discussions about how persuasive technologies ought to be designed responsibly. The ethics of persuasion has been an important issue in persuasive technology since it's early development [3] Important questions are: who benefits from the employment of a given persuasive technology?

© Springer International Publishing Switzerland 2015
T. MacTavish and S. Basapur (Eds.): PERSUASIVE 2015, LNCS 9072, pp. 196–201, 2015.
DOI: 10.1007/978-3-319-20306-5_18

Are persuasion strategies employed considered ethically responsible? As noted by Fogg [2] and others [3,4] there is a tension between persuasion and coercion or even manipulation. Spahn [4] defines this as the fundamental ethical question with regard to persuasive technologies. The relation between persuasion and autonomy is complex and a subject of discussion in many studies on ethics of persuasion [4,5].

To ensure ethically responsible design of persuasive technologies, guiding principles have been put forward by different authors [3,4]. The user should, for instance, always be informed about persuasion and should consent to being subjected to it [4]. Simply stated, as long as the user is 'free' to choose his goals and methods of persuasion of his own accord his autonomy is respected.

These principles hold when the individual has the ability to make an informed decision of his own. However, the ongoing development of persuasive technologies poses a challenge. Persuasive technologies are increasingly applied in a 'collective' setting, in which others, such as employers, stimulate or even mandate the use of persuasive technologies. For example, the oil-company BP has made activity trackers available to its staff [6]. In such collective situations it might be harder for the individual to make an autonomous choice about the goals he is being persuaded to, or whether he consent to the use persuasive technologies.

The expansion of persuasive technologies to new forms and contexts of application gives rise to new questions for designing ethically responsible persuasive technologies. We will discuss the application of persuasion in collective situations like the work environment (which we call **proliferation**), and discuss the **integration** of persuasive technologies with ambient intelligence and the internet of things [7].

We will describe the proliferation and integration of persuasive technologies using a number of examples. These examples show how persuasive technologies are used in different contexts, and can be used to explore the social and ethical impacts of these emerging applications of persuasion. We will conclude with a discussion of what is needed to safeguard autonomy in these new applications of persuasive technology.

2   Proliferation

As persuasive technologies move from research applications to the market, the range of contexts in which they are employed expands. Use scenarios of persuasive technologies tend to focus on the interaction between the user and the technology – i.e. an individual driver being persuaded to drive safer. But when we move to the market, the social context becomes more important. We cited the example of BP that has made Fitbit activity trackers available to its staff as part of its wellness program. Employees were challenged to join the 'Million Step Challenge' to earn wellness points which could be used for cuts in health insurance expenses [6]. BP is not alone; an increasing number of companies is stimulating the use of activity trackers by their employees and health insurers have initiated insurance schemes that promote the use of persuasive activity trackers for lower premiums. Compen, Ham & Spahn [5] describe an example of a persuasive technology for energy saving employed in a collective setting. Daimler Fleetboard is a system that uses GPS in trucks to enable fleet managers to analyze fuel consumption and driving style. This information is fed back to the truck drivers to persuade them to drive more fuel efficient. However, the fleet manager can also access the information for other goals than fuel saving [5].

In these new social contexts the provider of the technology (the employer or insurer) plays a crucial role when we want to assess whether the autonomy of the user is respected. In the case of BP, the fact that the user is offered the Fitbit as part of the company wellness program has influence on the users decision whether or not to use that technology, and on the extent to which he is able to choose his own goals.

These applications of persuasive technologies in a collective rather than an individual context, show that the proliferation of persuasive technologies gives rise to new questions. Who defines the goal and who benefits from the persuasion? Can the user still make an autonomous choice regarding the use of persuasive technology? This translates to the discussion of two dimensions in this paper: 1) the degree in which users agree to the goal of persuasion, and 2) the degree to which he can freely choose to use persuasive technology, see Table 1. We will argue that as we move to the bottom right corner of the table, persuasion becomes ethically problematic.

Table 1. Two dimensions of issues in emerging persuasive technologies

	Agreement on goal	No agreement on goal
Voluntary		
Mandatory		

2.1   Goals

To design an ethically responsible persuasive system, Spahn [4] notes that it should grant as much autonomy to the user as possible. For instance through setting his own goals, or by determining the persuasive strategies a system is allowed to use. In our two examples it becomes clear that in a collective situation the user will not always be able to determine his own goals. Rather, the provider – in this case the employer or fleet manager – determines the goals for the user.

The user and provider may share the same goals. The employee partaking in the wellness program will most likely be looking for ways to improve his health. And the driver using Fleetboard may have a shared interest in reducing his carbon footprint. Ideally, both parties would then profit equally, but their interests might also diverge. The actual goal of the fleet manager might not so much be reducing the carbon footprint, but saving money by maximizing fleet efficiency. What is promoted to the driver as a technology to increase sustainability, can be employed for other uses, like monitoring the behavior of the driver, his breaks and downtime [5]. This is also called *function creep*, a system put into place for one goal is repurposed for another goal. Had the driver known the Fleetboard system would also be used to monitor his behavior, he might not have consented to it.

When user and provider don't share the same goals, it is important whether the user is can refrain from using the persuasive system. For the Fleetboard driver this means that he would be able to stop participating in the program if he disagrees with the goals set by the provider. However if an employer would mandate its use, this would mean a violation of his autonomy. Persuasion would shift towards coercion since the user is persuaded to a goal he doesn't agree with. This brings us to our second dimension: the degree to which the use of a persuasive system is voluntary (2.2).

2.2   Voluntariness

When persuasion is offered in a collective setting this may affect the degree to which a user can voluntarily choose for persuasion. In the example of BP, the wellness program and the "Million Step Challenge" are voluntary. However, factors such as group pressure in a work environment, or implicit norms can influence the degree in which the user is truly able to make an autonomous choice. The inherent asymmetric power relationship between employers and employees impacts the user's level of autonomy. In addition, Morozov [10] asks if wellness programs with the added bonus of cuts in health expenses, can really be considered voluntary. He explains that for people on a tight budget it might not be much of a free choice, since they need to participate in order to qualify for indispensable health benefits.

As outlined above it is conceivable that a provider would mandate the use of a persuasive technology. An employer could mandate participation in the corporate wellness program, or a government could mandate a persuasive smart metering system. This can be considered an infringement of the autonomy of the user. This is especially problematic when the user and provider do not agree on the goal of persuasion. The question is whether the benefits are such that the infringement is justifiable. Where persuasion is mandated by a central agent – e.g. an employer, a health insurer or government body – critical scrutiny is necessary, as well as careful consideration of the ways in which autonomy can be respected. Mandatory persuasion should not be considered lightly. The Dutch Council for Social Development recently published an advice for the Dutch government in which it states that collective applications of persuasion or nudging should be approached cautiously, and require transparency about the methods of persuasion and an open discussion about the goals being pursued [9].

3   Integration

When considering emerging applications of persuasive technologies we also have to be aware of other developments in technology that intersect with persuasive technology. In 2003 Aarts and Marzano [10] projected their vision for the future of information technology entitled ambient intelligence. Technology would integrate with our surroundings and fade into the background. Everyday technologies would be able to communicate with each other and intelligently interact with users. Following their vision technology would become: embedded; environmentally aware; personalized; anticipatory; and adjustable to environment and user.

Developments around what is referred to as the Internet of Things are bringing the ambient intelligence vision a step closer to reality. The consumer market is seeing more 'smart' devices that are able to connect to the internet, are equipped with sensors, and can interact with the user or other devices. Examples are Philip Hue Lightbulbs, Nest Thermostats, smart TV's, and Apple's software platform HomeKit.

Persuasive technology can integrate or hatch on to these smart environments. This means they will also move into the background and become less explicit to the user. The networked nature of smart devices also enables persuasive technologies to connect and interact with these devices, enabling feedback to become multimodal. A scenario could be a persuasive system that is designed to help a user sleep better, it could comprise of an app and wristband measuring sleep quality, and could interact with the smart TV and smart lighting. Giving feedback via TV that the user should prepare to get to bed, and adjusting the lighting to a more sleep-inducing color.

The integration of persuasive technology with ambient intelligence raises new questions for ethically responsible persuasion. Maan et al [11] have shown that it is possible to influence people using low-cognitive light feedback. These types of *ambient persuasion* can enable situations in which the user is being influenced without consciously being aware of it. This limits the capability of the user to evaluate and reflect on the persuasion and its goals and whether he consents to those.

When things happen effortlessly and in the background, there are fewer naturally occurring moments of interaction between the user and the system to ensure the users consent. Therefore keeping the user informed is very important [12]. For instance when data transfers happen in the background it is important to inform the user about how data is collected and shared with other applications in a smart environment. Transparency requires extra effort in these situations.

This is not only important in securing consent and respecting the users autonomy, it is also important in keeping the system understandable for the user. The fact that technology becomes networked and these processes operate in the background can make a system hard to understand and to trust. Research in virtual training software suggest that designing technology as an *explaining agent* might help to inform users and establish trust [13].

4   Conclusion

We have discussed how the proliferation and integration of persuasive technology create challenges for the design of ethically responsible persuasive technology. We conclude that the social context in which persuasive technology is employed is becoming more important. When thinking about the ethics of persuasion we need to move beyond scenarios of user and technology and include the context of the provider of the technology. Methods like Value Sensitive Design and Participatory Design could provide a valuable way of taking these stakeholders into account [14].

As we have seen the provider is able to define goals or mandate the use of a persuasive technology, giving rise to new ethical dilemmas. We assert that mandatory persuasion should be avoided or approached cautiously. Open discussion and agreement on goals, methods and interests of user and provider should be ensured. Transparency about the interests of different stakeholders involved is essential. Compen, Spahn and Ham [5] plea for an 'information leaflet' to inform the user of methods and goals of a persuasive system. As more collective applications of persuasive technologies emerge - for instance in healthcare and insurance - research is needed on the role of these third parties as providers of persuasion and how they impact the users autonomy. Both designer and provider will have a responsibility here.

The integration of persuasive technology with ambient intelligence offers new possibilities for multimodal persuasive systems, but also create a more complex environment in which persuasion moves into the background. This complicates conscious deliberation and reflection by the user. In order to remain trustworthy a challenge lies in creating systems that can inform and explain their behavior to the user.

References

1. Behavioral Insights Team.: Applying behavioural insights to reduce fraud, error and debt. Cabinet Office, London (2012)
2. Fogg, B.J.: Persuasive Technology: Using Computers to Change What We Think and Do. Morgan Kaufmann, San Francisco (2002)
3. Berdichevsky, D., Neuenschwander, E.: Toward an Ethics of Persuasive Technology. Communications of the ACM 42, 51–58 (1999)
4. Spahn, A.: And Lead Us (Not) into Persuasion...? Persuasive Technology and the Ethics of Communication. Sci. Eng. Ethics. 18(4), 633–650 (2012)
5. Compen, N., Spahn, A., Ham, J.: Sustainability coaches. A better environment starts with your coach. In: Kool, L., Timmer, J., van Est, R. (eds.) Sincere Support: The Rise of the E-coach. Rathenau Instituut, The Hague (forthcoming)
6. Staywell Health Management.: Energy Company Generates Better Health For Employees. Staywell Health Management, LLC
7. Kool, L., Timmer, J., van Est, R.: E-coaching: from possible to desirable. In: Kool, L, Timmer, J., van Est, R. (eds.) Sincere Support: The Rise of the E-coach. Rathenau Instituut, The Hague (forthcoming)
8. Morozov, E.: To Save Everything Click Here. The Folly of Technological Solutionism. PublicAffairs, New York (2013)
9. Raad voor Maatschappelijke Ontwikkeling.: De verleiding weerstaan. Grenzen aan beïnvloeding van gedrag door de overheid. RMO, The Hague (2014)
10. Aarts, E., Marzano, S.: The New Everyday. Views on Ambient Intelligence. 010, Rotterdam (2003)
11. Maan, S.J., Merkus, B., Ham, J.R.C., Midden, C.J.H.: Making it not too obvious: the effect of ambient light feedback on space heating energy consumption. Energy Efficiency 4(2), 175–183 (2011)
12. Ikonen, V., Kaasinen, E., Niemela, M.: Defining Ethical Guidelines for Ambient Intelligence Applications on a Mobile Phone. Ambient Intelligence and Smart Environments, vol. 4, pp. 261–268. IOS Press (2009)
13. Harbers, M.: Explaining Agent Behavior in Virtual Training. PhD Thesis, Utrecht University (2011)
14. Davies, J.: Design Methods for Ethical Persuasive Computing. In: Proc. 4th Int. Conf. on Persuasive Technology, pp. 1–8. ACM, NY (2009)

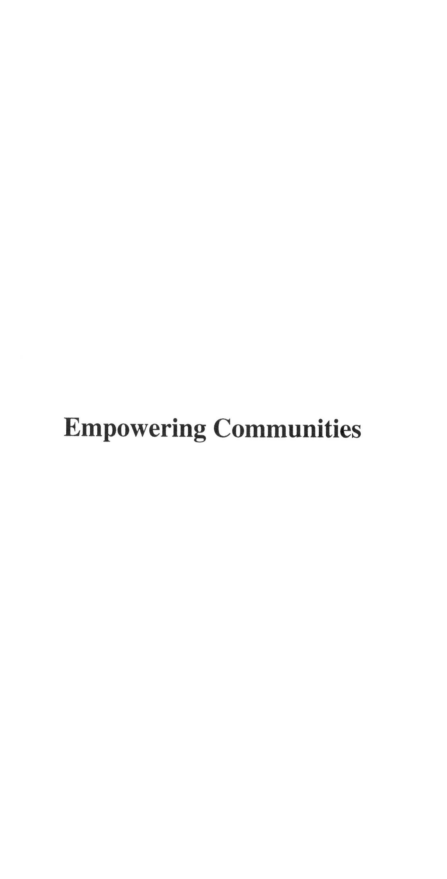

Empowering Communities

Influencing Retirement Saving Behavior with Expert Advice and Social Comparison as Persuasive Techniques

Junius Gunaratne[✉] and Oded Nov

New York University, New York, NY, USA
{junius,onov}@nyu.edu

Abstract. Numerous online communities and e-commerce sites provide users with crowd-based recommendations to influence decision making about products. Similarly, automated recommender systems often use social advice or curated knowledge provided by experts to give customers personalized product recommendations. Little, however, is known about the relative strengths of these approaches in repeated-decision scenarios. We used social comparison and an expert recommendation to examine the relative effectiveness of these methods of persuasion for users making repeated retirement saving decisions. We exposed 314 performance-incentivized experiment participants to a retirement saving simulator where they made 34 yearly asset allocation decisions in one of three user interface conditions. The gap between participants' retirement goal and actual savings was smallest in the expert advice condition and significantly better than the social comparison condition. Both conditions were significantly better than the control condition. In non-control conditions, users adjusted their behavior and achieved their saving goal more effectively.

Keywords: Retirement saving · Social comparison · Behavior change · Persuasive technology · Financial literacy

1 Introduction

Americans are estimated to hold $19.4 trillion in 401(k) retirement accounts [1] in which people make yearly decisions about how to allocate funds between a mix of assets. Theory-driven design of such interfaces can potentially help us understand and inform people who save for retirement, persuading them to make better saving decisions. Providing persuasive user interface design interventions at key decision points can improve investing behavior and avoid costs that hurt savers in the long-term.

We selected expert advice and social comparison as conditions to study because of their proven use in other research to influence and persuade users. When expert advice is available, people take into account such advice in their decision making [2]. In online communities individual decision making changes when individuals are exposed to aggregate decision data of an online community at large [3]. Studies have shown that changing people's retirement saving habits continues to be challenging due to factors such as status quo bias [4], and people end up losing a great deal of retirement income due to poor saving and investing habits. Given the persuasive pow-

© Springer International Publishing Switzerland 2015
T. MacTavish and S. Basapur (Eds.): PERSUASIVE 2015, pp. 205–216, 2015.
DOI: 10.1007/978-3-319-20306-5_19

er of expert advice and social comparison, we have two hypotheses with respect to how applying these methods of influence will affect the behavior of individuals saving for retirement: first, we expect that showing expert advice will motivate individuals to follow the expert advice over their own choices as individuals; second, we expect social comparison advice will influence decision making as individuals are likely to take into consideration the opinions of others—though this effect will be weaker than expert advice used as a means to influence decisions.

Recent studies show most Americans have underfunded retirement accounts [5]. Two aspects of retirement saving make it particularly difficult for non-experts: first, savers have to make repeated decisions about asset allocations that should decrease in risk over time, and understand the effects of multiple saving decisions over long periods. Second, most people do not assess risk properly [6]. In particular, a common mistake savers make is attempting to maximize returns or minimize volatility rather than reach a pre-determined saving goal [6].

While savers are advised to plan their savings towards reaching the goal of a comfortable retirement income, many often do not manage their retirement funds appropriately. For example, Samuelson and Zeckhauser [7] showed university faculty retirement contributions through TIAA-CREF retirement programs are rarely altered from their defaults leading to much lower long-term returns and unmet savings goals. Studies by the Employee Benefit Research Institute [8] show most Americans will have to work longer before retirement or spend far less once they enter retirement.

In response to these common difficulties and to motivate people to save in more effective ways, financial firms introduced target-date retirement funds in the late 1980s [9]. Target-date retirement funds, also known as lifecycle, dynamic-risk or age-based funds, provide a simple solution to automating asset allocation decisions. A saver invests into the target-date fund each year without having to make decisions about asset allocations and the target-date fund automatically rebalances allocations of asset types annually based on the saver's age or expressed level of risk. Financial companies often charge higher fees to manage target-date funds compared to having savers rebalance their retirement portfolio themselves: the fees a saver incurs in target-date funds range from 0.17% to 1.05% [10]. Over the long-term, these fees can add up to tens of thousands of dollars for the average saver.

Automated solutions for investing exist, but they often involve fees, require complex technical knowledge, or hide the underlying financial concepts individuals must learn to become effective investors. Automated retirement saving platforms, such as Wealthfront [11] and Betterment [12], charge consumers fees to use algorithms that automatically rebalance a recommended set of Exchange-Traded Funds to create optimized retirement portfolios. Automated retirement savings platforms help increase the transparency of underlying investments, but consumers are required to pay fees and it can be unclear how rebalancing occurs over time. Our motivation for using expert advice and social comparison as persuasive techniques to influence investing is to help people understand underlying risk by showing them how experts and groups are investing—which in turn persuades the individual to invest more appropriately.

Our objective is not to elicit more or less risky behavior, but rather, given a predetermined saving goal, to identify which interventions lead participants to take appropriate risks and stay on track toward their goal. We should note that increased proportion of stocks is not in itself more risky in the long run, since the alternative—allocating more to "safer" (but lower yield) assets—may lead to lower likelihood of achieving the goal and thus may not be effective in the long run. There are multiple ways to reach a retirement goal, and therefore the role of the interventions is to help users modify their behavior by suggesting a path to the goal.

Since investing is commonly done online in recent years, HCI research in behavior change and persuasive technology especially are well suited to study it, and inform and help people save for their retirement. Within the field of persuasive design and HCI, research specifically studying retirement saving is highly under-studied. In this study we contribute to persuasive design research by exploring the use of social comparisons and expert advice to help persuade users to make better retirement saving decisions.

2   Related Work

Prior research shows that social comparison strongly influences individual behavior. Drawing on social comparison theory, Chen et al [3] showed that when users of MovieLens, a movie rating online community, received information about others' contribution, users below the median increased their contribution, whereas those above the median did not decrease their ratings. Konstan and Riedl [2] demonstrated that providing expert information using algorithms can dramatically affect how recommender systems users make decisions. Schafer et al have shown that in e-commerce, providing hard-coded knowledge from expert or mined knowledge from consumer behavior leads to increases in sales [13].

In many financial contexts, people benefit from both expert advice and being able to compare themselves with others. Research in microfinance has shown that when lenders and borrowers have access to financial data of others they are more likely to adjust incorrect inferences, thus improving lender decisions and help those seeking loans [14]. In a study of crowd-sourced stock picks in online forums, Hill and Ready-Campbell [15] used a genetic algorithm approach to identify experts within the crowd. The online crowd that used expert advice performed better, on average, than the S&P 500 [15]. When more weight was given to the votes of the experts in the crowd, this increased the accuracy of the verdicts, improving performance yields. Both expert advice and social comparison "advice" have the potential to benefit savers and persuade them to make better decisions. With respect to design interventions used to influence decision making in the financial services domain, Teppan et al [16] investigated the impacts of the asymmetric dominance and compromise effect to influence the choice of bonds over stocks and vice versa.

Providing expert advice to change decision-making is not new. Design interventions have provided expert advice to users in areas such as healthcare informatics and environmental sustainability. Fogg's work in persuasive technology [17] has influenced research on how technology can be used to change behavior. Yun et al [18] used intervention techniques for encouraging energy conservation through the use of information dashboards. Similarly, Froehlich and colleagues [19] used immediate feedback that changed on a daily basis to promote environmentally sustainable behavior in water usage. These studies show that displaying timely feedback and information about deviating from a goal can affect individual behavior.

With respect to risk adjustment and investing, the notion of adapting portfolio allocations and adjusting for risk over time dates back to early research by Nobel laureate Robert Merton [20]. More recently, economists have studied the benefits and drawbacks of target-date funds extensively. Poterba et al [9] examined target-date fund asset allocation strategies and how age and stage of life can be used to optimize asset allocation decisions. Mitchell and Utkus [21] have shown that target-date retirement funds are becoming an implicit means of investment advice for employees since the choice architecture of fund selection has become so complex.

HCI researchers have explored how people manage and think about their money [22, 23], and how real-time information about simulated financial transactions leads to a better understanding of those transactions. Cramer and Hayes [24] studied financial literacy within classroom settings using ubiquitous computing technologies to track simulated financial transactions between students. Providing real-time information about simulated financial transactions gave students a stronger understanding of economic transactions versus merely discussing the concepts in the abstract. HCI applied to finance and economics shows that timely data, conveyed in such a way that is applicable to the present, help people better understand the impact of their decision making, thereby leading to better decision making. Gunaratne and Nov [25] studied how applying behavioral economic theory to retirement saving in an HCI context can improve reaching saving goals, but little other HCI research focuses on technology-mediated saving behavior and how design interventions can be used to persuade users to make better decisions with respect to personal finance.

3   Study

3.1   Setting

This study attempts to understand how to motivate individuals to make prudent decisions when dealing with a complex, long-term series of activities such as retirement saving where there is uncertainty regarding investment return performance. Building on prior work [24, 26, 27], we examine the effects of feedback relating to objectives, goals and deviating from those goals, on user saving behavior. In particular, we wanted to examine the effects of how to mitigate the effects risk has in influencing and motivating investors to be either too conservative or too aggressive when making investment decisions by applying persuasive techniques.

We examined the effects of expert advice and social comparisons, which changes with each subsequent participant and each passing saving year, on retirement users' behavior. We created an interactive retirement saving simulator that borrowed features from popular commercial retirement management systems (e.g., Vanguard and Fidelity Investments). We asked users to save $1.5 million over 34 years (2014-2048). A person who saves \$10,000 per year over 34 years with returns of 7.5% can expect to save about \$1.5 million. Returns of 7.5% are a typical rate of return for a mix of stocks and bonds.

In each simulation "year" participants allocated their yearly savings (\$10,000) among the three basic asset classes of stocks, bonds and cash, after exploring the implications of their decision using the simulator's interactive features. Stocks are the riskiest investment type, but provide the greatest return. Bonds are less risky, but provide a lower return. Cash has no risk and provides minimal return [28]. Once users clicked "submit" on their chosen yearly allocation of assets, they moved to the next simulation year. The interface then presented users with market behavior of the last year as well as their portfolio's performance (Figures 1-3). To make the market performance realistic, the simulator used (unknown to the users) the Dow Jones Industrial Average for stock data and the Fidelity Investment Grade Bond for bond data, both from 1980 to 2014. Actual market data from 1980 represented the simulated year of 2014, 1981 represented 2015, and so on, ending with the simulated year 2048, which used actual market data from 2014.

3.2   Reward Mechanism

We recruited users via Amazon Mechanical Turk and limited participation to U.S. users who did at least 100 Human Intelligence Tasks (HITs) prior to our HIT at an approval rate greater than 99%.

Following the approach of achieving a retirement goal rather than maximizing returns or evading risks [6], we rewarded taking goal-driven moderate risk. Consequently, users' compensation was based on a \$1.00 default pay and a maximum bonus of \$4.00 if they met the \$1.5 million retirement goal. Deviation from the goal either positively or negatively led to a proportionally lower bonus. This 4/1 bonus/default compensation ratio provides incentive to achieve the savings goal rather than maximizing returns with riskier behavior.

Retirement advisers recommend setting a savings goal based on a retirement replacement income and an appropriate level of risk rather than trying to maximize funds through risky investments. Risk tends to be especially important to mitigate the closer one gets to retirement. Meeting or exceeding a retirement goal is the core objective. However, missing a retirement goal can lead to loss of income in retirement. Given fluctuations in the stock market, experts recommend being more conservative in investing the older one gets. Certainly, one can continue to be aggressive and put substantial investments into stocks throughout one's lifetime, but if the stock market plunges close to a retirement date there are few ways to recover the losses. For such reasons retirement advisers encourage diversification in stocks and bonds, shifting a greater portfolio allocation towards bonds the older one gets. In other words, investors should take risk when they are young, but be risk averse when they are old. Therefore setting a retirement goal is important, but taking too much risk to attempt to exceed that retirement goal is imprudent.

3.3   Experimental Conditions

Following a between-subjects experimental design, 314 users took part in the experiment. Their average age was 34.1 and 45.7% were women. They were divided between the expert advice group (103 users), the social comparison group (109 users) and the control group (101 users).

To match common retirement saving user interfaces we presented to users the asset allocation, the overall value of the user's investments over time, the current year, and the year of retirement. To help participants understand how changing asset allocations can affect goal outcomes, we provided an interactive feature enabling users to check the potential outcomes of asset allocation alternatives prior to starting the simulator.

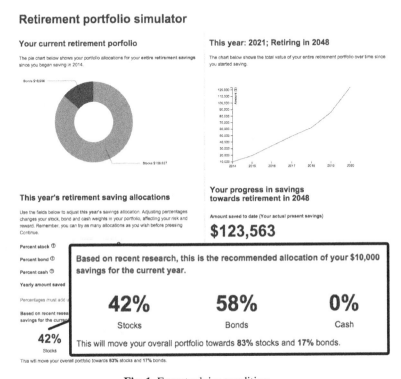

Fig. 1. Expert advice condition

In the condition emphasizing adaptive *expert advice* (Figure 1), we used a target-retirement formula [29, 30] that is typically used to determine stock and bond asset allocations based on an individual's age. Most financial firms use this formula as the primary basis for determining stock and bond allocations in a target-date retirement fund. For the purpose of this study we applied the formula in such a way to ensure the final amount a participant would save if she followed the formula exactly would be near $1.5 million. To convey this as expert advice to participants we stated: *"Based on recent research, this is the recommended allocation of your $10,000 savings for the current year."* Following this statement we showed recommended yearly percentage allocations of stocks, bonds and cash, followed by how this would affect the overall balance of the entire retirement portfolio. This condition aimed to convey an expert opinion to participants. We expected participants to follow the expert advice, though they were free to make any allocation choice they deemed fit to achieve the $1.5 million goal.

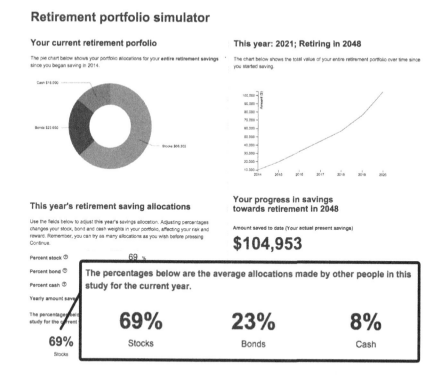

Fig. 2. Social comparison condition.

The *social comparison* condition (Figure 2) displayed the average yearly asset allocation percentages other participants in the study used for the current saving year. To convey this to users we stated: *"The percentages below are the average allocations made by other people in this study for the current year."* The asset allocations shown to users varied since each subsequent participant would change the average asset allocations presented. We expected showing percentages in this light would serve to anchor participants' asset allocations decisions, but would not influence participants as strongly as expert advice. To seed average asset allocations for the initial participants we used data from a prior study that captured asset allocation percentages, but in the prior study we did not reveal those percentages to participants.

The *control condition* (Figure 3) presented a user interface similar to that of a typical online retirement savings firm (such as Fidelity or Vanguard) where asset class distributions accompany a historical investment performance chart. In addition to these charts, users can modify retirement saving allocations for the current year by altering the percent of stocks, bonds and cash.

We recorded gaps between users' actual savings and their goal ($1.5M), as well as the number of asset allocation changes during the simulation. We compared these data across the experimental conditions using ANOVA and a Bonferroni post-hoc test. Another measure, less susceptible to outliers, we used for comparing saving performance across conditions, was users' likelihood of reaching a final saving amount within a 10% range of their goal. This comparison was made using a Pearson chi-square test.

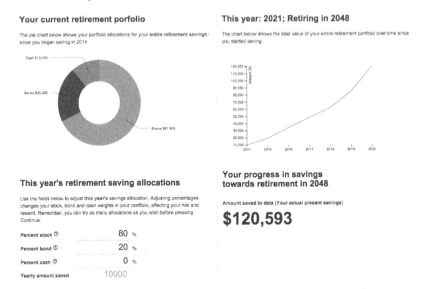

Fig. 3. Control condition

4   Results

The results of the ANOVA ($F_{2,310}$=15.39; p<0.001) and post-hoc test revealed that the gap between participants' goal and actual savings (see Table 1 and Figure 4) was smallest, on average, in the expert advice condition ($74,792) and significantly smaller than in the social comparison condition ($110,085). Both gaps were significantly smaller (p<0.01) than the gap in the control condition ($154,806). In addition, the difference between the expert advice and the social comparison conditions was significant (p<0.05).

Users' likelihood of reaching a final saving amount within a 10% range of their goal (Pearson chi-square=34.23; df=2; p<0.01) also differed significantly between the experimental conditions: the likelihood of reaching this range among users in the expert advice condition (93.2%) was significantly higher (p<0.01) than the likelihood of social comparison users to reach the same range (77.1%). Furthermore, the likelihood of reaching the 10% range among social comparison was significantly higher (p<0.01) than that of users in the control condition (58.4%). Users also differed in their allocation change behavior: those in the expert advice and social comparison conditions made, on average, significantly more adjustments to their asset allocations than the control group (24.0, 20.7 and 16.2 respectively; p<0.01).

Table 1. Differences from the control group: *significant at p<0.01

Condition	Mean gap from goal ($)	Average number of asset allocation changes	Likelihood of ending up within 10% range of saving goal (%)
Expert advice	74,792* (SD=71,583)	23.96* (SD=9.02)	93.2*
Social comparison	110,085* (SD=109,579)	20.66* (SD=10.16)	77.1*
Control	154,806 (SD=121,695)	16.24 (SD=11.62)	58.4

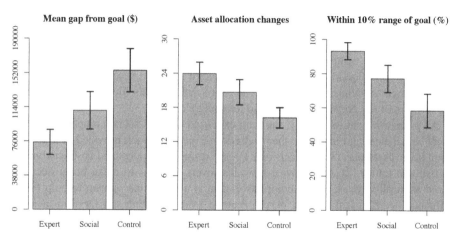

Fig. 4. Comparison between experimental conditions. Error bars represent a 95% confidence interval

5   Discussion and Conclusion

Small changes in interactive user interface design can lead to differences in how people approach saving and persuade them to mitigate risk. Participants in the study most closely reached their savings goal when using the expert advice interface condition, followed by the social comparison interface condition. The control condition, similar to current popular retirement saving interfaces, was least effective. In both the expert advice and social comparison conditions participants made more asset allocation changes than the control condition.

In the expert advice condition, we showed participants that research recommended specific asset allocation decisions to correctly balance their retirement portfolio. These recommendations used a commonly used target-fund asset allocation formula that financial firms use. Consistent with prior research [2, 3, 13], this framing of information as expert advice (asset allocation advice provided by a formula [29, 30]), was likely to influence participants, and make them adjust their allocations more frequently than others. Participants focused on their retirement goal guided by an expert opinion rather than maximizing their return (a more risky strategy [6]).

The weaker performance of the social comparison condition relative to the expert advice condition may be explained by two factors: first, participants who see peer advice may perceive the advice as a suggestion that may be correct or incorrect, as opposed to validated advice, and only loosely follow other participants; and second, average asset allocations that affect the final retirement goal amount are generated by the participants themselves, and therefore perpetuate others' mistakes common to retirement investing, such as allocating too little towards stocks at the beginning of one's career and too much when approaching retirement. However, some participants are probably familiar with good practices to follow for retirement investment portfolio allocation. These informed participants may skew the overall averages towards the correct portfolio allocations. This is similar to how experts surfaced in Hill and Ready-Campbell's study in online investment forums [15]. The existence of these experts within the crowd would account for why the social comparison condition outperformed the control condition. The social comparison condition outperforming the control condition also shows that being able to see what peers are doing provides an advantage to acting alone without such information. This illustrates the power of the wisdom of the crowd [15] compared to acting alone.

As prior work shows [3, 13], showing expert advice and social comparison data to users can change and influence their behavior. Expert feedback provided at a decision point helps users make better decisions. People struggle to understand abstract concepts of risk and return [21], and advice provides savers a means to make better decisions about asset allocations. Social comparison data is a useful mechanism to help further influence decision-making and prevent people from deviating too far from a mean, which can be helpful with respect to staying on track for retirement saving. These techniques are especially useful in the context of personal finance and retirement saving where longitudinal studies of retirement saving by Thaler and Benartz [4] have shown that it is difficult to motivate and persuade people to make sound financial decisions over time. The findings are also consistent with HCI research by Froehlich et al [27] and Bauer et al [31] which show that timely, relevant feedback is provided to users at a decision point to help them make better, more informed decisions.

In future work we would like to study how combining both expert advice and social comparison affects persuasion of a user interface including how individuals perceive the advice of a single expert versus multiple experts. We also envision allowing users to control the yearly saving amounts to study how saving is influenced by risk.

Our application of persuasive design to retirement saving has important design implications: government and private financial institutions who regulate and manage retirement saving can help the public by applying these concepts to interactive user interfaces design for retirement saving. In particular, displaying information with actionable and easily digestible expert advice, and social comparison data to motivate people to stick to norms. In our study we found these two means to present data to have effects. Such an approach carries minimal cost to financial institutions, and can help non-expert investors make informed decisions. Savers benefit by being able to manage retirement portfolios independently at a lower cost than a target-date fund.

References

1. Dougherty, C.: Retirement Savings Accounts Draw U.S. Consumer Bureau Attention. In Bloomberg
2. Konstan, J.A., Riedl, J.: Recommender systems: from algorithms to user experience. User Modeling and User-Adapted Interaction 22(1-2), 101–123 (2012)
3. Chen, Y., et al.: Social Comparisons and Contributions to Online Communities: A Field Experiment on MovieLens. American Economic Review 100(4), 40 (2010)
4. Thaler, R.H., Benartzi, S.: Save More Tomorrow: Using behavioral economics to increase employee saving. Journal of Political Economy 112, S164–S187 (2004)
5. Helman, R., et al.: The 2014 Retirement Confidence Survey: Confidence Rebounds—for Those With Retirement Plans. Employee Benefit Research Institute
6. Merton, R.: The Crisis in Retirement Planning. Harvard Business Review 92(7), 42–50 (2014)
7. Samuelson, W., Zeckhauser, R.: Status Quo Bias in Decision Making. Journal of Risk and Uncertainty 1(1), 7–59 (1988)
8. Individual Account Retirement Plans: An Analysis of the 2007 Survey of Consumer Finances, With Market Adjustments to June 2009. Employee Benefit Research Institute (2009)
9. Poterba, J., et al.: Lifecycle Asset Allocation Strategies and the Distribution of 401(k) Retirement Wealth, NBER: NBER (2006)
10. Vanguard Target Retirement Funds (October 5, 2014, https://investor.vanguard.com/mutual-funds/target-retirement/.
11. Wealthfront, http://www.wealthfront.com
12. Betterment, http://www.betterment.com
13. Schafer, J.B., Konstan, J.A., Riedl, J.: E-Commerce Recommendation Applications. Data Min. Knowl. Discov. 5(1-2), 115–153 (2001)
14. Yum, H., Lee, B., Chae, M.: From the wisdom of crowds to my own judgment in microfinance through online peer-to-peer lending platforms. Electron. Commer. Rec. Appl. 11(5), 469–483 (2012)
15. Hill, S., Ready-Campbell, N.: Expert Stock Picker: The Wisdom of (Experts in) Crowds. Int. J. Electron. Commerce 15(3), 73–102 (2011)
16. Teppan, E.C., Felfernig, A., Isak, K.: Decoy effects in financial service E-sales systems (2011)
17. Fogg, B.J.: Persuasive Technology: Using Computers to Change What We Think and Do. In: Jonathan, G., Jakob, N., Stuart, C. (eds.) Science & Technology Books, p. 224 (2002)
18. Yun, R., et al.: Sustainability in the workplace: nine intervention techniques for behavior change. In: Proceedings of the 8th international conference on Persuasive Technology. Springer-Verlag, Sydney (2013)
19. Froehlich, J., et al.: The design and evaluation of prototype eco-feedback displays for fixture-level water usage data. In: Proceedings of the SIGCHI Conference on Human Factors in Computing Systems. ACM, Austin (2012)

20. Merton, R.C.: Lifetime Portfolio Selection under Uncertainty: The Continuous-Time Case. The Review of Economics and Statistics 51(3), 247–257 (1969)
21. Mitchell, O., Utkus, S.: Target Date Funds in 401(k) Retirement Plans, National Bureau of Economic Research (2012)
22. Vines, J., Dunphy, P., Monk, A.: Pay or delay: the role of technology when managing a low income. In: Proceedings of the SIGCHI Conference on Human Factors in Computing Systems, Toronto, ON, Canada (2014)
23. Kaye, J.J., et al.: Money talks: tracking personal finances. In: Proceedings of the 32nd Annual ACM conference on Human Factors in Computing Systems. ACM (2014)
24. Cramer, M., Hayes, G.R.: The digital economy: a case study of designing for classrooms. In: Proceedings of the 12th International Conference on Interaction Design and Children, pp. 431–434. ACM, New York (2013)
25. Gunaratne, J., Nov, O.: Informing and improving retirement saving performance using behavioral economic theory-driven user interfaces. In: Proceedings of the SIGCHI Conference on Human Factors in Computing Systems. ACM, Seoul (2015)
26. Yun, R., Scupelli, P., Aziz, A., Loftness, V.: Sustainability in the workplace: nine intervention techniques for behavior change. In: Berkovsky, S., Freyne, J. (eds.) PERSUASIVE 2013. LNCS, vol. 7822, pp. 253–265. Springer, Heidelberg (2013)
27. Froehlich, J., et al.: The design and evaluation of prototype eco-feedback displays for fixture-level water usage data. In: Proceedings of the SIGCHI Conference on Human Factors in Computing Systems, pp. 2367–2376. ACM, Austin (2012)
28. Commission, U.S.S.a.E. Invest Wisely: An Introduction to Mutual Funds [cited 2014], http://www.sec.gov/investor/pubs/inwsmf.htm
29. TIAA-CREF Lifecycle Funds: Methodology and Design, TIAA-CREF Asset Management (2014)
30. Ibbotson, R.G., et al.: Lifetime Financial Advice: Human Capital, Asset Allocation, and Insurance. Research Foundation Publications. The Research Foundation of CFA Institute, 95 (2007)
31. Bauer, J.S., et al.: ShutEye: encouraging awareness of healthy sleep recommendations with a mobile, peripheral display. In: Proceedings of the SIGCHI Conference on Human Factors in Computing Systems, pp. 1401–1410. ACM, Austin (2012)

A System Development Life Cycle for Persuasive Design for Sustainability

Moyen M. Mustaquim$^{(\boxtimes)}$ and Tobias Nyström

Uppsala University, Uppsala, Sweden
{moyen.mustaquim,tobias.nystrom}@im.uu.se

Abstract. The impact of a system development lifecycle (SDLC) often determines the success of a project from analysis to evolution. Although SDLC can be universally used design projects, a focused SDLC for a specific complex design issue could be valuable for understanding diverse user needs. The importance of sustainability elevation using a persuasive system is not new. Previous research presented frameworks and design principles for persuasive system design for sustainability, while an SDLC of sustainable system development also exists. However, at present no SDLC for persuasive design aiming for sustainability is evident, which was proposed in this paper. An existing sustainable SDLC established earlier by the authors was taken as the reference framework. A cognitive model with established persuasive design principles was then analyzed and mapped within the context of the reference framework to come up with the resulting life cycle. Finally, extensive discussions and future work possibilities were given.

Keywords: Sustainability · SDLC · Persuasive System Design · Cognitive model · Persuasive system design for Sustainability · Life cycle for persuasive system design

1 Introduction

The search for solutions to solve the eminent problem to reach a balance and achieve a sustainable future is pervasive in research [15]. The research field of computer science has also participated in this quest, e.g. green IT and sustainable human-computer interaction. The design of different interaction processes and the system is important, since badly designed systems can contribute to social and environmental degradation [32]. The design phase of a system is often considered to be the core of information systems research since it could be considered the construction of a socio-technical system—the artificial [31]. A computer-mediated persuasive system is thus a socio-technical system created with a specific purpose in a defined context based on certain assumptions. The pattern of existing persuasive technology has been criticized in recent years as not being adequate for sustainable system-design solutions [4], [19]. The nature of persuasive system aiming for sustainability has been limited within a certain scope of interests and therefore a call for expanding the possibilities of using large-scale system design and long-term design problems were identified to be the

© Springer International Publishing Switzerland 2015
T. MacTavish and S. Basapur (Eds.): PERSUASIVE 2015, LNCS 9072, pp. 217–228, 2015.
DOI: 10.1007/978-3-319-20306-5_20

most important upcoming challenges for the individual sustainable human-computer interaction (HCI) researchers and the sustainable HCI community as a whole [4]. Also, since there is a considerable difference between green design and green engineering, a building of knowledge for the green-design domain, originating from green engineering, is important and to fill this gap is a challenge for the designers. For promoting sustainability goals, both green design and green engineering are important and the role of persuasive design has already been known to be an effective and powerful design strategy for green-design issues. However, while the possibilities and scopes of sustainability need to be broadened for an effective use of persuasive design, it is at the same time important to realize what the appropriate and right design procedure could be, because a design process can become more complicated for the designers as the complexity and size of a problem increases. Selecting the right methodologies would therefore play a vital role for an organization to be successful by means of their design in terms of productivity; the demands along with a fast and predictable return on investment. System development life cycle (SDLC) is a type of model that could play a critical role in the development of complex systems. Building an appropriate SDLC is difficult for a specific type of information system (IS) design since it involves and requires careful preparation and administration to guarantee the standard and the quality of an end design that delivers a robust, effective, and efficient system that ensures what it is supposed to do. Nevertheless, doing this successfully could help IS designers and analysts to compare different parameters and factors of the designed system to take critical decisions, such as selecting between different available design options. Expenses like time and cost usually play a major role in the development of IS and proper SDLC would estimate these factors properly for the effectiveness and efficiency of an organization's design policy.

With the demanding nature of complex persuasive system design for sustainability, it would be appropriate to have a specific SDLC that could ensure a reduction of complexity during the design process, resulting in a successful end design for the users. Although an eight-step design process of persuasive design was presented by Fogg [12] that was more like some general guidelines and was established from different practical industrial design success demonstrations. While Fogg [12] played the part of a pioneer and major contributor to persuasive design, designers were still not specifically informed of what should be a general design flow of persuasive design. With several guidelines and design structures along with a few evident design principles [3], [6], [20], [23], [28], an SDLC for persuasive design with sustainability goals could not be found to be described by researchers in academia or to be used by practitioners to date. This was the underlying rationale behind this research paper, in which we have proposed an SDLC for persuasive system design for sustainability, and the formulated underlying research question of this paper is thus: 'What are the appropriate design phases that need to be associated in a persuasive system design aiming for sustainability?' To answer this research question two previously established theoretical frameworks were selected and used as a basis on which to constitute our theoretical framework, for which an SDLC for a persuasive system for sustainability was proposed in a methodological form.

This paper is divided into six sections. A concrete background in Section 2 introduces the notions of a persuasive system and sustainability along with SDLC. The background of the selected theoretical frameworks in this paper is then presented, followed by the proposed SDLC for persuasive design for sustainability in Section 3, in which different phases of the proposed life cycle are briefly described. Discussions are given in Section 4 and finally a future work direction is addressed in Section 5 followed by the conclusion in Section 6.

2   Background

2.1   Persuasive Design and Sustainability

Based on Festinger's cognitive dissonance theory [10], persuasion as an instrument to change people's attitudes and behavior is a well-explored research field in psychology [34]. 'Persuasive design' is the designing of experiences to influence people's behavior [11]. Computers can be used as persuasive technology (a study labeled by Fogg as 'captology' based on an acronym derived from 'Computer As Persuasive Technologies' [13]) to support persuasive design. Persuasion is defined by Fogg as "an attempt to change attitudes or behavior or both (without using coercion or deception)" [13]. The belief in the power of persuasive information systems mediated by computers is firmly set by the collective research from Festinger [10]. Oinas-Kukkonen [26] showed, in research on the behavior change support system (BCSS), that the persuasive system-design (PSD) model is a state-of-the-art vehicle for designing and evaluating BCSSs. A PSD with a sustainability goal could be made to alter individual users' behavior and to impact a larger part of society. Sustainable HCI has, since 2007, been an active research area of HCI [8]. The persuasive research in the sustainable HCI community is mainly about shaping people's behavior through a system. Computer-mediated persuasive systems could also play an important role in healthcare [17] and may be considered to facilitate personal sustainability. Recent research about developing a persuasive system displays a goal setting to make the user behave in a sustainable manner and reduce their use of resources like water or electricity, or to drive in a more eco-friendly way [10], [14], [18]. One problem could be the top-down selection of measurements by the designers to calculate the users' behavior [4].

Sustainability could be derived from the conception of the World Commission on Environment and Development (WCED) regarding sustainable development: "… that it meets the needs of the present without compromising the ability of future generations to meet their own needs" [35]. Sustainability thus works by reversing or minimizing the effect and impact of different human-induced processes. Sustainability can be seen as a complex and dynamic problem, not only linked to the environment but also a way to better understand the possible complexity to use the quadruple bottom line (QBL). QBL relates sustainability to environmental/practical, personal/spiritual, and social needs with which economic concerns—the economic is not seen as natural condition of being a human but as a human construction—mediate the ability to satisfy these three needs [33]. This implies a need of a holistic view regarding sustainability. In previous research conducted by Nyström and Mustaquim [24] the importance of a holistic view of sustainability is emphasized in order to be able to capture this mentioned complexity of sustainability and the multiple dimensionalities that must be considered in the design of a system to make it stand a chance of successfully reaching sustainable goals.

2.2   System Development Life Cycle (SDLC)

Many different system development methodologies exist and the SDLC is one of them. An SDLC can be used together with different development models, e.g. the classical waterfall model, the joint application model, and rapid application development (RAD). Due to the complexity of system development, the predictive waterfall model has emphasized the use of iterative lifecycle models [22]. The models can be mixed into hybrids, e.g. something that seems to be more prevalent than the concept of methodology in the traditional systematic sense [21]. For the ease of understanding this, in this paper the classic waterfall model introduced by Royce [29] is used. However, with several models the methodological complexities arise and it might be necessary to use multiple models for addressing different complex design issues in a system-design setup. The development of unique SDLC for a focused system-design problem, e.g. persuasive design, could thus be beneficial as it would reduce different complexities associated through the use of multiple models. For example, Pollard et al. blended SDLC with Information Technology Service Management (ITSM) life cycle concepts [27]. The main feature of SDLC is the use of different phases that are used in the system development process. The number of phases can vary, but often consist of: feasibility study, systems investigation, analysis, design, development, implementation, and maintenance [2]. Once the deliveries from one phase are reached, the next phase can begin or an iterative process may be initiated [2]. The process of design could be simplified into three main activities: "the need identification", "the development of a solution", and "the implementation of the solution" [7].

2.3   Theoretical Background

A cognitive dissonance model (based on PSD) aimed at persuasive design for sustainability was developed and presented by Mustaquim and Nyström [24]. The model includes five principles: equitability, inclusiveness, optimality, privacy, and transparency, which have an impact on three persuasive factors identified by Fogg [11]: motivation, ability, and triggers that work in a bidirectional way. By including equitability in the design, potential users would contribute to the thinking concerning the design process and designing inclusiveness can manifest possibilities that the system will facilitate regarding a group rather than an individual. One example is to make things more fun and engaging, as in gamification with the goal of changing consumers' consumption behavior [16]. Targeting the optimum design would make an end system inclusive and would increase the possibility of customizing for gaining the most possible effect. The other two principles—privacy and transparency—will follow and are crucial to guaranteeing a successful persuasive system, since the user must trust and be fully aware of the content and the possible results that their interactions will give, thereby guaranteeing that they feel secure to use and give information to the system.

The developed framework for SDLC [25] is composed of three phases: definition, development, and operation. In the definition phase the analysis and design is made and it is important to consider the simplicity and flexibility that would maximize the system benefits and targets. It is important to be aware of the difficult balance of requirements for the future, since too little will make the system lack capabilities and be future proof, although on the other hand too many requirements will make the system too complex and expensive to construct and maintain in the future. The development phase includes implementation and maintenance and in this the practice of design for all is of uttermost importance since with a maximization of additional users who are involved in the process, the better the system will be and will have an increased possibility to reach sustainability targets. In the development phase important tradeoffs must be considered, e.g. functionality versus cost and time. Also important synergies must be identified that could be combined with properties and considerations taken from the definition phase. The operation phase consists of maintenance and planning and of importance here is the sustainability impact-assessment, since it will measure the outcome of sustainability and decide the direction and future of the system. It will also be concerned with long-term intergenerational issues that will influence the development to tackle newly discovered problems facing the sustainable IS.

3   Proposed System Development Life Cycle

As mentioned in Section 2.3, our theoretical foundation for proposing an SDLC for persuasive system design for sustainability was based on two previous research frameworks. The design principles and cognitive dissonance model by Mustaquim and Nyström [24] was the first one and a sustainable system development life cycle (SSDLC) proposed by Nyström and Mustaquim [25] was the second theoretical basis. These were reflected in proposing an SDLC in this paper on the basis of the classical SDLC. The proposed SDLC was shown in Figure 1. Different phases associated with the proposed life cycle were explained and discussed in this section along with the context of classical SDLC.

Motivation. The motivation phase could be compared with the definition phase of the SSDLC in parallel with the development life cycle that was shown in Figure 1. Different phases are associated with the analysis and design phase of the classical SDLC. Minimization of resources in design was included here as stages of procedure, since resources for developing systems are always scarce and tradeoff decisions are always necessary. Understanding the individual behavior of the user group is important for reasoning what sustainability could achieve in a focused user group. What sustainability is for most users might be simply switching towards some green behavior in the form of a low-hanging fruit while the appeal through the design for sustainability could mean a lot more than this and might make a larger impact towards sustainability and may impact different levels, such as the community or organizations, and not merely at an individual level. At the same time, fulfilling the need of the users has also to be accomplished through the design. On the other hand, it is not possible to achieve sustainability by focusing on individuals, since often a systematic and thorough change is needed to reach a sustainable set goal. Individuals could be biased and motivated towards a certain sustainability action, while they see that other users of the same system are practicing that too. This could be connected with making the system 'fun' and users can compete or collaborate towards a set sustainable goal. Therefore the motivation stage of the persuasive design for sustainability is critical and involves deep knowledge and an understanding of users and their requirements, analyzing users' individual needs, combining mainstream users and their require-ments together to focus on them as a bigger group to solve the problem as a whole, and finally finding the different possibilities of solving the addressed problem. Main-taining consistency in design has always been a big challenge for the designers, who therefore need to be benefited by sufficient information of sustainability from the be-ginning of the design process, and the motivation stage of the proposed life cycle can initiate this task. Over time, designers can rely on a certain service which could be based on the motivation-stage analysis of different types of system design and thereby they can consult and share experiences with other experts or designers facing similar design challenges. Different types of motivational forces could be compared and ben-chmarked against each other and perhaps it would be possible to find a better practical solution that can be implemented when sustainability goals are set in a similar con-text, e.g. a similar approach that enterprise resource-planning systems use to standard-ize their platforms and offer standard solutions for companies.

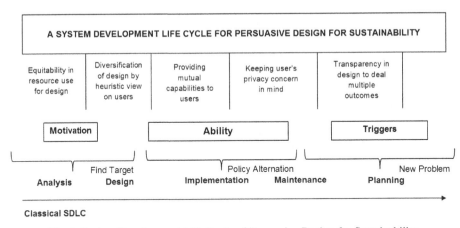

Fig. 1. System Development Life Cycle of Persuasive Design for Sustainability

Ability. The ability phase could be compared with the development phase in the SSDLC, and may be correlated to implementation and maintenance in the classical SDLC. By practicing design for all it would be possible to deliver a system that brings mutual capabilities to different users, independent of their prior knowledge, different physical needs, e.g. color blindness or limited vision, or difference in learning style, i.e. abilities, and would thus impose an easy way to interact with the system and max-imize their chance of active use and participation. The more users that a system can maintain as active the better, since users can compare and work together to overcome challenges in sustainability and may reach a set sustainability goal. The system should therefore be easy to modify and reconfigure, to fit individual needs; something that could be guaranteed by iteration of the previous stage. The more users that use the system the better, since their different abilities can be detected and the strengths and weaknesses of the system can be found. Problems could be solved in an appropriate way. Trust is always an important issue for users and the transparency of how collected data will be handled is central to building a trust and thereby creating the user interaction with the system. Different options should be possible for the user to choose from since individuals have different preferences and the features of the system could require different needs of keeping user data private. For a healthcare system designed for persuasion of behavior towards sustainability on a personal level, the privacy could be of uttermost importance and even regulated by laws. On the other hand, in other settings the sharing of data among users could be important and might enhance the ability to participate and help each other towards a sustainable goal. Since a combination of technology and behavior design result persuasive technology, it is very important to remember that individuals might have a different threshold level for their behavior to be modified. This is particularly important for the ability phase since it would define the micro or macro persuasion in design since any required policy alternation based on user capabilities and privacy could create value through the overall end design or generate certain features in design to persuade.

Triggers. The trigger phase is analogous to the operation phase of the SSDLC, and is comparable with planning in the classical SDLC. The design should be ready for different outcomes and the transparency of the design plays an important role in enabling this. Since the design of the artificial is a constructed socio-technical system made for persuasion towards a set sustainability goal and is a complex system, the outcome can be difficult to predict. Systems should therefore be designed to be prepared for this. Some unwanted side-effects could occur, e.g. if a system to make it easier to drive vehicles is energy-efficient by updating the traffic route, to have as few traffic stops as possible and avoiding the traffic jam. This system for efficient driving could in one way make it more enjoyable to drive, the effect could be for users to drive more, and then the set sustainability goal will not be reached. This kind of unwanted outcome could be dealt with if the design is transparent and the system could be modified, and also might count other parameters. The user behavior thus needs to be persuaded a little to make it possible to reach the set sustainability goal; in this example, perhaps by including the total driven mileage when assessing the user's behavior. The behavioral, cognitive, and emotional aspects of a design should thus be properly realized by users. Therefore a challenge is to present a design in which the persuasion could take place in the form of an optimum and appropriate user experience for enhanced usability. These issues are very important to consider in the planning phase. These design issues are, however, very contextual in nature. This means that the type of user experiences necessary for achieving a sustainable goal could be totally independent in nature for two different persuasive design problems. Consequently, persuasive technology is often thought to be working as a catalyst to change the behavioral environment and hence impact the change of the behavior of the users of a system. So, the planning phase would also focus on identifying new problems, which would then be taken into consideration as a next-design problem. This also is therefore a step associated with the trigger stage. Whether the new problem should be solved by keeping users in a non-coercive PSD category or if the design should work as a trigger for users

intentionally, in an adoptive or interactive and easy or difficult way, etc. should be completely taken into consideration while identifying new problems in this phase of the life cycle. This should be done by also exploring the causes for which the identified problems could not be solved, based on those design criteria.

4   Discussions

Designing a socio-technical system like a persuasive system for sustainability is important, since it is going to try to make an impact by bringing about changes and is not only trying to make sense of the world, as Carlsson et al. [5] denoted to be the core of design-science research. The established SDLC of Persuasive Design for Sustainability was an effort to introduce a novel methodology that could be used to design solutions that confront the problems of developing a persuasive system that changes people's behavior towards a set goal like sustainability. While the call for the compulsion of sustainable HCI research on the environmental sphere of sustainability is inevitable, Dourish [9] pointed out the need of accompanying sustainable HCI research through different theories and concepts for broadening its context. The proposed methodology in the form of a life cycle for persuasive design could thus be seen as one of such accompanying frameworks to impose on existing work and design relating to a persuasive design for sustainability. Three phases of the suggested SDLC are important and have different properties and challenges that need to be solved. No almighty solution that is working in all different contexts will ever be found, as sustainability is a very complex and contextual issue. One of the strengths of the proposed SDLC is that it would help designers and system analysts to look into the subjective criteria for sustainable goals instead of objective criteria, which, according to Huber and Hilty [16] often is the case and thus critical for persuasive technology. Several important subjective criteria like deep thinking, wide collaboration, respecting values of users, preventing users from acting on values, improving relationships between technology and sustainable social change, etc. and their importance in persuasion for sustainability through advancing the sustainable HCI research was addressed by Silberman et al. [30]. We believe that the practice of our proposed SDLC would be able to address these issues for improving sustainability goals through persuasive design. Nevertheless, it is very important to understand the different outcomes that the choice of the sustainability goal will have on the development and efficiency and effectiveness of the development process, as well as the management of the running system. It is central to acknowledge the importance by keeping in mind that the persuasive system must not be static, but instead must be able to meet new technological trends, user preferences, and changes in the collected knowledge about sustainability and its effects. We believe that the proposed SDLC methodology has these features addressed and could thus be used in the long run to persuade people towards the set sustainability goal.

Our theoretical reference frameworks [21, 22] are structured on an advanced concept of universal design (UD), in which the notion of UD was used beyond the scope of its traditional practice-accessibility. Therefore the concept of UD could be used to expose a new dimension in persuasion by expanding its traditional concept. UD could add new values in generating new design principles for persuasive design. For instance, understanding simplicity, intuitiveness, and reduced effort during the use of persuasive systems could be redefined in the persuasion context, which in turn could help in developing new cognitive models for persuasive design. Such an attempt was demonstrated in our reference framework, in the work of Mustaquim and Nyström [24]. Based on this it would be possible to establish new driving factors as design parameters through the practice of the proposed life cycle in a specific design setup.

About the utility of our proposed SDLC, it is still highly theoretical and contextual at this stage of the research. No doubt that persuasion is a complex phenomenon and sustainability also is a delicate issue. Combination of these two could be more delicate in different cases and the proposed SDLC could be used to ease such complexities. For example, Aleahmad et al. [1], discussed the impact of direct and indirect persuasion on sustainable attitudes. When it is necessary to result in this kind of complex persuasion through the design, then the proposed SDLC could be useful for identifying proper user needs and thus could contribute towards achieving sustainability through a successful system design. Also, even though persuasive technology could be a powerful tool for engaging stakeholders with sustainable behavior it is still important that they are already aware and convinced about the importance of sustainability, since failure to do so would make them not to choose a persuasive technology to use [1]. The proposed SDLC could be a key tool in this respect for handling these types of issues throughout its different phases and thereby make sure that the end design would be ready to be accepted by users.

Ethics have always been an important issue in discussing persuasive design. While achieving sustainability goals through design is important, it is also significant to remember that any higher power in design decision should not be misused to initiate unwanted impacts on user actions for any commercial success only for organizations. The proposed SDLC could be used to identify sensitive issues and factors in design in the direction of subsidizing the ethical aspects of design in persuasion for sustainability.

Further, the tendency of quickly switching to a green solution and changing human behavior towards green materials through persuasive design is often seen as a quick methodological fix towards achieving sustainability, which should really be prevented from occurring since this is and should not be the only perception of sustainability or sustainable action. The proposed life cycle would be able to realize other different issues that could be associated with a focused sustainability problem. It could then be solved using persuasive system design to be identified truly as persuasion towards sustainability goals. The research question addressed in the introduction section could thus be answered here by stating that one way to successfully design persuasive systems for sustainability could be to follow the proposed SDLC. And yet, system designers alone should not be expected to be benefited by the use of the proposed life cycle to claim the end design to be successful, since, as mentioned earlier, sustainability is a multifaceted complex issue and active involvement of different stakeholders from our collective society is centrally focused on the optimistic change of attitude towards this issue through the persuasive design.

5   Future Research

The proposed SDLC opened up some interesting research opportunities worth mentioning. First of all, this life cycle could be followed to design a program intending persuasion for sustainability. Then it could be compared with a system that was developed without following this process. The feasibility of using the proposed life cycle could then be realized. Likewise, systems designed by following two different processes could go through usability studies to see the impact of a design process on the end sustainability goal. New methodologies could thus be formulated for shaping the success of the proposed SDLC. Secondly, the context of sustainability could be realized in an improved way through the practice of this life cycle. Subsequently changing user behavior through design is not enough only in persuasion; what other factors could be important to consider in the design could be realized in different phases of the design process. Finally, the proposed life cycle could give system designers a new way of looking into the evaluation of sustainability. Since new entities of sustainability could be realized during the design process, they could also be evaluated later for measuring sustainability. On the other hand, new entities would be able to contribute towards developing or improving design principles for persuasive design.

6   Conclusions

This paper has considered reflecting through two previously established frameworks of a cognitive dissonance model for persuasive design for sustainability and an SDLC process in design for sustainability. These frameworks were analyzed and mapped together to formulate a new SDLC, pointing in the direction of persuasive system design for sustainability. The new framework was then explained and discussed within the context of persuasive system design aiming for sustainability. Despite the fact that changing the user's behavior or actions towards sustainability is concerned with what the concept of classical persuasive design is built on, within the context of sustainable HCI this perception is rapidly taking a shift. At the same time, available technologies are peaking, fast improving and altering. This reality will force and lead organizations that are facing new, tougher competitions and challenges in design. A proper SDLC, in hand as a systematic methodology, could be a fit within the existing structure of organizations, making it easier for them to identify the right problems faster and to answer their internal demands on different design solutions. The underlying philosophy behind the pillar of this paper—universal design—should also thus be mainstreamed, escaping from its traditional practice and one of such examples is shown in this paper and its reference to theoretical frameworks. With the trending shift of sustainable HCI and persuasive design for sustainability together with the research towards large-scale design problems and design for everyday use, the proposed SDLC in this paper could be highly promising in contributing to and supporting organizations and designers, focusing upon issues like persuasive design for sustainability. The proposed persuasive design life cycle of sustainability in the form of a methodology thus demands empirical verification for further interesting results.

References

1. Aleahmad, T., Balakrishnan, A.D., Wong, J., Fussell, S.R., Kiesler, S.: Fishing for sustainability: the effects of indirect and direct persuasion. In: CHI 2008 Extended Abstracts on Human Factors in Computing Systems (CHI EA 2008), pp. 3021–3026. ACM, New York (2008)
2. Avison, D.E., Fitzgerald, G.: Where now for development methodologies? Communications of the ACM 46(1), 78–82 (2003)
3. Beilan, G., Yen, D.C., Chou, D.C.: A manager's guide to total quality software design. Industrial Management & Data Systems 98(3), 100–107 (1998)
4. Brynjarsdóttir, H., Håkansson, M., Pierce, J., Baumer, E., DiSalvo, C., Sengers, P.: Sustainably unpersuaded: how persuasion narrows our vision of sustainability. In: Proceedings of the SIGCHI Conference on Human Factors in Computing Systems, CHI 2012, pp. 947–956. ACM, New York (2012)
5. Carlsson, S.A., Henningsson, S., Hrastinski, S., Keller, C.: Socio-technical IS design science research: developing design theory for IS integration management. Information Systems and e-Business Management 9(1), 109–131 (2011)
6. Cervone, H.F.: The system development life cycle and digital development. OCLC Systems & Services: International digital library perspectives 23(4), 348–352 (2007)
7. Connell, J., Brice, L.: Rapid Prototyping. Datamation 30(13), 93–100 (1984)
8. DiSalvo, C., Sengers, P., Brynjarsdóttir, H.: Navigating the terrain of sustainable HCI. Interactions 17(4), 22–25 (2010)
9. Dourish, P.: Print this paper, kill a tree: Environmental sustainability as a research topic for human-computer interaction. Technical Report LUCI-2009-004 from the Laboratory for Ubiquitous Computing and Interaction at UC Irvine (2009)
10. Festinger, L.: A theory of cognitive dissonance. Stanford University Press, Stanford (1957)
11. Fogg, B.J.: A Behavior Model for Persuasive Design. In: Proceedings of the 4th International Conference on Persuasive Technology, Persuasive 2009. ACM, New York (2009)
12. Fogg, B.J.: Creating persuasive technologies: an eight-step design process. In: Proceedings of the 4th International Conference on Persuasive Technology, Persuasive 2009. ACM, New York (2009)
13. Fogg, B.J.: Persuasive Technology: Using Computers to Change What We Think and Do. Morgan Kaufmann, Boston (2003)
14. Froehlich, J., Findlater, L., Ostergren, M., Ramanathan, S., Peterson, J., Wragg, I., Larson, E., Fu, F., Bai, M., Patel, S., Landay, J.A.: The design and evaluation of prototype eco-feedback display for fixture-level water usage data. In: Proceedings of the SIGCHI Conference on Human Factors in Computing Systems, CHI 2012, pp. 2367–2376. ACM, New York (2012)
15. Glavic, P., Lukman, R.: Review of sustainability terms and their definitions. Journal of Cleaner Production 15(18), 1875–1885 (2007)
16. Huber, M.Z., Hilty, L.M.: Gamification and Sustainable Consumption: Overcoming the Limitations of Persuasive Technologies. In: Hilty, L.M., Aebischer, B. (eds.) ICT Innovations for Sustainability. AISC, vol. 310, pp. 367–385. Springer, Heidelberg (2014)
17. Kelder, S.M., Kok, R.N., Ossebaard, H.C., Van Gemert-Pjnen, J.E.W.C.: Persuasive System Design Does Matter: A Systematic Review of Adherence to Web-Based Interventions. Journal of Medical Internet Search 14(6), 17–40 (2012)

18. Kjeldskov, J., Skov, M.B., Paay, J., Pathmanathan, R.: Using mobile phones to support sustainability: A field study of residential electricity consumption. In: Proceedings of the SIGCHI Conference on Human Factors in Computing Systems, CHI 2012, pp. 2347–2356. ACM, New York (2012)

19. Knowles, B., Blair, L., Walker, S., Coulton, P., Thomas, L., Mullagh, L.: Patterns of persuasion for sustainability. In: Proceedings of the 2014 Conference on Designing Interactive Systems, DIS 2014, pp. 1035–1044. ACM, New York (2014)

20. Kydd, C.T.: Understanding the information content in MIS management tools. MIS Quarterly 13(3), 277–290 (1989)

21. Lang, M., Fitzgerald, B.: New branches, old roots: A study of methods and techniques in Web/hypermedia systems design. Information Systems Management 23(3), 62–74 (2006)

22. Larman, C.: Applying UML and Patterns: An Introduction to Object-Oriented Analysis and Design and Iterative Development, 3rd edn. Prentice Hall, Upper Saddle River (2005)

23. McDowall, R.D.: The systems development life cycle. Chemometrics and Intelligent Laboratory Systems 13(2), 121–133 (1991)

24. Mustaquim, M., Nyström, T.: Designing Persuasive Systems For Sustainability – A Cognitive Dissonance Model. In: Proceedings of the European Conference on Information Systems (ECIS) 2014. AIS Electronic Library, Tel Aviv (2014)

25. Nyström, T., Mustaquim, M.: Sustainable Information System Design and the Role of Sustainable HCI. In: Proceedings of the 18th International Academic MindTrek Conference (MindTrek 2014). ACM, New York (2014)

26. Oinas-Kukkonen, H.: A foundation for the study of behavior change support systems. Personal Ubiquitous Computer 17(6), 1223–1235 (2013)

27. Pollard, C.E., Gupta, D., Satzinger, J.W.: Teaching Systems Development: A Compelling Case for Integrating the SDLC with the ITSM Lifecycle. Information Systems Management 27(2), 113–122 (2010)

28. Rodríguez, L.C., Mora, M., Martin, M.V., O'Connor, R., Alvarez, F.: Process models of SDLCs: Comparison and evolution. In: Syed, M.R., Syed, S.N. (eds.) Handbook of Research on Modern Systems Analysis and Design Technologies and Applications, pp. 76–89. IGI Global (2008)

29. Royce, W.W.: Managing the development of large software systems. Proceedings of IEEE WESCON 26(8) (1970)

30. Silberman, M.S., Nathan, L., Knowles, B., Bendor, R., Clear, A., Håkansson, M., Dillahunt, T., Mankoff, J.: Next steps for sustainable HCI. Interactions 21(5), 66–69 (2014)

31. Simon, H.: The Sciences of Artificial, 3rd edn. MIT Press, Cambridge (1996)

32. Stegall, N.: Designing for sustainability: A philosophy for ecologically intentional design. Design Issues 22(2), 56–63 (2006)

33. Walker, S.: The Spirit of Design: Objects, Environment and Meaning. Routledge, London (2011)

34. Wood, W.: Attitude change: Persuasion and social influence. Annual Review of Psychology 51(1), 539–570 (2000)

35. World Commission on Environment and Development (WCED): Our Common Future. Oxford University Press, London (1987)

Conforming to an Artificial Majority: Persuasive Effects of a Group of Artificial Agents

Cees Midden, Jaap Ham[(✉)] and Joey Baten

Human-Technology Interaction, Eindhoven University of Technology, P.O. Box 513,
5600 MB, Eindhoven, The Netherlands
{c.j.h.midden,j.r.c.ham}@tue.nl

Abstract. In this paper we propose a new perspective on persuasive technology: *Persuasive effects of a group of artificial agents.* We argue that while effects of single social agents have been corroborated, understanding of persuasion by multiple agents in a group setting is very limited. In the current research, we argue that conformity effects could occur not only with human majorities, but also with artificial majorities consisting of smart agents or computers. Two studies were conducted to investigate the conformity effect of group pressure on participants' comparative judgments of lengths of lines, based on the classic Asch paradigm. Group pressure by human majorities was compared with pressure by majorities of boxed PC's and of artificial virtual agents. Results indicated that normative pressure is limited to human majorities, while informational pressure can also be exerted by artificial majorities. This research revealed that applying majorities of artificial agents opens up a new domain of persuasive technology.

Keywords: Conformity · Artificial agent · artificial majority · persuasive technology · Persuasive agents · Groups of artificial agents

1   Introduction

Artificial virtual agents are becoming popular rapidly and are applied in various contexts (e.g., the internet, home appliances, telephone systems, and cars). People interact with artificial agents frequently, and probably more often the near future. This raises many questions about people's behavior and responses in such encounters. Artificial virtual agents (AVA's, also labelled Embodied Conversational Agents, see [13]) are virtual humans generated by a computer, represented in many ways, often having humanlike appearances, features, looks, and speech.

Artificial agents have been employed as persuasive systems as well. They are able to perform all kinds of supportive tasks (e.g., providing warnings, instructions). Recent research indicated that persuasive agents can be powerful social influencers. For example, own previous work demonstrated that AVA's that employed social feedback (e.g., by expressing social approval or disapproval) had stronger persuasive effects than persuasive technology that employed non-social factual feedback [1]. For example, research [2] showed that social embodiment (a social robot versus a computer

© Springer International Publishing Switzerland 2015
T. MacTavish and S. Basapur (Eds.): PERSUASIVE 2015, LNCS 9072, pp. 229–240, 2015.
DOI: 10.1007/978-3-319-20306-5_21

giving feedback) increases the persuasive effects of energy consumption feedback. These effects demonstrated that artificial agents can exert social influence on human users similar to social influence in human-human interaction. Moreover this research showed that some kind of social cueing is needed to create these effects. However, the extent of social cueing needed seemed limited, that is, effects were achieved with rather simple cues. This finding is also supported the media equation hypothesis (e.g.,[3]), that showed that people tend to relatively mindlessly apply social rules and expectations to computers.

So, research suggested social feedback by AVA's might be effective, but is limited to effects generated by single agents and thereby only covered a part of human social influence processes. Many social psychological studies demonstrated the power of influence exerted among group members [4]. This raises the question whether human users are also sensitive to group pressure as exerted by AVA's operating as (artificial) group members. In the current research, we extend the persuasive potential of artificial agents by exploring the persuasive effects of multiple agents in a group setting. In social psychology social influence by group pressure is referred to as conformity (see [4]).

1.1   Conformity

Conformity is the process by which an individual shapes his or her behavior to make it consistent with group norms [4]. For example when a person smokes cigarettes because other group members do so, the group member is exhibiting conformity. Conformity has been extensively studied in groups consisting of humans, largely initiated by the seminal work of Solomon Asch [5]. Group norms emerge because group members in an uncertain situation exchange judgments and develop common norms [6].

Participants in Asch's experiments believed to be part of an experiment on perceptual judgment. They were asked to sit down in a group with six other people. The task of each group member was to say which of three black lines on a card was the same length as a line on another card. Only one of the three lines was similar to the one on the other card. The others were clearly different. Members of the group gave their judgments in sequence. Only the group member on the sixth position was a real participant. The other group members were confederates, instructed to give false answers. Asch's results showed that most (about 3 out of 4) people went along with the clearly false majority answers. Furthermore results showed that individuals gave almost completely accurate answers when answers were anonymous. Clearly this type of group pressure effects may extend to other more important situations in all kinds of domains like health, safety, sustainability, political behavior, altruism and so on.

Asch's findings were replicated many times. We investigated whether these group pressure effects hold for group majorities consisting of *artificial* agents. Given human tendencies to interact with artificial agents in a more or less social way, people might be sensitive to the judgments of a group majority consisting of artificial agents. Research investigating this issue seems limited. In [8] the majority existed of computers. Instead of humans providing an answer, each computer screen showed the answer for three seconds and participants were told that the computers generated the answer based on a simple algorithm. The focal task was however rather different from the

Asch-studies: participants had to mentally rotate and match 3D-objects. Results showed that participant's error rate increased in both human and computer conditions compared to the control condition. Moreover, in the human condition the errors increased more compared to the computer condition, although both groups were rated as equally reliable.

Possibly, different processes were occurring. [9] proposed that two kinds of social influence can be distinguished: Normative social influence (occurring when a person conforms in order to be accepted or liked by others) and informational social influence (the tendency to accept information obtained from another as evidence; [9]).

When comparing the human condition versus the computer condition in the study by [8], it could be that humans generated a higher normative social influence than computers. However, the study did not test explanations for the observed differences. Because of the different task structures the results were not directly comparable to those using the Asch-paradigm. In the current research we tried to shed light on these underlying mechanisms of conforming to an artificial majority.

1.2   The Current Research

Study 1 examined whether social influences could also occur due to group pressure by AVA's. We argued that in line with media equation studies and related research, conformity responses to artificial majorities could occur. Extending our research (e.g., [1]; [2]) we expected AVA's that show one or more social cues could be more effective in evoking conformity reaction than smart systems lacking these cues. The latter situation was actually the case in the Berns et al study, who used plain computer systems. To allow for direct comparison of our findings to those of Asch and colleagues, we used the classic conformity paradigm of Solomon Asch [5] and accordingly replaced the majority of humans by a majority of AVA's or PC's. The study tested whether conformity would occur when the majority consisted of humans, AVA's or PC's.

2   Study 1

2.1   Method

Participants and Design. A total of 74 male students of Eindhoven University of Technology (M = 22.5, SD = 2.5) participated in the study and each participant received a payment of €5 for participation. The study had a 1-factor design with 4 levels representing types of group pressure (type of group pressure: no pressure (control), majority of humans, majority of PC's, majority of AVA's). The dependent variable was the number of critical errors. Critical errors are errors in which the majority uniformly provided a wrong answer. In the case of the control group the participants received no answers of the other stooges around the table.

Apparatus. The stimulus was presented as black lines against a white background, on a computer display. A neutral white background was shown prior to the tasks. The comparison lines were numbered 1, 2 and 3 from left to right and had the same length as in the Asch [5] experiments. A group size of 5 was utilized in accordance with the findings by Asch [5] showing that larger group sizes did not change conformity. In addition, the study of Berns et al. [8] also used a group size of 5. The stooges were male students with respectively the same age, in order to be similar as the participants being tested.

Procedure. In this experiment, we used the experimental procedure as used by Asch [5]. The stimulus was projected on a screen opposing the side of the table where no one was seated. Completely as in [5], participants had to indicate which of the three lines was the longest in 18 trials, while the stooges answered incorrectly on 12 of these (the critical trials). The participants were always seated in the fourth position, so they would give their answer after the first three stooges, but before the last stooge.

Before the experiment started the participants and the stooges would sign an informed consent form. The participants and stooges were given a brief instruction about what they had to do after the consent form. Then the group performed a task in which a presented line had to be compared with three other lines. The standard and comparison lengths, the order in which they appeared, the responses of the majority, and the type of error were identical to the experimental procedure that Asch (1956) used.

In condition 1, the control group, the participants had to write down their answers on a (paper) answer sheet paper (next to the corresponding task number) without communicating their answer with the other group members, while four male stooges did the same task. In the three other experimental conditions the experiment leader recorded the answers of the participants who needed to announce their answer publicly.

In condition 2, the stooges were 4 male persons, who were instructed in advance by the experimenter and were aware of the goal of the experiment. They were also instructed which answer to give per round. The first stooge would announce his answer and the other stooges would repeat his answer when it was their turn. At the start of the experiment, the stooges asked two questions in order to create the impression to the participant that they were naive as well. One would ask what date it was today, and another stooge would ask a verifying question about the assignment.

In condition 3, a majority of four identical boxed PC's was used to influence the participants. After the comparison lines were shown each computer and the participants publicly announced their answers when it was their turn to respond. The displays were visible for the real participant. Each computer had a webcam to suggest the capability of the computer to perceive the stimulus. The computer displays were black until the computer had to give a response. Then the computers showed by means of their answer a corresponding white number 1, 2 or 3 on the screen against the black background for 3 seconds, after which the screen turned black again.

In condition 4, a majority of AVA's was used to influence the participants, which were shown on computer displays (see Figure 1). Each AVA was shown on a display that pointed towards the participant. The AVA's were created with use of Haptek software (Haptek, 2013). All AVA's were different males, and only their head and shoulders were shown. Each AVA had a neutral expression and moved his head and eyes slightly. The answers of the avatars were recorded before the experiments started and each avatar was voiced by a different male person. Similar to condition 3 a web-cam to each computer was attached to stimulate the capability of the computer to see the stimulus. After the comparison lines were shown each AVA and the participants would publicly announce their answer when it was their turn to answer.

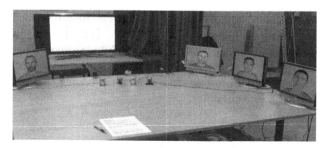

Fig. 1. The experiment setup in condition 4, showing a majority of AVA's

After finishing the tasks, in all conditions, the participants (and also stooges, if present) completed two questionnaires (a funneled debriefing task that inquired amongst others for perceived influence of other group members, cf. Asch [5], and a second questionnaire that measured level of anthropomorphism [10]).

2.2   Results

Manipulation Checks. Two participants indicated being familiar with the experiments by Asch [5] and were excluded from further analysis. Two persons in the PC's condition and one person in the AVA's condition were excluded because they did not complete the questionnaire. Based on work by [10], a measure of anthropomorphism was constructed. Based on the fit statistics of Rasch analysis 22 items were selected for scale construction [10]. The result was a 22-tems scale measuring the level of anthropomorphism ranging from 1 to 22. Participants perceived the PC's and AVA's as equally human-like, based on the Anthropomorphism scale. The mean score of AVA's (M = 11.6, SD = 2.5) was higher than of PC's (M = 10.7, SD = 3.3), but this difference did not reach significance t(33) = -.912, NS.

Testing Hypotheses. Level of conformity, the main dependent variable, was constructed based on the number of conformity errors made by participants during the 12 critical trials. A conformity error was an error in which the participant followed the majority while the majority answer was faulty. The experiment consisted of twelve critical trials and therefore the range consisted of values between zero (fully independent) and twelve (fully yielding).

In order to test H1 and H2 we conducted a 4 (type of group pressure: Control, Humans, PC's, AVA's) x 1 factor ANOVA. The results showed a significant effect F(3, 8) = 5.36, p =.02 of type of group pressure (Control, Humans, PC's, AVA's). A post-hoc Tukey test indicated that participants who did not receive social pressure produced significantly less errors (M = .24, SD = .54, p = .01) than participants who had received social pressure from other human group members (M = 1.45, SD = 2.2). In addition, in the human majority condition participants produced significant more errors than PC's (M = .38, SD = .81, p = .05) and AVA's (M = 0, SD = 0, p = .02). In line with the findings by Asch, these results provided evidence that a majority of humans produced conformity effects compared to the control group and also generated more conformity than a majority of AVA's or PC's. No statistical differences were found between the control group, the PC group and AVA group. Thus, these results did not provide evidence in support of the hypothesis that a majority of AVA's showing strong social cues would generate more conformity among humans than a majority of PC's with weak social cues.

2.2.1   Qualitative Exploration of Results

The funneled debriefing answers presented an understanding of what the participants were experiencing, whether they knew the purpose of the experiment and whether they were consciously aware that they conformed towards the group judgments. Interestingly, in the AVA's and PC's conditions participants did not seem to be worried about what the group was expecting while in the humans condition almost everyone seemed to express concern and many felt doubts and tendencies to follow the group In the PC's group very few errors occurred. The non-conformers were questioning the algorithm or indicated that the computers were trying to influence them. They hardly showed doubts about their answers. On the other hand some participants expressed doubts. One person said: "Because they are computers you think that you could be wrong" and in the AVA condition: "Maybe the majority is right. They are with 4 people." These examples indicate that at least part of the participants experienced group pressure also in the PC and AVA-conditions, although not always enough to generate conformity behavior.

2.3   Conclusions and Discussion Study 1

Our results showed that participants conformed to a group majority consisting of humans and did so more than in the PC and AVA groups, which supports hypothesis 2. However, our results did not show conformity behavior in groups with `PC's or AVA's. This result seems contrary to the results of Berns et al. (2005) in which participants showed conformity to PC-groups. In the human majority group an overall conformity level of 12% was found as the overall error rate. This is less than in the classic Asch-experiments [5] in which the overall conformity amounted to around 30%. Of course many factors may have played a role in this difference including cultural factors (e.g., a fifty years' time difference), psychological factors (e.g. engineering students vs social science students) and situational factors. One factor in the latter category may have been that quite a few participants had some hunch about the purpose of the experiments, which might have stimulated their independence.

Our results indicated that people conformed less when a majority existed of technological systems instead of human, irrespective of its representation as boxed PC or artificial virtual agent. These results support the conclusion that the socialness of artificial agents, which has been demonstrated in other contexts, may not be strong enough to elicit powerful normative influence in a group setting. One reason may have been that the difference between the boxed PC's and the AVA's was not big enough. At least, he manipulation check showed no significant difference in the level of anthropomorphism between the technological conditions. Participants rated the PC's and AVA's as equally human-like. This is in itself remarkable given the substantial differences between the two conditions. One factor may have been the measurement of anthropomorphism. The direct questioning about human-likeness may affect available measures of anthropomorphism [10]. Anthropomorphic responses seem to work at a rather implicit level and may even remain unacknowledged by persons when asked (see also [3]). Our qualitative results point in a similar direction. Participant's verbal reactions showed indications of anthropomorphism, for example when participants in the PC's and AVA's groups used quotes where they referred to the technology as people. However, our findings suggest that the AVA's with additional social cues like speech and humanoid appearance, created no additional group pressure. In line with the Reeves and Nass findings, the weak social cues of the PC's may have been sufficient to provoke similar social responses as the stronger social cues of the AVA's. Moreover, our own research, a study by [2], demonstrated that one social cue may be sufficient while additional cues may not strengthen the effect. Another possible explanation could be that the level of presence of the AVA's was too low to exert social influence. In [2] and [1] a social robot was physically present while the AVA's in our study were, for experimental reasons, only virtually present on a display. One could speculate that this more constrained level of presence limited the effect of the AVA group, but did not affect the PC-effect.

Furthermore the experiment of [8] differed in an important way with the experiments by Asch [5] and ours, which concerned the task difficulty level. Participants had a more difficult task in the study by Berns et al. [8] in which they had to mentally rotate and match a 3D-object. This greater task difficulty could be a reason why people would conform towards the group of computers as the available information was more ambiguous. Task difficulty is related to the distinction made by [9] between informational group pressure and normative group pressure, which suggests that single group members may conform to a group majority either because they feel pressure not to deviate from the norms set by the group majority or feel an internal pressure to conform to the group judgments, because these seem to represent a social reality. This social reality becomes particularly relevant when the objective reality is less obvious, thereby creating uncertainty for the individual. So, a task that creates ambiguity about the right answer could stimulate informational social influence. In the study by [9] participants conformed more when the answer possibilities were only shown for 3 seconds, thereby raising doubts about the correct answer

Finally, we conjectured that the used setup did not exert sufficient pressure in the technological conditions. The webcams pointed mainly towards the line stimuli and therefore might have failed provoking the impression that the participants were being watched and evaluated by the group. As a consequence, one could argue that participants remained their anonymity to a larger extent, thereby possibly reducing group pressure.

The main goal of study 2 was to test the role of conformity due to information influence. In addition, we followed up on the current discussion by implementing some adjustments of our experimental set-up.

3   Study 2

In the previous study participants changed their behavior when under group pressure by humans, while almost no conformity occurred when the majority consisted of AVA's or PC's. In study 2 we will follow up on these findings by investigating possible explanations for the results of study 1 and attempt to understand why participants were not influenced by the AVA's.

First, we argued that informational pressure could be more important for agents to generate conformity than normative pressure. Possibly normative pressure is not likely happening with the current type of agents and the relations that people have with agents. [8] showed that increasing the task difficulty, thereby enhancing informational pressure, increased conformity. [7] found that increasing the task difficulty in computer mediated communication increased conformity. The study by Berns et al. [8] who showed conformity effects of a PC group included a more difficult task than ours. Possibly, a more difficult task could provoke conforming behavior in our study.

Second, based on our discussion of study 1, we assumed that some elements of the setup of the study might have flawed an adequate comparison of the human vs artificial majorities. The level of social pressure might have been too low, first because the webcams pointed towards the stimuli and possibly kept the participants too much anonymous. This effect could have been enhanced by the only virtual presence of our agents. For study 2 we adjusted the experimental set-up of study 1 by adding monitoring capabilities of the AVA's and PC's through the use of extra webcams that pointed towards the participant. These webcams were supposed to provide a salient social cue of participants being watched (see also [11]).

On the basis of this modification of setting 1 we tested again hypothesis 1:

H1.2: A majority of AVA's showing strong social cues will generate more conformity among humans than a majority of PC's with weak social cues.

Secondly, we hypothesized that the level of informational pressure could make a difference to create conformity effects:

H2.2: A majority of AVA's or PC's will generate (more) conformity among human participants when the judgmental task is more demanding, thus creating more conformity based on informational pressure.

3.1   Method

Participants and Design. A total of 98 male students of the TU/e (mean age = 21.88, SD = 2.38) participated in the experiment . Participants received a payment of €5.00 for their participation. Eleven participants stated being familiar with the experiments by Asch (1956) and were excluded from further analysis. In order to test our hypotheses a 2 (task difficulty: low difficult vs high difficulty) x 3 (type of group pressure: Control, PC's, AVA's) factorial design was applied. Like in study 1, the dependent variable was the number of conformity errors a participant made during the 12 critical trials. In the case of the control groups the participants received no pressure.

Apparatus. Similar apparatus was utilized as in study 1 with minor modifications. One modification was adding four webcams to the PC's and AVA's condition. These webcams would point towards the participant in order to provoke the impression that the participants were being watched and judged by the PC's or AVA's.

Furthermore, task difficulty level was manipulated. In the 'low difficulty' condition the set-up was similar to the Asch [5] set-up In the 'high difficulty' task condition the comparison lines were only shown for 0.35s. This duration was based on a pilot study to assess the right level of ambiguity.

3.2   Results

Anthropomorphism Level. First of all, we assessed whether participants perceived the AVA's as more human-like than the PC's. Anthropomorphism was measured similarly to the procedure in Study 1. A 2x2 factorial ANOVA (task difficulty: low difficulty vs high difficulty; type of group pressure: PC's vs. AVA's) showed a marginal significant main effect of type of group pressure, $F(1, 0.3) = 4.47$, $p = .058$; no main effect of task difficulty (low, high), $F(1, 0.7) = 10.01$, p= .40 and no interaction effects, $F(1, 1) = 13.81$, $p = .33$. Thereby this result suggested that our manipulation of type of group pressure was quite successful.

Testing Hypotheses. In order to examine H2.1 and H2.2 we conducted a 2x3 factorial ANOVA: task difficulty (low difficult vs high difficulty by type of group pressure (Control, PC's, AVA's). The dependent variable was the number of conformity errors a participant made during the critical trials. We found two significant main effects; type of group pressure (Control, PC's, AVA's), $F(2, 9) = 7.84$, $p < .001$ and task difficulty (low, high), $F(1, 81) = 70.76$, $p < .001$. These results showed that the AVA's and PC's were able to exert more group pressure in comparison with the control group. Furthermore, results showed that our task manipulation was effective. In the high difficulty condition we found more conformity than in the low difficulty condition. Posthoc Tukey comparisons of the three types of pressure indicated that the control group (M = .33, SD = 0.6) showed less conformity than AVA's-condition (M = 1.31, SD =1.67), $p < 0.01$ and PC's-condition (M = 1.18, SD = 1.56), $p = 0.03$. Comparison between the AVA's and PC's showed no significant difference. These results provided no evidence in support of Hypothesis 2.1 that a majority of AVA's would generate more conformity among humans than a majority of boxed PC's.

In addition, we found a significant interaction effect between type of group pressure and task difficulty, $F(2, 8) = 7.36$, $p < .001$. Posthoc Tukey comparisons of the six types of interactions indicated that in the high difficulty task condition more conformity occurred in the AVA's condition (M= 2.53, SD = 1.50), $p < 0.01$ and PC's condition (M = 2.9, SD = 1.55), $p < 0.001$) compared to the control group (M = 0.66, SD = 0.72). These effects did not occur in the low difficulty conditions. In the low difficulty task condition no differences were found between the control group (M = 0, SD = 0), the AVA-group (M = 0, SD = 0), NS, and the PC-group (M = 0.07, SD = 0.07). These results supported H2.2 suggesting that a majority of AVA's or PC's would generate conformity among human participants when the judgmental task is more demanding, thus creating more conformity based on informational pressure.

3.3   Conclusions and Discussion study 2

Results of Study 2 provided no evidence in support of Hypothesis 2.1 as our results showed no differences in conformity between the AVA's group and the PC's group. Furthermore, participants largely kept their independence when facing a clearly faulty majority of PC's or AVA's under low task difficulty. Also, under high task difficulty no difference was found between the AVA and PC groups as conformity occurred alike. It seems that the presence of strong social cues versus weak social cues made no difference on conformity since the AVA's and PC's group did not differ compared to the control group. So apparently AVA's and PC's did not exert effective normative pressure. Moreover, our results showed that almost nobody expressed concern about how the other group members would feel about their answers.

By contrast, our results demonstrated that under high task difficulty AVA and PC majorities could exert group pressure and induce conformity, which was in support of H2.2. This result under high task difficulty conditions indicates that informational group pressure occurred. That is participants were using the inputs of the other group members to develop and validate their own judgments.

4   General Discussion

In sum, results showed that a majority of AVA's and a majority of PC's created a similar overall conformity effect among participants when the participants had to perform a relatively difficult task. While human majorities were able to create normative pressure and supposedly informational pressure, our data suggest that a group of artificial agents can alter humans answers by exerting informational pressure.

While these results learn us about the group influences that can be exerted by groups of artificial agents, our results also raise new questions. Study 1 showed AVA's limit in using normative pressure suggesting that they are not equally able to generate the feeling that norms exist or are expected to be followed. Our studies could not fully analyze reasons why that would be the case. However, in contrast to most other studies on social agency and social responses to artificial agents (see introduction), the power of the agents in our study was dependent on the degree to which they were perceived by participants as a *group*. Possibly this group feeling was not sufficiently present. Future research might investigate explanations for why an artificial majority is less powerful in exerting normative pressure than a human majority. A challenging question would be whether the perception of being in a group of artificial members could be enhanced by introducing (subtle) cues of group behavior like informal social interaction. Similarly to the issue of making agents social, the question could be raised whether social cues at the group level could generate a group feeling.

Apparently these cues will be different from the ones at the level of individual agents. These cues did not create the group behavior we expected on the basis of human group majorities. Moreover, we found similar overall conformity between the AVA and PC groups indicating participants did not respond differently toward the two groups with artificial group members differing in human-likeness at the individual level. This could be explained by media equation studies showing that the most simple computer systems were able to elicit social responses and research that showed that adding a second social cue to a system with one cue did not enhance persuasive effects [2]. At the psychological level, the distinction between a boxed computer providing text messages and a human-like face of a speaking artificial agent seems not significant. Although the current results are based on the stimulus materials of the current study, our finding fit to the Media Equation hypothesis and earlier findings.

This explanation is in line with the result that in spite of obvious differences between the PC-condition and the AVA condition, our measure of Anthropomorphism did not reveal any subjective differences. This suggested that AVA's and PC's had similar anthropomorphism levels and were perceived as equally human-like. Still we argue that questionnaires that ask explicitly about anthropomorphic responses may be inaccurate and that more unobtrusive measures seem desirable.

While we did not find indications of normative pressure by artificial majorities, we did find that these groups were able to exert informational pressure. This was most clearly demonstrated in Study 2, that showed that when a judgmental task is demanding, conformity occurs also when the majority consists of article members. In a more general sense this means that when reality is ambiguous, conformity tends to occur based on informational pressure, and individuals seem to seek for the most valid interpretation. Informational pressure is important, because it controls de development of converging views on reality. While normative pressure may lead to conformity behavior, it does not necessarily lead to mental change. Informational pressure on the other hand includes internal pressure to conform to group judgments, because these seem to represent a social reality. In that perspective informational pressure may lead to a deeper and possibly also more persistent change.

Research on the persuasive effects of groups of artificial agents has just started. Theory is needed on the features of artificial groups that influence conformity levels going beyond individual characteristics of agents, just as better measuring instruments, studies of relevant characteristics of human participants (e.g., gender, loneliness).

To conclude, we believe that the use of agents at the group level offers ample opportunities to enhance persuasive processes. Human beings are sensitive for social influence exerted by groups of persons. Developing groups of artificial agents that have a similar potential seems a great challenge for researchers and designers of persuasive systems.

Aknowledgements. We thank Niels Kleemans and Gerrit Nijrolder for the contributions to Study 1.

References

1. Midden, C., Ham, J.: Social influence of a persuasive agent: the role of agent embodiment and evaluative feedback. In: Conference Proceedings of Persuasive, Claremont, USA (2009)
2. Vossen, S., Ham, J., Midden, C.: What makes social feedback from a robot work? Disentangling the effect of speech, physical appearance and evaluation. In: Ploug, T., Hasle, P., Oinas-Kukkonen, H. (eds.) PERSUASIVE 2010. LNCS, vol. 6137, pp. 52–57. Springer, Heidelberg (2010)
3. Reeves, B., Nass, C.: The media equation. Cambridge University Press, NY (1996)
4. Cialdini, R.B., Trost, M.R.: Social influence: Social norms, conformity, and compliance. In: Gilbert, D.T., Fiske, S.T., Lindzey, G. (eds.) The Handbook of Social Psychology, 4th edn., vol. 2, pp. 151–192. McGraw-Hill, New York (1998)
5. Asch, S.E.: Studies of Independence and Conformity: I. A Minority of One Against a Unanimous Majority. Psychological Monographs: General and Applied 70(9) (1956)
6. Moscovici, S.: Social influence and conformity. In: Lindzey, G., Aronson, E. (eds.) Handbook of Social Psychology, vol. 2, pp. 347–412. Random House, New York (1985)
7. Rosander, M., Eriksson, O.: Conformity on the Internet – The role of task difficulty and gender differences. Computers in Human Behavior 28, 1587–1595 (2012)
8. Berns, G.S., Chappelow, J., Zink, C.F., Pagnoni, G., Martin-Skurski, M.E., Richards, J.: Neurobiological correlates of social conformity and independence during mental rotation. Biological Psychiatry 58(3), 245–253 (2005)
9. Deutsch, M., Gerard, H.B.: A study of normative and informational social influences upon individual judgment. The Journal of Abnormal and Social Psychology 51(3), 629–636 (1955)
10. Ruijten, P.A.M., Bouten, D.H.L., Rouschop, D.C.J., Ham, J., Midden, C.J.H.: Introducing a Rasch-Type Anthropomorphism Scale. In: Proceedings of the 9thACM/IEEE International Conference on Human-Robot Interaction. IEEE Press (2014)
11. Midden, C., Ham, J.: The Illusion of Agency: The Influence of the Agency of an Artificial Agent on its Persuasive Power. In: Bang, M., Ragnemalm, E.L. (eds.) PERSUASIVE 2012. LNCS, vol. 7284, pp. 90–99. Springer, Heidelberg (2012)
12. Cassell, J., Bickmore, T., Campbell, L., Vilhjálmsson, H., Yan, H.: Conversation as a System Framework: Designing Embodied Conversational Agents. In: Cassell, J., Prevost, S., Churchill, S.J. (eds.) Embodied Conversational Agents. MIT Press (1999)

A System's Self-referential Persuasion: Understanding the Role of Persuasive User Experiences in Committing Social Web Users

Michael Oduor[✉] and Harri Oinas-Kukkonen

Oulu Advanced Research on Software and Information Systems,
Faculty of Information Technology and Electrical Engineering,
University of Oulu, P.O. Box 3000, 90014, Oulu, Finland
{michael.oduor,harri.oinas-kukkonen}@oulu.fi

Abstract. This paper discusses how social web platforms try to influence user interactions. We explain this influence from the perspective of persuasion context analysis and provision of persuasive user experiences. Additionally, the paper introduces and expounds on the concept of self-referential persuasion and illustrates its application through discussion and analysis of preliminary results of a survey (N=57) on the use of the social web. The persuasive systems design (PSD) model is utilized to analyze the social influence aspects through analysis of the persuasion context and the subsequent persuasive user experiences.

Keywords: Social web · platform · Social influence · Persuasive systems design · Self-referential persuasion · Persuasive user experience · Humanized web.

1   Introduction

Our contemporary web can be described as the era of the social web, and the future web is becoming even more humanized [16]. The social web platforms provide ecosystems of related elements comprising of both digital and traditional media that leverage the personal relationships embodied in social networks [22, 27]. Thus re-transforming the World Wide Web (WWW) to what it was initially created for "a platform to facilitate information exchange between users" [24]. In the social web user participation and user-generated content in a collaborative and open environment plays an essential role [20].

There are many kinds of information technologies available that have been developed for online collaboration and sharing of user-generated content, and many of these technologies share similar features such as creation of user profiles that disclose whom the user is in contact with, access to others contacts lists, customization of user profiles, private messaging, discussion forums, media uploading, integration with other applications [3, 12] amongst others. In this type of activity, one of the major challenges is how to motivate and encourage different stakeholders and particularly end-users to keep contributing to the operational environment [16]. Especially as users are no longer passive recipients of information and they are increasingly taking

© Springer International Publishing Switzerland 2015
T. MacTavish and S. Basapur (Eds.): PERSUASIVE 2015, LNCS 9072, pp. 241–252, 2015.
DOI: 10.1007/978-3-319-20306-5_22

part in all aspects of value creation [21]. We refer to this as an *information system's self-referential persuasion* where users can not only participate in the co-creation of value, but also leave their own identity into the system [22] and are persuaded to keep using it more.

In overall, this paper examines how users interact via social web channels and it sheds light on the inherent features of social networking technologies that purposefully aim at influencing user behaviors. The background stems from a persuasive technology domain, which describes how interactive computing systems have an impact on users' thoughts and consequently lead to a change in their behavior [9, 17]. Persuasive systems design is a growing research area, which has attracted a lot of interest recently. Illustrative examples of research include using persuasive system design models for analyzing carbon management systems [6] or systems for weight management [29] and avoidance of alcohol abuse [15] as well as for studying adherence in the use of health behavior change support systems [14] amongst many others.

The specific focus of this paper, a system's self-referential persuasion, is illustrated through analysis of preliminary results of an Internet survey (N=57) on the use of the social web. The survey covered topics such as reasons for joining a particular platform, the types of platforms used, use history and the kind of information primarily shared in the social web sites. Our analysis also explored the differences between certain categories and demographics of the respondents. An inherent feature in all social web platforms is their appeal to human need for interaction as the basic reason for doing activities online–even though these activities may be different for different people–remains the same [23]. Understanding social influence requires one to understand fundamental aspects of human behavior and these social web platforms with their focus on supporting social interaction–through social design–[7, 16, 23] seem to embody this and should be examined from a social-technical perspective [7].

The rest of the paper discusses other related work and the conceptual underpinning in persuasive systems design (section 2). Section 3 describes the survey methodology, followed by the analysis and results in section 4, which presents data on the importance (from the end-users' viewpoint) of the various features. We conclude by discussing the implications of the findings for persuasive systems design of social web platforms.

2   Related Work

To place our research in context, the current section will be based on two interlinked perspectives related to the social web. These perspectives are persuasive systems design, in particular for understanding the persuasion context, and provision of persuasive user experiences, in particular for committing users.

2.1   The Persuasion Context

Although not related to the social web only, such underlying features as simplicity of use, wide reach and easy accessibility provide social web platforms with an ideal context for influence; also many of the persuasive techniques applied in other computing systems are equally applicable in these platforms [9]. Additionally, many persuasive strategies and software features can be applied in them. Technological influence depends on whether one is interacting through–computer-mediated communication– or with–human-computer interaction [9]. For example, instant message for people in different locations is interaction through and where a technological product, such as an activity band, is a participant in the interaction and can proactively seek to motivate and influence is interaction with technology.

Oinas-Kukkonen and Harjumaa's [17] persuasive systems design (PSD) model for designing and evaluating persuasive systems suggests that before one is able to implement any of the desired persuasive software features, seven essential postulates behind persuasive systems must be understood. These postulates relate to accessibility and reach, ease of use, making and enforcing of commitments, attitudes and persuasion strategies, sequential nature of persuasion, the ideal moments for initiating persuasive features and openness [17].[1]

Inherent in the above postulates and the PSD model are social psychological theories on attitude change, influence, learning and so forth that help to explain human behavior in different circumstances. Therefore, when developing persuasive systems it is relevant to consider the applicable theories such as the elaboration likelihood model (ELM) [19] which is a theory on attitude change that describes two distinct routes to information processing and persuasion; Bandura's [1, 2] social learning and social cognitive theories which provide a framework for understanding, predicting and changing human behavior and state that people learn new behaviors by studying (the consequences), observing and then replicating the actions of others; and Cialdini's [4, 5] studies on influence which show how formulating requests in certain ways can trigger automatic compliance response from individuals.

After acknowledging the persuasion postulates, the context for persuasion is analysed. *Persuasion context* analysis comprises of recognizing the intent of persuasion, the persuasion event, and the strategies in use [17]. Acknowledging the intent includes determining, who the actual persuader is. Since computers don't have any intentions of their own, the source of persuasion in a system is always one of those who create, distribute, or adopt the persuasive technology [8]. Analyzing the intent also covers defining the change type [18]. The outcome/change design matrix [18] defines the three potential, successful voluntary outcomes of behavior change support systems as formation, alteration, or reinforcement of attitudes, behaviors, or compliance.

As for understanding the persuasion event, the contexts of use, the user, and the technology should be recognized [17]. The use context covers the characteristics of the problem domain in question, the user context includes the differences between the individuals, and the technology context addresses the technical specifications of a system. Finally, identifying the persuasion strategies includes attempting to analyze the persuasive message that is being conveyed and the route, whether direct or indirect, that is used

---

[1] After this step, the development can commence into designing actual software features, which are categorized by the PSD model as primary task, computer-human dialogue, credibility and social support features. [19]

to reach the persuadee–the end-user [17]. It is important to realize that the persuasion context can be fleshed out as software architecture [cf. 28].

2.2   Persuasive User Experiences

The social web platforms as spheres of influence focus on the consumers' user experience and expand media choices so as to capture reach, intimacy, and engagement [21]. The social web has conjured radical new ways of interacting and presented an unparalleled opportunity for people to network [13]. This is mainly because of it being a platform that provides tools and documentation to enable creation of applications that can be embedded within the respective environments [3, 7, 13, 20, 24].

Interaction online also depends on the medium used, which defines and helps to frame the message. Communication media as explained by the social presence theory differ according to the degree of "social presence". That is, the state of being present between two communicators using a social medium [25]. Some communication media have a higher degree of social presence, for example, characters in virtual environments, whereas others have a lower degree of social presence, for example, e-mail, and audio. The higher the degree of social presence the more a communication medium is viewed as sociable, warm and personal and the larger the social influence that communicators-people interacting with the media-have on one another [24, 25].

One of the most important directions for the future web is providing persuasive user experiences for the masses of users, particularly when people who are not on an organization's payroll still contribute to its success; these users must be motivated, encouraged and persuaded [16]. From persuasive system's point of view, we call this a system's self-referential persuasion. The phases of the behavior chain related to this and referred to in [10] are discovery, superficial involvement and (true) commitment. Discovery and superficial involvement are concerned with becoming aware of a web service by learning about it from friends, for example, and deciding to try it by setting up an account. When trying to understand the platforms, which are already very well known by a large audience, analyzing persuasive strategies for commitment is needed. The success witnessed by the growth of the platforms has hinged on persuading users to perform certain inherently social behaviors. These include, creating value and content that others can consume, staying active and loyal through repeated visits to the site and involving others to use the service by inviting them to be friends and sharing information and links–both social and formal [10].

Fogg [11] explains that the software components and particularly their design can explain how technology creates a persuasive experience (designed to change attitudes and/or behaviors) making the creation and delivery of target behaviors and persuasive goals easier and much faster. Although there are many uses and goals for social web platforms, the main persuasion goals can be broken down to: (1) encourage users to create a personal profile (cf. creating value and content); (2) invite and connect with friends (cf. involving others); (3) respond to others' contributions (cf. creating value and content); and (4) regularly access the site (cf. staying active and loyal) [12].

The stages of the behavior chain and corresponding persuasion goals above have been further elaborated on in [23] where various methods for developing social websites have been discussed. These include the importance of considering the users primary goal–the intent, the social objects that enable interaction and features, which are possible actions that can be done as derived from the goals and social objects [23]. More recently, Sleeper et al. [26] explore users' behavior-change goals for using the social web platforms. This provides insights to their perceptions of how their lives are affected and informs on tools that can be used to help users achieve the desired behavior change goals [26].

3   Survey Methodology

There have been numerous studies on how social web platforms are used and some such as [3, 13, 21, 24] that discuss the various categories of these platforms and the reasons for joining them[2] were used to generate the list of those included (for user selection) in the survey. As Morris et al. [12] have noted, other than catching up on personal information and current activities (of social ties), many users are utilizing their social web sites as sources of information and productivity. Thus we conducted a survey to explore users' platform preferences, their interactions, the information they primarily share and the features they found most useful. The survey was primarily based on PSD model principles [17] and persuasion goals [10, 12] as these studies discussed features and their target behaviors, which was an important consideration for our study.

3.1   Data Collection

The online survey of social web users in Finland was conducted between December 2 and December 23, 2014. The data was collected using an online survey and analysis tool called Webropol. According to the statistics given by the tool, the total number of visitors was 110 of which 57 responded; thus, the effective survey response rate was 52% (57/110) – albeit a small sample size. All these were valid for further analysis. Prior to publishing the survey online, a pilot test was conducted with 8 (2 senior scholars and 6 doctoral students) participants. Based on the results of the pilot test some questions and Likert scale options were modified.

3.2   Survey Content

In addition to collecting basic demographic and background information about participants' use of social web platforms, the survey asked a number of questions related to reasons for joining a particular platform, satisfaction with the use of the various platforms and the features present in them. Additionally, we requested users to self-report on what they primarily use social websites for and after selecting a particular platform(s), what they share in these platforms. Participants were also asked to rank a set of features found in most social web platforms in order of importance and these were

---

[2] This was based on the idea of object-centered sociality - http://bit.ly/1oL6JfM - where there are social objects (also discussed in [23]) (work, hobby, friendship etc.) that connect people.

compared to the satisfaction ratings on the same. As with most self-reported data, there is potential for inherent mistakes that the reader should bear in mind.

3.3   Respondent Characteristics and Usage Statistics

There were more male (61.4%) than female respondents, a majority (86%) of the respondents also had a university degree and were mostly (56.1%) in the 25-34 year age range. Detailed characteristics are presented in Table 1. The survey also asked users which social web platforms they mostly used (Table 2) from a given list with an open text option to add extra if not given.

Table 1. Respondent characteristics

Demographics		Frequency	Percentage
Gender	Male	35	61.4%
	Female	22	38.6%
Age	Less than 24	13	22.8%
	25 - 34	32	56.1%
	35 or older	12	21.1%
Marital status	Married	11	19.3%
	In a relationship	20	35.1%
	Single	26	45.6%
Education	High school	6	10.5%
	Vocational training	2	3.5%
	Bachelor's degree	21	36.8%
	Master's degree	23	40.4%
	Other advanced	2	3.5%
	Doctoral degree	3	5.3%

Table 2. Percent of respondents who reported the frequency of access (of 52 Facebook, 47 Youtube, 38 Wikipedia, 37 Linkedin and 31 Twitter users)

Service	Few times a day	Once a day	A few times a week	Once a week or less
Facebook	59.6%	19.2 %	9.6%	5.8%
YouTube	40.4%	25.5 %	25.5%	8.5%
Wikipedia	18.4%	26.3%	31.6%	25.7%
Twitter	12.9%	16.1%	35.5%	34.7%
Linkedin	5.4%	8.1%	18.9%	67.5%

4   Data Analysis and Results

Opinions, level of satisfaction and agreement and the frequencies were reported on 5-point Likert scale, where 5 = the most positive (e.g. strongly agree) and 1 = negative value (e.g., strongly disagree). Participants' responses to what they primarily use the platforms for were coded after first reviewing all the responses and then reading them again to assign them to the respective categories (reason for joining).

4.1   Information Sharing and Use of the Social Platforms

The reasons people had for joining or using the various social platforms were investigated. These reasons (for joining) were divided into five main categories with a sixth option–Other–given for user input. Table 3 shows the categories, their prevalence and examples by categorization of the usage of the social websites.

Table 3. Reason for joining and platform use

Reason	N (%)	Percent	Social platform use
For networking	35 (61.4)	30.4 %	To connect with people, share online resume
For entertainment	31 (54.4)	27.0 %	Music, chat, share photos
Suggestion (friend/family)	28 (49.1)	24.3%	Social updates
Interest in a topic	15 (26.3)	13.0%	Seeking information, news updates
To support a particular cause	3 (5.3)	2.6%	Share information on organizations, local events, news etc.
Other	3 (5.3)	2.6%	Mainly for work-related purposes

The most popular reasons for joining, *networking, entertainment* and *suggestion* all involve a social aspect where users are mainly interested in sharing information with those they already know [11, 12] and consequently to also meet others. This also corresponds with most responses given to the question "*What do you primarily use social web sites for?*" which consisted of communication and connecting with old friends. Additionally, most of the information shared on the various platforms (mainly social networking sites) is of a personal nature or links related to ones' interests. With continuous technological development extending the functionality of the various platforms, both social and professional boundaries have recently become blurred [13] and all or most of the forms of use above could be simultaneous and within one environment.

4.2   Feature Satisfaction Ratings

In the survey there was a question measuring 'user satisfaction' (from 1 very dissatisfied to 5 very satisfied) which consisted of 12 features found in the social platforms. Initially they were 13, but one was removed (open-text input) after testing because it resulted in the greatest increase in alpha. The scale had a high level of internal consistency as determined by a Cronbach's alpha of 0.865. A summary of the satisfaction ratings is presented in Table 4.

The features with the highest satisfaction ratings included: *inviting and connecting with friends* (M=3.89, SD=0.92), *responding to posts and updates* (M=3.89, SD=1.064), *uploading content* (M=3.74, SD=0.955), *private communication* (within the platforms) (M=3.7, SD=1.085), *creating* (M=3.67, SD=1.075), and *editing profile* (M=3.35, SD=1.142), and *forming groups* (M=3.56, SD=0.866). An independent samples t-test was conducted to compare satisfaction with the features in males and females. There was no significant difference in the scores for male (M=3.49, SD=0.64) and female (M=3.42, SD=0.68) conditions; t (55)=0.36, p = 0.721. A one-way between subjects ANOVA was also conducted to compare the effect of age and level of education on satisfaction. There was no significant effect of age and level of education on satisfaction remembered at the p<.0.05 for the three conditions [F (2, 54) = 4.94 p=0.26] and [F (7, 49) = 1.61 p=0.16]. These results suggest that gender, age and education do not have an effect on satisfaction with the features and the difference in means is likely a result of chance.

Table 4. Summary of feature satisfaction ratings

	Mean	Min	Max	Range	Max / Min	Va-riance	N of Items
Means	3.463	2.930	3.895	.965	1.329	.109	12

4.3 Feature Rankings

In addition to satisfaction ratings, users were also asked to rank (1=least, 13=most) the features in order of importance. Thus, a higher score corresponded to a higher importance ranking. The features ranked most important were (apart from newsfeed) similar to those users were most satisfied with though the ranking order differed slightly. These were (in descending order): *private communication* (M=9.23, SD=3.89), *editing profile* (M=8.89, SD=3.26), *inviting and connecting with friends* (M=8.74, SD=3.44), *creating profile* (M=8.32, SD=3.51), *responding to posts and updates* (M=8.02, SD=3), *newsfeed* (M=7.91, SD=3.25) and *uploading content* (M=6.18, SD=3.19). Again an independent samples t-test was conducted to compare ranking of the highest ranked feature (private messaging) in males and females. As before, there was no significant difference in the scores for male (M=9.5, SD=3.91) and female (M=8.82, SD=3.9) conditions; t (55)=0.63, p = 0.533. A one-way between subjects ANOVA was also conducted to compare the effect of use history on ranking (of private communication). Consistent with other findings above, there was no significant effect for the three conditions [F (2, 54) = 1.1 p=0.34]. These results suggest that gender and use history do not have an effect on the feature rankings and the difference in means is likely a result of chance and not due to the manipulation of the grouping variables. It is possible though that a larger sample size might reveal different results with greater variance in the rankings between groups.

5 Self-referential Persuasion in Social Web Platforms

This paper is about a system's self-referential persuasion, i.e. the system's persuasive intent being to refer to itself so that users stay as part of its ecosystem–and are persuaded to frequently use it, even though the system may not necessarily be persuasive in itself. We have presented data from a survey of 57 social web users on the social platforms used, the information shared and the platforms features' usefulness. The data provides valuable insights on the features users consider important and the information they primarily share, which can somewhat be linked to their reason(s) for registering to or frequently using any particular platform.

However, when interpreting the findings, it is important to bear in mind the limitations of our mostly highly educated survey demographic and the sample size that could have had an effect on the significance of some results. It is possible that a larger sample could have led to different findings. Additionally, the survey mainly focused on the features in general without considering the specifics of platform. Although, we did ask users to rank the features based on the one they used most frequently. This information could be used to compare the differences in rankings and satisfaction level (if any) between users of different platforms, which we have not done in this study. We also did not collect respondents' contact details denying us an opportunity for follow up questions that could provide additional insights. Furthermore, in creating persuasive user experiences via technology, user actions determine whether the systems meet their intended purpose [28]. Therefore, supplementing the study with a more extensive survey/multiple surveys to compare differences in user responses over time, use of system logging data and/or interviews to explore certain findings in greater detail are potential avenues for further research. Another avenue for further research that is especially important for persuasive systems design is exploring of unintended consequences from the developers point of view and the gap between their intentions and users' behavior.

The results provide support for the claim put forward by [10] that users creating value and content as well as involving others lead to their staying active and loyal. The features that enable this include: *creating and editing profiles, inviting and connecting with friends, responding to posts and updates, uploading content, newsfeed, and* a result not previously considered is that users value the possibility to *privately communicate* within these social platforms. As most of previous research [7, 11, 13, 20, 21, 23, 24] emphasize the collective, interactive, and interconnected nature of the social web, person-person push communication akin to email is also considered important by users (especially in social networks like Facebook). These features can more precisely be categorized as self-presentation, connecting, communication and regular access.

Creating and editing the profile is a form of self-presentation and enables users to portray a favorable image of themselves and leave their own identity into the system [22]. The other features are of a social nature and they reflect the need for interaction; the extent to which is dependent on the purpose and medium used [7]. The social web is at the core of people's and businesses' online presence today because it typifies and has a subsequent influence on the current culture of fast information sharing, synchronous communication and interconnectedness [cf. 16]. The possibility to connect with friends or other like-minded individuals is what makes interactions in the social web intriguing. As people primarily utilize the platforms to share their thoughts, views, successes and/or failures, interaction over user-generated content and their responses form the core of such services.

People are more satisfied especially when they see others responding positively to their posts or updates [12]. This pattern of user behavior makes the service more valuable by creating content that others can consume (e.g., videos, polls, breaking news, photos, and links) and form discussions around and adds value to the service [10]. This is also reflected by some of the user responses on what they primarily share. For example, *"my mood, funny pictures, interesting news articles, commenting different events, professional information, links to music videos or inspirational content, status updates concerning my own personal life and photographs"* and so forth. The varying forms and degrees of system use can be explained by the persuasion context, particularly the use context which classifies users according to their usage patterns and familiarity with the respective systems [17]. Users are also frequently reminded of on-going activities through emails (which were ranked lowly compared to the other features) and the newsfeed that provides a snapshot of other users' posts and messages encouraging regular access. Nowadays, the growth of mobile devices has also facilitated regular use as these services can be accessed while on the move and at any moment.

6   Conclusions

This paper has shed light through a survey (N=57) of social web users on the features, which aim at committing social web users into their platforms so that they keep regularly accessing these systems. The key in this system's self-referential persuasion is that these services provide persuasive user experiences, which are able to capture and maintain users' interest on the content provided, thus enhancing frequent visits. Inherent in the persuasive elements are social psychological approaches, which form the basis for crafting the user experiences. That is, even though technology is not the centermost factor it enables and helps in realization of the persuasion intent. Moreover, even if the features in the investigated social web platforms were still relatively limited in terms of persuasive potential, this study suggests that social web platforms are prone to persuasion–they have been built for behavior change in mind.

Acknowledgements. This is part of OASIS research group of Martti Ahtisaari Institute, University of Oulu. The study was partly supported by the SalWe Research Program for Mind and Body (grant 1104/10), the SEWEB research project on Sensors and Social Web (40027/13, 40028/13), and the Someletti research project on Social Media in Public Space (grant 1362/31), all provided by Tekes, the Finnish Funding Agency for Technology and Innovation.

References

1. Bandura, A.: Social-learning Theory of Identificatory Processes. In: Goslin, D.A. (ed.) Handbook of Socialization Theory and Research, pp. 213–262. Rand McNally, Chicago (1969)
2. Bandura, A.: Social Cognitive Theory. In: Vasta, R. (ed.) Annals of Child Development Six Theories of Child Development, vol. (6), pp. 1–60. JAI Press, Greenwich (1989)
3. Boyd, D., Ellison, N.: Social network sites: Definition, History, and Scholarship. Journal of Computer-Mediated Communication 13(1), 11 (2007)
4. Cialdini, R.: Descriptive Social Norms as Underappreciated Sources of Social Control. Psychometrika 72(2), 263–268 (2007)
5. Cialdini, R.: Influence: The psychology of persuasion. HarperCollins Publishers, New York (2007)
6. Corbett, J.: Designing and Using Carbon Management Systems to Promote Ecologically Responsible Behaviors. Journal of the Association for Information Systems 14(7), Article 2 (2013), http://aisel.aisnet.org/jais/vol14/iss7/2
7. de Moor, A.: Conversations in Context: A twitter Case for Social Media Systems Design. In: Proceedings of the 6th International Conference on Semantic Systems, Graz, Austria, pp. 1–8 (2010)
8. Fogg, B.J.: Persuasive Computers: Perspectives and Research Directions. In: Proceedings of the SIGCHI Conference on Human Factors in Computing Systems (CHI), pp. 225–232 (1998)
9. Fogg, B.J.: Persuasive Technology: Using Computers to Change what we Think and Do. Morgan Kaufmann Publishers, San Francisco (2003)
10. Fogg, B.J., Eckles, D.: The Behavior Chain for Online Participation: How Successful Web Services Structure Persuasion. In: de Kort, Y.A.W., IJsselsteijn, W.A., Midden, C., Eggen, B., Fogg, B.J. (eds.) PERSUASIVE 2007. LNCS, vol. 4744, pp. 199–209. Springer, Heidelberg (2007)
11. Fogg, B.J.: Mass Interpersonal Persuasion: An Early View of a New Phenomenon. In: Oinas-Kukkonen, H., Hasle, P., Harjumaa, M., Segerståhl, K., Øhrstrøm, P. (eds.) PERSUASIVE 2008. LNCS, vol. 5033, pp. 23–34. Springer, Heidelberg (2008)
12. Fogg, B.J., Iizawa, D.: Online Persuasion in Facebook and Mixi: A Cross-cultural Comparison. In: Oinas-Kukkonen, H., Hasle, P., Harjumaa, M., Segerståhl, K., Øhrstrøm, P. (eds.) PERSUASIVE 2008. LNCS, vol. 5033, pp. 35–46. Springer, Heidelberg (2008)
13. Hansen, D.L., Shneiderman, B., Smith, M.A.: Analyzing Social Media Networks with NodeXL: Insights from a Connected World. Morgan Kaufmann Publishers, Burlington (2011)
14. Kelders, S.M., Kok, R.N., Ossebaard, H.C., Van Gemert-Pijnen, J.E.W.C.: Persuasive system design does matter: a systematic review of adherence to web-based interventions. Journal of Medical Internet Research 14(6) (2012)
15. Lehto, T., Oinas-Kukkonen, H.: Persuasive Features in Web-based Alcohol and Smoking Interventions: A Systematic Review of the Literature. Journal of Medical Internet Research 13(3), e46 (2011)
16. Oinas-Kukkonen, H., Oinas-Kukkonen, H.: Humanizing the Web: Change and Social Innovation. Palmgrave Macmillan, Basingstoke (2013)
17. Oinas-Kukkonen, H., Harjumaa, M.: Persuasive Systems Design: Key Issues, Process Model, and System Features. In: Communications of the Association for Information Systems (24:28), pp. 485–500 (2009)
18. Oinas-Kukkonen, H.: A foundation for the study of behavior change support systems. Personal and Ubiquitous Computing 17(6), 1223–1235 (2013)

19. Petty, R.E., Cacioppo, J.T.: The Elaboration Likelihood Model of Persuasion. In: Berkowitz, L. (ed.) Advances in Experimental Social Psychology, pp. 123–205. Academic Press, New York (1986)
20. van Zyl, A.S.: The Impact of Social Networking 2.0 on Organizations. Electronic Library 27(6), 906–918 (2009)
21. Hanna, R., Rohm, A., Crittenden, V.L.: We're all connected: The power of the social media ecosystem. Business Horizons 54(3), 265–273 (2011)
22. Gupta, M., Li, R., Yin, Z., Han, J.: Survey on social tagging techniques. ACM SIGKDD Explorations Newsletter 12(1), 58–72 (2010)
23. Porter, J.: Designing for the social web. New Riders Publishing Thousand Oaks, CA (2010)
24. Kaplan, A.M., Haenlein, M.: Users of the world, unite! The challenges and opportunities of Social Media. Business Horizons 53(1), 59–68 (2010)
25. Lowenthal, P.R.: The evolution and influence of social presence theory on online learning. In: Kidd, T.T. (ed.) Online Education and Adult Learning: New Frontiers for Teaching Practices, pp. 124–139. IGI Global, Hershey (2010)
26. Sleeper, M., Acquisti, A., Cranor, L.F., Kelley, P., Munson, S.A., Sadeh, N.: I Would Like To.., I Shouldn't.., I Wish I..: Exploring Behavior-Change Goals for Social Networking Sites. In: CSCW. Vancouver, BC (2015)
27. Oinas-Kukkonen, H., Lyytinen, K., Yoo, Y.: Social Networks and Information Systems: Ongoing and Future Research Streams. Journal of the Association for Information Systems 11(2), 61–68 (2010)
28. Oduor, M., Alahäivälä, T., Oinas-Kukkonen, H.: Persuasive software design patterns for social influence. Personal and Ubiquitous Computing 18(7), 1689–1704 (2014), doi:10.1007/s00779-014-0779-y
29. Lehto, T., Oinas-Kukkonen, H.: Explaining and Predicting Perceived Effectiveness and Use Continuance Intention of a Behavior Change Support System. Behaviour and Information Technology 34(2), 176–189 (2015), doi:10.1080/0144929X.2013.866162

Advancing Typology of Computer-Supported Influence: Moderation Effects in Socially Influencing Systems

Agnis Stibe[(✉)]

MIT Media Lab, Cambridge, MA, USA
`agnis@mit.edu`

Abstract. Persuasive technologies are commonly engineered to change behavior and attitudes of users through persuasion and social influence without using coercion and deception. While earlier research has been extensively focused on exploring the concept of persuasion, the present theory-refining study aims to explain the role of social influence and its distinctive characteristics in the field of persuasive technology. Based on a list of notable differences, this study outlines how both persuasion and social influence can be best supported through computing systems and introduces a notion of computer-moderated influence, thus extending the influence typology. The novel type of influence tends to be more salient for socially influencing systems, which informs designers to be mindful when engineering such technologies. The study provides sharper conceptual representation of key terms in persuasive engineering, drafts a structured approach for better understanding of the influence typology, and presents how computers can be moderators of social influence.

Keywords: Influence typology · Computer-moderated · Persuasive technology · Computer-mediated · Computer-human · Socially influencing systems

1 Introduction

Persuasive technologies are commonly engineered to change behavior and attitudes of users through persuasion and social influence without using coercion and deception [9]. Both persuasion [22] and social influence [11] have been studied as concepts in behavioral, cognitive, and social psychology for long time. Evidently, they both exert capacity to alter human attitude and behavior, but each of them employs specific attributes to achieve that through face-to-face communication and presence in the physical world [3], [21].

While computers are becoming ubiquitous as tools, media, and social actors, it is necessary to clarify how the concepts of persuasion and social influence can be engineered in computing systems [9], [29]. More importantly, before designing such persuasive systems, scholars and practitioners should be aware of how each concept can be operationalized and what consequences each design component can bear [28].

According to Fogg [9], people can respond socially to computer products, which opens the door for social influence aspects [29] to exert their powers of motivating and persuading users. Thus, computers can be perceived as social entities or actors

© Springer International Publishing Switzerland 2015
T. MacTavish and S. Basapur (Eds.): PERSUASIVE 2015, LNCS 9072, pp. 253–264, 2015.
DOI: 10.1007/978-3-319-20306-5_23

that influence people on their own [28]. This happens when people make inferences about social presence [26] in persuasive technology through social cues, such as physical (face, eyes, body, movement), psychological (personality, similarity, feelings), language (spoken language, praise, language recognition), social dynamics (dialogues, reciprocity), and social roles (authority, doctor, teacher). Although it broadens understanding of computers as social actors, such discussion is focused on perceiving computers as individual entities with human-like characteristics rather than means for computer-supported influence that originates from other users [29].

To address this gap, the present research aims at clarifying the role of social influence [17], [25], [27], [33] and its distinctive qualities in the field of persuasive technology (Section 2). Based on these differences, this paper outlines how the concepts of persuasion and social influence can be best supported through computing systems (Section 3). Further, the notion of interpersonal computer-moderated influence is introduced, its place among other relevant types of persuasion is defined, and its specific role in the realm of persuasive technology is explained (Section 4). Lastly, the paper discusses implications of this research for scholars and designers of socially influencing systems (Section 5), and provides final conclusions (Section 6).

2   Socio-Psychological Foundation

Concepts of persuasion and social influence are often used interchangeably when describing a phenomenon of behavioral or attitudinal change that is caused by other people. Although persuasion and social influence can achieve the same goal of shaping human attitude and behavior, research in social psychology (Table 1) demonstrates that both concepts have notable differences in character and encompass distinct properties [14], [16].

According to Wood [31], *persuasion* typically includes detailed argumentation that is presented to people in a context with only minimal social interaction (e.g. one-to-one or one-to-many verbal persuasion), whereas *social influence* is usually enabled and facilitated by more complex social settings (e.g. many-to-one or many-to-many social contexts). O'Keefe [21] has argued that persuasion mainly relies on and is built upon reasoning and argument to shift attitudes and behavior of individuals towards a desired agenda, but social influence is commonly driven by the behavior and actions of surrounding people.

An additional perspective by Cialdini [3] has proposed that persuasion works by appealing to a set of deeply rooted human drives and needs, such as liking, reciprocity, consistency, authority, and scarcity. At the same time, humans look for social proof as a source of influence, and rely on the people around them for cues on how to think, feel, and act. In earlier work, Cialdini together with Goldstein [4] also claimed that social influence is a psychological phenomenon that often occurs in direct response to overt social forces. Finally, in recent collaborative work with Guadagno and Ewell [11], Cialdini specified that social influence refers to the changing of attitudes, beliefs, or behavior of an individual because of real or imagined external pressure.

Table 1. Persuasion and social influence in social psychology literature

Reference	Persuasion	Social Influence
Cialdini [3]	Works by appealing to a set of deeply rooted human drives and needs, such as liking, reciprocity, consistency, authority, and scarcity.	Humans look for social proof, therefor rely on the people around them for cues on how to think, feel, and act.
Guadagno et al. [11]		Refers to the changing of attitudes, beliefs, or behavior of an individual because of real or imagined external pressure.
O'Keefe [21]	Mainly relies on and is built upon reasoning and argument to shift attitudes and behavior of individuals towards a desired agenda.	Commonly driven by the behavior and actions of surrounding people.
Petty and Cacioppo [22]	Two basic routes to persuasion. One is based on the thoughtful consideration of arguments central to the issue, whereas the other is based on peripheral cues.	
Rashotte [23]	Focuses merely on written or spoken messages sent from source to recipient.	Defined as change in thoughts, feelings, attitudes, or behavior of an individual that results from interaction with another individual or a group.
Wood [31]	Typically includes detailed argumentation that is presented to people in a context with only minimal social interaction.	Usually enabled and facilitated by complex social settings.

Petty and Cacioppo [22] have argued that there are two basic routes to persuasion. One route is based on the thoughtful consideration of arguments central to the issue, whereas the other is based on peripheral cues in the persuasion situation. Rashotte [23] has defined social influence as change in thoughts, feelings, attitudes, or behavior of an individual that results from interaction with another individual or a group.

2.1   Persuasion

Persuasion is broadly defined as the action of causing someone to do something through reasoning or argument [21-22]. According to Rashotte [23], current research on persuasion focuses merely on written or spoken messages sent from source to recipient. This research is based on the assumption that people process messages carefully whenever they have motivation and ability to do so. Modern persuasion research is mainly dominated by studies employing either the elaboration likelihood model (ELM) [22] or heuristic-systemic models (HSM) [8].

2.2   Social Influence

Social influence is broadly defined as the capacity to have an effect on the behavior of someone in a social context. In general, social influence is naturally and instantly present in most social contexts of everyday life. According to earlier research [27], the study of social influence is central to social psychology and essential to understand group dynamics and intergroup relations. Historically, the research on social influence covers a broad range of topics, from persuasion and attitude change [31], to compliance and conformity [4], to collective action and social change [18]. Social influence is the process by which people really change their behavior depending on interaction with others who are perceived to be similar, desirable, or expert [23].

2.3   Understanding Distinctive Characteristics

Earlier discussion on persuasion and social influence creates an understanding that both paradigms are present in settings with two or more people that lead to behavioral or attitudinal changes in one or many of them. However, it is also important to clarify the distinctive characteristics of the two paradigms so that researchers and designers would be able to implement them in a proper way and study their effects on human behavior in a rigorous manner. Social psychology research on persuasion and social influence (Table 1) suggest numerous aspects that differentiate the two, therefore further discussion focuses only on the four main distinctive characteristics that are categorized in Table 2, i.e. the *origin*, the *driver*, the *impact*, and the *direction*.

Table 2. Distinctive characteristics of persuasion and social influence

	Persuasion	Social Influence
Origin	Intention or agenda	Presence of other people
Driver	Reasoning or argument	Behavior of surrounding people
Impact	Controlled and guided	Unpredictable and ambient
Direction	Push	Pull

Origin. Persuasion generally originates either from an *intention* to change an attitude and behavior of an individual or from a broader agenda of shaping what crowds of people think and do. In contrast, social influence effects occur and persist in the *presence* of other people around an individual.

Driver. According to earlier definitions [21], persuasion mainly relies on and is built upon *reasoning* and argument to shift attitudes and behavior of individuals towards a desired agenda, whereas social influence is commonly driven by the behavior and *actions* of surrounding people.

Impact. For persuasion to exert a desired impact on an individual through consistent reasoning and argumentation, it has to be performed in a *controlled* and guided manner. But, social influence primarily depends on the presence of other people and their behavior in a given social environment, therefore making its impact *unpredictable* and reliant on a particular context.

Direction. Prior research demonstrates that persuasion by definition operates as *push* mechanism that communicates an intended agenda with supportive arguments through guided approach, i.e. a persuader intentionally attempts to shapes the behavior and attitudes of receivers. Whereas in case of social influence, an individual is rather *picking* up an influence from a particular social context, i.e. individuals acquire sense of influence from surrounding people and their behavior.

3   Influence Typology

Computer-supported influence holds considerable promise as a topic of research [10]. Prior research in the realm of persuasive technology [9] has distinguished three relevant types of persuasion [13], i.e. interpersonal persuasion, computer-mediated persuasion, and human-computer persuasion. To advance this research area, the aforementioned types have been adjusted and are further discussed as: interpersonal *face-to-face (FTF)* influence, interpersonal *computer-mediated (CME)* influence, and *computer-human (CHU)* influence, respectively.

Based on the distinctive characteristics of persuasion and social influence (Table 2) and the ways in which both can be supported through computing systems, this paper outlines the existence of another type, namely interpersonal *computer-moderated (CMO)* influence, and explains its place and role within the realm of computer-supported influence (Fig. 1). More elaborate comparison of the four types of influence is provided in Table 3.

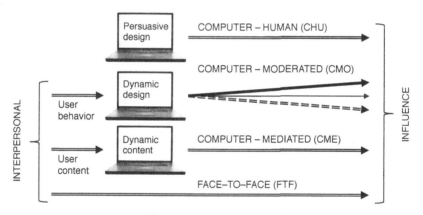

Fig. 1. Influence typology

3.1   Interpersonal Face-to-Face (FTF) Influence

According to Wilson [30], interpersonal influence can take place during an interaction of two or more people, involving verbal and non-verbal forms of behavior, personal feedback, and coherence of behavior. Further, this type of influence is termed as face-to-face (FTF) [20] to distinguish it from computer-supported influence (Fig. 1).

3.2   Interpersonal Computer-Mediated (CME) Influence

Interpersonal influence can also take place through various computing technologies, such as emails, mobile messaging, video chats, etc. In this case, the chosen technology serves as a mediator of interpersonal influence without any additional agenda to affect its users. Therefore, this type of influence is termed as interpersonal computer-mediated (CME) influence (Fig. 1) [11-12] and it can be well operationalized through fixed content (FC) and dynamic content (DC) components that are further explained in Section 4.1 and presented in Table 4.

Prior research also exposes that scholars have been active in studying interpersonal CME persuasion [15], [24], and its comparison to interpersonal FTF persuasion for many years. For example, Di Blasio and Milani [7] found that computer-mediated discussion could possibly activate the central route of persuasion [22] more easily than face-to-face interaction. This knowledge can be instrumental to explore more granular differences between the two types of influence.

Table 3. Comparing the four types of influence

	Interpersonal			Computer-human (CHU)
	Face-to-face (FTF)	Computer-mediated (CME)	Computer-moderated (CMO)	
Origin	Human	User	User behavior	Designer
Description	People can influence each other in the physical world.	Users can influence each other through computers.	Computers can amplify, decrease, or reverse influence based on the presence (or absence) of other users and their behavior.	Computers can influence users when designed to do so.

3.3   Computer-Human (CHU) Influence

Computer-human (CHU) influence is very different from both types of interpersonal influence previously discussed, i.e. FTF and CME, because it is based on the notion that computers can be designed to perform the role of social actors [9], and thus they can have capacity to influence users independently of interpersonal relationships with other users (Fig. 1). For this reason, the CHU influence can be better operationalized through the fixed design (FD) component, which is described in Section 4.1 and presented in Table 4.

Earlier research provides different collections of techniques and principles that can be useful for designing and evaluating persuasive technologies. For instance, the behavior change technique taxonomy contains 93 hierarchically clustered techniques to build an international consensus for the reporting of behavior change interventions [19]. According to Fogg [9], there are various theory-driven persuasive principles that can be incorporated into the design of computers to improve their persuasiveness. Many principles and techniques by definition and design can support the CHU influence, but not all of them. Those principles that are primarily dependent on behavior of other users rather fall under the interpersonal computer-moderated (CMO) influence, as discussed further in the next section.

3.4   Interpersonal Computer-Moderated (CMO) Influence

Interpersonal computer-moderated (CMO) influence is distinct from all other types of influence described above with its unique characteristic of being able to amplify, decrease, or reverse the persuasion effect through computing technology depending on the presence (or absence) of other users and their behavior.

Interpersonal CMO and CME influences differ, because the latter serves as a mediator without affecting interpersonal influence, while the effects of the former can fluctuate depending on the actual behavior of other concurrent users. In other words, the role of a computer in the interpersonal CME influence is mainly to mediate interpersonal persuasion, whereas in case of the interpersonal CMO influence, the role of a computer is to facilitate the effects of social influence though the dynamic design (DD) component, further described in Section 4.1 and exhibited in Table 4.

As it can be observed from Fig. 1, interpersonal CMO influence also substantially differs from CHU influence, because the latter is not supposed to receive any input from other users, thus the CHU influence is solely based on the intentions that its designers have preset in the interfaces of the computing technology (the FD component). Another way to better understand the nature of the interpersonal CMO influence and how it differs from the interpersonal CME influence is to think about the common attributes of moderation and mediation in social psychological research [2].

4   Computer-Supported Influence

Computing technologies increasingly penetrate various aspects of everyday life. This advancement continuously expands ways of how people can be reached, thus experience persuasion or social influence through human-computer interaction [10] and computer-mediated communication [10].

According to Wilson [30], communication via computer is intrinsically less suitable for persuading as compared to face-to-face interaction, because of deficiencies to transmit non-verbal cues and limited number of utilizable strategies. At the same time, computers can be designed to play the role of a social actor [9], which means that they are capable not only to mediate persuasive communication but also support persuasion and social influence through intentionally designed computer software and interfaces [13].

4.1   Components

Before designing persuasive technologies [9] and socially influencing systems [29], it is very important to understand the main components of how computers can support influence (Table 4). The two main components of computing systems, which are directly exposed to users through interfaces, are *content* (e.g., texts, photos, sounds, videos) and *design* (e.g., layout, navigation, colors, features). Both components can be operationalized either as *fixed* or *dynamic*.

Table 4. Components of computer-supported influence

	Content	Design
Fixed	(FC)	(FD)
	Preset by developers and owners	Preset by designers
	Supports CHU influence	Supports CHU influence
Dynamic	(DC)	(DD)
	Generated by users	Evolving through user behavior
	Supports interpersonal CME influence	Supports interpersonal CMO influence

Historically, computer systems were often built with fixed design that was preset by designers and fixed content that was predefined by system developers and owners. With the overall technological advancement, computer systems are becoming more social and dynamic by both allowing users to contribute own content and displaying their interactions with the systems.

Through clearer understanding of the four components, the designers of computer systems become better equipped with ways of how both persuasion and social influence can be operationalized more effectively.

Based on the distinctive characteristics of persuasion and social influence (Table 1), the likelihood of support for both concepts was assessed and reported for each component in Table 4. That is, if an intention is to persuade users through computing systems, then the *fixed content (FC)*, *fixed designed (FD)*, and *dynamic content (DC)* components are suitable in achieving that. However, if an aim is to leverage social influence through socially influencing systems [29], then the DC and *dynamic design (DD)* components can yield favorable results.

In this case, if a system is implemented with fixed design and fixed content so that users can see only outcomes of their own actions, then the chances for social influence to play a role in the given context are very limited. Of course, the fixed components can contain preset messages conveying social influence aspects, e.g. social normative statements [5], but their effects can decline over time, as they do not change. Nevertheless, dynamic content and dynamic design expand user interaction and enable them to see what others are doing. In that way, both dynamic components open up multiple ways for social influence to occur and affect users.

4.2 Operationalization

The concepts of computer-supported influence can be operationalized in many ways depending on a given context and intended behavior change. To give an example, imagine a situation where a person is concerned about his health conditions and has decided to exercise more by jogging each morning. As part of this plan, the person installs a mobile application intentionally designed to help achieve the target behavior change. First, the mobile app enables a jogger to check weather conditions, and secondly, enables users to see how many others are jogging at that moment (Fig. 2). The counter of joggers is an operationalization of the DD (dynamic design) component from Table 4, as it purely depends on the behavior of other users.

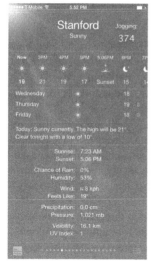 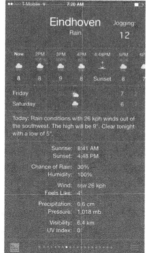 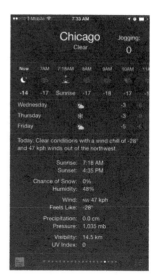

Fig. 2. Example of an interpersonal computer-moderated influence: on the left, nice weather in Stanford and 374 are jogging; in the middle, bad weather in Eindhoven and only twelve are jogging; on the right, cold and windy weather in Chicago and no one is jogging outside

If the weather conditions are great in Stanford and the counter shows that 374 people are currently jogging outside (Fig. 2, left), then the user would experience increased motivation to go out and exercise together with others. Instead, the heavy rain and the comparative low number of joggers on the streets and in the parks of Eindhoven (Fig. 2, middle) would most likely to decrease the motivation of a user to step outside. Now, imagine a situation when there is one extremely cold and windy morning in Chicago (Fig. 2, right). The alarm clock rings, the user opens the application and notices the bad weather conditions, which naturally affects the motivation for jogging that morning. Now what? The user looks at the number of others jogging at that exact moment. Quite simply, a zero joggers in the picture would discourage the individual from jogging that morning, a small number would make the user hesitant, but a large number of other joggers would still give an extra boost to the motivation.

This example demonstrates how the behavior of other users can increase, decrease, or reverse the persuasive effect of a mobile application that is complemented with the design principle of social facilitation [32], which represents social influence. In a similar manner, it can be easily illustrated how other social influence design principles would end up having the same pattern. The competition principle [6] that is implemented as a top, for example, would amplify its persuasive potential only as long as an individual has competitive position among other users. Whenever the individual falls behind the competition, this principle naturally loses its capacity to influence.

5   Discussion

This theory-refining research highlights the importance and necessity to continue studying various facets of persuasion and social influence in the realm of persuasive technology. The substance of this paper demonstrates that both concepts maintain distinctive qualities, and therefore their nature has to be better understood before making an attempt to design and implement them in computing technologies.

The contribution of this paper is fourfold. First, the paper provides a comparison of persuasion and social influence that clarifies the nature of both concepts in a structured manner. Second, the paper outlines four components of how computers can support persuasion [21-22] and social influence [11], [23]. Third, the influence typology is presented and, forth, extended with an introduction of interpersonal computer-moderated (CMO) influence.

Overall, the outcome of this research effort demonstrates that there are various ways that persuasion and social influence can be facilitated through computing technologies, but a positive effect is not always guaranteed. In the case of the interpersonal CMO influence, intended effects can be amplified, decreased, or reversed depending on the presence (or absence) of other users and their behavior.

5.1   Implications for Designers

The designers of persuasive technologies should be very careful when designing interpersonal computer-moderated (CMO) influence, which is mainly about implementing aspects of social influence. In order to avoid possibly negative effects of the interpersonal CMO influence, the designers of persuasive technologies can and oftentimes should incorporate specific rules and triggers to control for the likelihood of unwanted effects occurring. If such control mechanisms were in place, another kind of an implementation could be deployed as long as necessary. For example, when the number of joggers on the streets of Chicago (Fig. 2) drops below twenty, instead of reporting a low number, the mobile app can show an average number of joggers at that time of day which is aggregated over the last month or over ten other days with similar weather conditions.

5.2   Future Research

This research provides additional evidence that the theoretical work on persuasive technologies and socially influencing systems has potential for further research initiatives. In the next steps, each aspect of social influence has to be further studied separately and rigorously in line with related theories from social psychology. Then these aspects need to be designed, implemented, and tested to assess thresholds of when interpersonal computer-moderated (CMO) influence begins to shift its effect from amplifying to decreasing and from decreasing to reversing. Conducting such studies is highly important, as they would contribute to more detailed understanding of how and when socially influencing systems [29] are gaining, losing, or reversing their capacity to affect user involvement, participation, and engagement [28].

6   Conclusions

The present study explained the role of social influence and its distinctive characteristics in the field of persuasive technology. Based on the unique differences between persuasion and social influence, this paper described ways of how both concepts can be best supported through computing systems.

The study introduced the notion of interpersonal computer-moderated (CMO) influence and defined its place within the influence typology. Compared to the other types, the CMO influence firmly relies on four distinguishing characteristics of social influence, namely origin, driver, impact, and direction. By definition, the CMO influence can amplify, decrease, or reverse an intended effect on users, therefore designers of socially influencing systems [28] should be mindful when engineering them.

To summarize, this research outlined a sharper conceptual representation of the key terms in persuasive engineering, drafted a structured approach for better understanding of the influence typology, and presented how computers can be moderators of social influence. Consequently, future research attempts can be directed towards formalizing and operationalizing the influence typology, and advancing the methodology for socially influencing systems [29].

References

1. Angst, C.M., Agarwal, R.: Adoption of Electronic Health Records in the Presence of Privacy Concerns: the Elaboration Likelihood Model and Individual Persuasion. MIS Quarterly 33(2), 339–370 (2009)
2. Baron, R.M., Kenny, D.A.: The Moderator-Mediator Variable Distinction in Social Psychological Research: Conceptual, Strategic, and Statistical Considerations. Journal of Personality and Social Psychology 51(6), 1173 (1986)
3. Cialdini, R.B.: Influence: The Science of Persuasion. HarperCollins Publishers Inc., New York (2009)
4. Cialdini, R.B., Goldstein, N.J.: Social Influence: Compliance and Conformity. Annu. Rev. Psychol. 55, 591–621 (2004)
5. Cialdini, R.B., Kallgren, C.A., Reno, R.R.: A Focus Theory of Normative Conduct: A Theoretical Refinement and Reevaluation of the Role of Norms in Human Behavior. Advances in Experimental Social Psychology 24(20), 1–243 (1991)
6. Deutsch, M., Gerard, H.B.: A Study of Normative and Informational Social Influences upon Individual Judgment. Journal of Abnormal and Social Psychology 51(3), 629 (1955)
7. Di Blasio, P., Milani, L.: Computer-Mediated Communication and Persuasion: Peripheral vs. Central Route to Opinion Shift. Computers in Human Behavior 24(3), 798–815 (2008)
8. Eagly, A.H., Chaiken, S.: The Psychology of Attitudes. Harcourt, New York (1993)
9. Fogg, B.J.: Persuasive Technology: Using Computers To Change What We Think And Do. Morgan Kaufmann, San Francisco (2003)
10. Gass, R.H., Seiter, J.S.: Persuasion: Social Influence, and Compliance Gaining, 5th edn. Pearson/Allyn & Bacon, Boston (2013)
11. Guadagno, R.E., Ewell, P.J., Cialdini, R.B.: Influence. In: Cooper, C.L. (ed.) Wiley Encyclopedia of Management, pp. 3–5. John Wiley & Sons (2014)

12. Guadagno, R.E., Muscanell, N.L., Rice, L.M., Roberts, N.: Social Influence Online: The Impact of Social Validation and Likability on Compliance. Psychology of Popular Media Culture 2(1), 51 (2013)
13. Harjumaa, M., Oinas-Kukkonen, H.: Persuasion Theories and IT Design. In: de Kort, Y.A.W., IJsselsteijn, W.A., Midden, C., Eggen, B., Fogg, B.J. (eds.) PERSUASIVE 2007. LNCS, vol. 4744, pp. 311–314. Springer, Heidelberg (2007)
14. Haslam, S.A., McGarty, C., Turner, J.C.: Salient Group Memberships and Persuasion: The Role of Social Identity in the Validation of Beliefs (1996)
15. Hong, S., Park, H.S.: Computer-Mediated Persuasion in Online Reviews: Statistical Versus Narrative Evidence. Computers in Human Behavior 28(3), 906–919 (2012)
16. Hovland, C.I., Janis, I.L., Kelley, H.H.: Communication and Persuasion. Psychological Studies of Opinion Change (1953)
17. Kiesler, S., Siegel, J., McGuire, T.W.: Social Psychological Aspects of Computer-Mediated Communication. American Psychologist 39(10), 1123 (1984)
18. Lewin, K.: Group Decision and Social Change. In: Newcomb, T.M., Hartley, E.L. (eds.) Readings in Social Psychology, pp. 330–344. Holt, Rinehart, and Winston, NY (1947)
19. Michie, S., Richardson, M., Johnston, M., Abraham, C., Francis, J., Hardeman, W., Eccles, M.P., Cane, J., Wood, C.E.: The Behavior Change Technique Taxonomy (v1) of 93 Hierarchically Clustered Techniques: Building an International Consensus for the Reporting of Behavior Change Interventions. Annals of Behavioral Medicine 46(1), 81–95 (2013)
20. O'Keefe, B.J., Shepherd, G.J.: The Pursuit of Multiple Objectives in Face-to-Face Persuasive Interactions: Effects of Construct Differentiation on Message Organization. Communications Monographs 54(4), 396–419 (1987)
21. O'Keefe, D.J.: Persuasion: Theory and Research. Sage, Newbury (1990)
22. Petty, R.E., Cacioppo, J.T.: The Elaboration Likelihood Model of Persuasion. Advances in Experimental Social Psychology 19, 123–205 (1986)
23. Rashotte, L.: Social influence. The Blackwell Encyclopedia of Social Psychology 9, 562–563 (2007)
24. Sassenberg, K., Boos, M., Rabung, S.: Attitude Change in Face-to-Face and Computer-Mediated Communication: Private Self-Awareness as Mediator and Moderator. European Journal of Social Psychology 35(3), 361–374 (2005)
25. Sassenberg, K., Ionas, K.I.: Attitude Change and Social Influence. In: Oxford Handbook of Internet Psychology, 273 (2007)
26. Short, J.A., Williams, E., Christie, B.: The social psychology of telecommunications. Wiley, London (1976)
27. Smith, J.R., Louis, W.R., Schultz, P.W.: Introduction Social influence in action. Group Processes & Intergroup Relations 14(5), 599–603 (2011)
28. Stibe, A.: Socially Influencing Systems: Persuading People to Engage with Publicly Displayed Twitter-based Systems. Acta Universitatis Ouluensis (2014)
29. Stibe, A.: Towards a Framework for Socially Influencing Systems: Meta-Analysis of Four PLS-SEM Based Studies. In: MacTavish, T., Basapur, S. (eds.) Persuasive Technology. LNCS, vol. 9072, pp. 171–182. Springer, Heidelberg (2015)
30. Wilson, E.V.: Perceived Effectiveness of Interpersonal Persuasion Strategies in Computer-Mediated Communication. Computers in Human Behavior 19(5), 537–552 (2003)
31. Wood, W.: Attitude Change: Persuasion and Social Influence. Annual Review of Psychology 51(1), 539–570 (2000)
32. Zajonc, R.B.: Social facilitation. Science 149, 269–274 (1965)
33. Zimbardo, P.G., Leippe, M.R.: The Psychology of Attitude Change and Social Influence. Mcgraw-Hill Book Company (1991)

Author Index

Printed in the United States
By Bookmasters